Rural Health - Investment, Research and Implications

Edited by Christian Rusangwa

Published in London, United Kingdom

Rural Health - Investment, Research and Implications
http://dx.doi.org/10.5772/intechopen.104166
Edited by Christian Rusangwa

Contributors
Kidus Yenealem Mefteh, Oluwafunmiso Adeola Olajide, Jean Ross, Samuel Mann, Kate Emond, Abu Macavoray, Moinina Nelpheson Kallon, Joseph A. Bunting-Graden, Roland Suluku, Umar Nain, Gaylord Ngaboyeka, Eméry Likaka, Espérant Kiangana, Rizanda Machmud, Finny Fitry Yani, Feri Mulyani Hamid, Yuniar Lestari, Irvan Medison, Emilzon Taslim, Bestari Jaka Budiman, William Maepa, Heather Helpard, Lori E. Weeks, Mark Shephard, Susan Janet Matthews, Corey Markus, Emma de Courcy-Ireland, Lauren Duckworth, Isabelle Haklar, Ellen Kambanaros, Tamika Regnier, April Rivers-Kennedy, Grant White, Min Jung Cho, Eva Haverkort, Bamdev Subedi, Alain Casseus, Chery Maurice Jr, Kenia Vissieres, Tracy L. McClair, Charlotte Warren, Pooja Sripad, Linneth Nkateko Mabila, Patrick Hulisani Demana, Tebogo Maria Mothiba, Josie Crawley, Rachel Parmee, Marion Okoh-Owusu, George Kojo Owusu, Celia Brown, Frank Baiden

First published in London, United Kingdom, 2023 by IntechOpen
IntechOpen is the global imprint of INTECHOPEN LIMITED, registered in England and Wales, registration number: 11086078, 5 Princes Gate Court, London, SW7 2QJ, United Kingdom

British Library Cataloguing-in-Publication Data
A catalogue record for this book is available from the British Library

Additional hard and PDF copies can be obtained from orders@intechopen.com

Rural Health - Investment, Research and Implications
Edited by Christian Rusangwa
p. cm.
Print ISBN 978-1-83768-598-1
Online ISBN 978-1-83768-599-8
eBook (PDF) ISBN 978-1-83768-600-1

For EU product safety concerns:
IN TECH d.o.o., Prolaz Marije Krucifikse Kozulić 3, 51000 Rijeka, Croatia,
info@intechopen.com or visit our website at intechopen.com.

Meet the editor

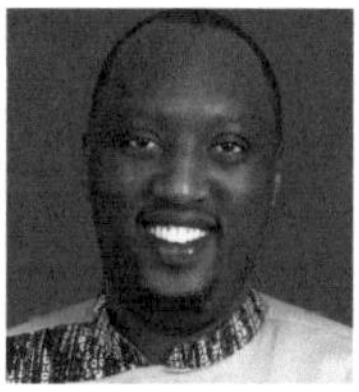

Dr. Christian Rusangwa serves as the Director of Technical Assistance at Muso Health, where he leads the organization's vision for improved access to primary and community health care with speed and quality in Mali and the Ivory Coast. He also worked for Partners in Health as Deputy Chief Medical Officer in charge of Chronic Care and Health System Strengthening. Dr. Rusangwa has supported district health systems that serve more than 1,000,000 people. In addition, Dr. Rusangwa oversaw the technical and financial support of a cancer center of excellence in Butaro, Rwanda, the only center in the region to provide free cancer diagnosis and care. He is a global health and operational research expert pushing for access to health care for all.

Contents

Preface

In the quiet corners of our world, far from the bustling cityscapes and the relentless pace of urban life, lies a treasure trove of experiences, challenges, and opportunities that often go unnoticed and unaddressed. This book, *Rural Health – Investment, Research and Implications*, is an exploration into the heart of rural communities and the intricate web of factors that shape the health and well-being of their inhabitants.

Rural areas, with their expansive landscapes and close-knit communities, offer a unique lens through which we can examine the broader landscape of health care, research, and the socioeconomic implications that flow from it. The purpose of this book is not merely to spotlight the healthcare disparities that exist between rural and urban populations but to delve deep into the core issues that perpetuate these disparities and to offer a roadmap for meaningful change.

Our journey begins with a recognition of the undeniable truth that rural health is an integral part of the larger global health landscape. It is a cornerstone upon which the health of nations is built and yet it often struggles in the shadows of its urban counterpart. Rural areas are home to a diverse array of cultures, lifestyles, and economies, each with its own set of health challenges and solutions waiting to be discovered.

As we embark on this exploration, we are guided by three pillars: investment, research, and implications. Investment is the bedrock upon which any meaningful change in rural health must be built. Without the necessary resources, infrastructure, and financial support, the health disparities that persist in rural communities will continue to widen. But investment alone is not enough; it must be informed by rigorous research. The chapters within this book weave together the latest findings, innovative methodologies, and insightful analyses to shed light on the intricacies of rural health. Finally, we delve into the implications of our discoveries, examining the ways in which they can shape policies, healthcare practices, and the lives of those residing in rural areas.

This book is the culmination of the collective efforts of researchers, healthcare professionals, policymakers, and community members who are dedicated to improving the health and well-being of rural populations. It serves as both a testament to the progress that has been made and a call to action for the work that lies ahead. It is a reminder that rural health is not a peripheral concern but a central pillar of our society's overall well-being.

In the pages that follow, you will find a rich tapestry of insights, stories, and perspectives that paint a vivid picture of rural health in all its complexity. We hope that this book will not only inform but inspire action—a renewed commitment to investing in rural health, conducting groundbreaking research, and recognizing the profound implications that extend far beyond the countryside. Together, we can bridge the gap and ensure that rural health is no longer an afterthought but a thriving, integral part of our global healthcare landscape.

As we embark on this journey, we invite you to join us in the exploration of *Rural Health – Investment, Research and Implications*. It is our sincere hope that through the pages of this book, you will gain a deeper understanding of the challenges and opportunities that lie within rural communities and be inspired to contribute to the betterment of rural health worldwide.

A special acknowledgment goes to those who contributed intellectual materials and editorial efforts to make this book possible.

Christian Rusangwa
Muso Health
Abidjan, Ivory Coast

Section 1

Addressing Community Health Issues: Experiences from the Field

Chapter 1

Lessons Learned from Implementing a Community Health Worker-Initiated Referral Strengthening Intervention in Haiti: A Mixed-Methods Program Case Study

Alain Casseus, Kenia Vissieres, Tracy L. McClair, Chery Maurice Jr, Charlotte Warren and Pooja Sripad

Abstract

Referral processes linking communities to facilities are under-appreciated and lack evaluation, particularly in humanitarian settings. Community health workers or agents de santé communautaire polyvalent (ASCPs) in Haiti refer communities to health facilities for a range of services. This program case study assessed implementation of a public-private referral strengthening intervention within on-going community health programming, including a triplicate referral form, supportive training, and follow-up structures. We applied mixed methods to describe referral trends using routine programmatic data, factors affecting implementation and referral completion through a pre-intervention referred patient survey (n = 525), meeting observations, and interviews with ASCPs, supervisors, and key stakeholders (n = 88). We found that the intervention demonstrates little influence on referral trends, but qualitatively enhances the referral process for ASCPs and supervisory stakeholders in Haiti. It improves supervision relationships and shows promise for enhanced community-integrated patient monitoring systems – when supported by financial support and non-governmental and governmental partners, but is vulnerable to sociopolitical, geographic, and insecurity challenges preventing referral completion. Integrating intervention activities within existing programming and scaling the triplicate referral form in Haiti can strengthen the national ASCP curricula. Globally, we suggest adapting the triplicate referral form as a promising job-aid and data-reporting tool within community health worker programs.

Keywords: community health workers, community-based referral, case study, referral processes, Haiti

1. Introduction

Referral processes linking communities to facilities for an array of health services, though critical are often under-appreciated and challenging to measure globally. In part this is due to measurement gaps given limited community inputs into integrated health information systems and the challenges of monitoring referral completion [1–3]. Facilitating linkages through functional referral and counter-referral mechanisms demands that community health workers (CHWs) are able to correctly identify when to refer patients; patients are able to access the referral facility; and the referral facilities provide sufficient counter-referral information to patients for follow-up with CHWs in their communities [4]. Global estimates of adherence to referral guidelines, defined broadly as both CHW adherence to guidelines and referral completion by patients, range from 9 to 83% [4]. Few studies have evaluated the effectiveness and comprehensiveness of CHW referral in low- and middle-income country (LMIC) settings, nor assessed the influence of context and programming on CHW-activated referral processes and completion [2, 3, 5].

Exploring referral processes in the context of expanding community health programming to support CHWs as they reduce service coverage gaps and improve outcomes is critical. In countries like Haiti that struggle with frequent political transition, decreasing economic resources, and environmental and disease outbreaks, all of which have left it with the worst health indicators in the Western Hemisphere, CHWs are often the only source of care for many [6–9]. Haiti's ratio of physicians and nurses to individuals is 2.5 and 1.1 to 10,000, respectively, has led CHWs, to serve as the primary health workforce in delivering care and counseling to communities [10]. CHWs in Haiti, known as agents de santé communautaire polyvalent (ASCPs) make approximately 100 home visits per month during which they provide direct services (e.g. medicines, vaccination, and some family planning methods), health education, and referrals. ASCPs link communities to health facilities for a range of services by referring for a variety of health issues: tuberculosis, HIV, malnutrition, women's health, maternity care, child health, non-communicable diseases, mental health, and other emergencies. ASCPs refer patients to facilities for care as needed and document referrals in paper-based registers. Generally, the referral process involves ASCPs interacting with individuals in the community and referring, and at times, accompanying clients to the appropriate facility – a dispensary, health center or hospital, and following up with the clients once they return home. Sociopolitical and contextual factors influence ASCP-initiated referral processes [11]. To-date, however, documentation of how to strengthen referral processes in practice is weak in the absence of data reporting tools to aid ASCPs and their supervisors, among other factors.

This program case study describes learnings from the introduction of a public-private referral strengthening intervention, consisting of the introduction of a triplicate referral form and supportive programmatic structures. We draw on multiple perspectives – ASCPs, ASCP supervisors, and key policy/program stakeholders to assess how the referral strengthening intervention (e.g. introduction of a triplicate referral form and associated-trainings for adoption) affected the community-initiated referral process in all sites. Referral "completion", in our study, refers to whether a patient who was referred by an ASCP for a service went to a facility received the intended service. We investigate:

- Did the referral strengthening intervention affect the referral trends?
- How did the referral strengthening intervention affect referral processes?

- What factors affected implementation of the intervention?
- What factors affect referral completion?

2. Program development and adaptation

2.1 Program development and description

Zanmi Lasante (ZL), a non-governmental local organization in Haiti has been working in community health for decades in collaboration with the Ministère de la Santé Publique et de la Population (MSPP). Under the Integrating Community Health Partnership (2016–2020), ZL supported the MSPP in the introduction and orientation of ASCPs in Central and Artibonite regions, through the development and implementation of a comprehensive curricula. The curricula included five modules: Organization of Health Services, the ASCP Work Process, Health at Different Life Stages, Prevention and Control of Common Diseases, and ASCP Actions in Crisis Situations. Despite the various contextual disruptions including political volatility and generalized insecurity, ZL supported implementation of curricula, integrated with on-going programming efforts, over 4 years, to inform scaling a ASCP capacity-building approach country-wide.

Within this program context, in 2018, there was recognition of the need to further strengthen and support referral and counter-referral processes embedded within the ASCP's core functions. ZL, in collaboration with the Department de la Promotion de la Sante et Protection de l'Environnement in the MSPP, developed and implemented a triplicate referral form, a related training, and a supportive feedback mechanism to pilot as a tool for tracking and enhancing referrals, referral completion, and follow up. The triplicate referral form – comprised of three carbon copy slips that can be shared with clients, CHWs and health facilities – allows for better documentation around health areas that ASCPs normally counsel and refer (**Figure 1**). Following a week-long training in November 2019 in Mirebalais, the triplicate referral forms were implemented across Central and Artibonite Departments, including in Mirebalais, Le Petit Rivière Artibonite (PRA) and Verrettes communes. Upon referral of a client to a facility, an ASCP documented the referral in his/her register, provided a referral sheet to the client, and shared in aggregate a monthly referral report to their supervisor. The feedback mechanism, coordinated by ZL program managers, included health teams discussing referral challenges and enablers during on-going monthly meetings between a community health nurse (program oversight), ASCPs, and their supervisors.

Several adaptations affected program development and application. First, while initially a technological component (digital triplicate referral form) to complement the paper-based form was explored, various organizational, political, and logistical challenges prevented its integration. Second, a Community Health Nurse and Auxiliary Nurse intended to review and cross-reference ASCP registers and reports with the referral lists at the dispensaries, health centers, and hospitals to identify complete and incomplete referrals. However, in practice, only referrals made – rather than completed– were able to be checked. Third, COVID-19 pandemic-related restrictions prevented feedback sessions to occur at in their anticipated frequency –four sessions were held before lockdowns ensued; not all three communes resumed sessions as the pandemic wore on. These restrictions, along with persisting socio-political

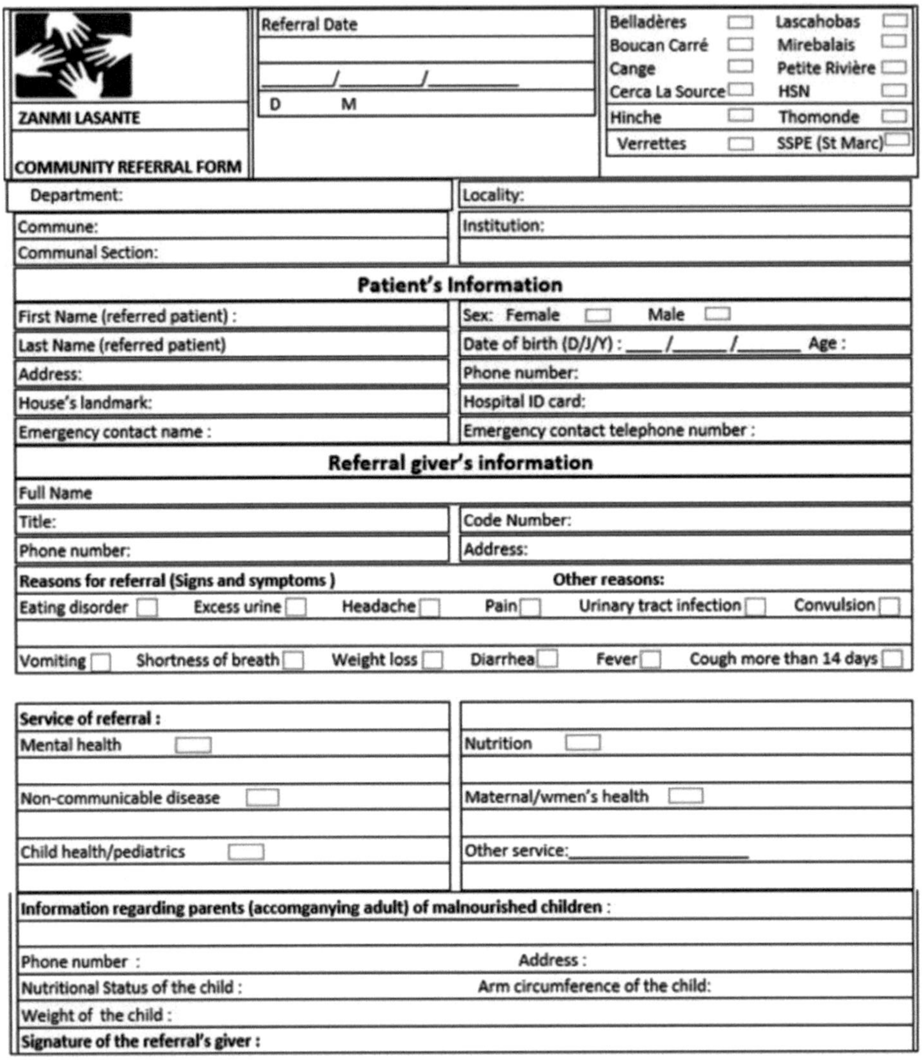

ZANMI LASANTE

COMMUNITY REFERRAL FORM

Referral Date

______/______/______

D M

Belladères ☐ Lascahobas ☐
Boucan Carré ☐ Mirebalais ☐
Cange ☐ Petite Rivière ☐
Cerca La Source ☐ HSN ☐
Hinche ☐ Thomonde ☐
Verrettes ☐ SSPE (St Marc) ☐

Department: | Locality:
Commune: | Institution:
Communal Section:

Patient's Information

First Name (referred patient) : | Sex: Female ☐ Male ☐
Last Name (referred patient) | Date of birth (D/J/Y) : ___/____/____ Age :
Address: | Phone number:
House's landmark: | Hospital ID card:
Emergency contact name : | Emergency contact telephone number :

Referral giver's information

Full Name
Title: | Code Number:
Phone number: | Address:

Reasons for referral (Signs and symptoms) **Other reasons:**

Eating disorder ☐ Excess urine ☐ Headache ☐ Pain ☐ Urinary tract infection ☐ Convulsion ☐

Vomiting ☐ Shortness of breath ☐ Weight loss ☐ Diarrhea ☐ Fever ☐ Cough more than 14 days ☐

Service of referral :
Mental health ☐ | Nutrition ☐
Non-communicable disease ☐ | Maternal/wmen's health ☐
Child health/pediatrics ☐ | Other service:____________

Information regarding parents (accomganying adult) of malnourished children :

Phone number : Address :
Nutritional Status of the child : Arm circumference of the child:
Weight of the child :
Signature of the referral's giver :

Figure 1.
Triplicate referral form used in Haiti (English version).

fluctuations and insecurity in Haiti, prevented the application of some of our original learning tools (e.g., survey with referred patients) in a formal evaluation.

2.2 Learning tools

Our program case study draws on quantitative and qualitative data sources to learn about the piloting process of the triplicate referral form in practice. Trends in referrals across the three communes were ascertained through routine programmatic referral tracking data, including registers and referral reports verified by health teams. Factors associated with referral completion were assessed by self-report through 525 referred patients surveyed in a pre-intervention assessment and qualitatively from ASCPs following implementation. Semi-structured monthly meeting observational check-lists recorded by trained research assistants qualitatively informed how supervisory

Participant type	Pre-intervention	Post-intervention
ASCPs	24	23
Supervisory stakeholders	15	13
Community health policy/program stakeholders	10	3
Total	49	39

Table 1.
In-depth interview sample.

processes affected the community-activated referral mechanisms. Eighty-eight in-depth interviews with ASCPs, ASCP supervisors, and community health policy/program stakeholders, conducted before (n = 49) and after (n = 39) the implementation, provided rich perspectives on the referral processes, completion and related factors (**Table 1**).

3. Piloting

3.1 Did the referral strengthening intervention affect the referral trends in all sites?

Referral data from ASCP records indicate that over 12 months of active implementation from December 2019 to November 2020, referrals by ASCP in the Central and Artibonite Departments were similar (**Figure 2**). Referrals appear slightly higher in the Central Department, with a slight increase over time in both groups. There is a notable spike in referrals in September 2020 in the Artibonite Department and dips in referrals, across all sites, in April and November 2020, notably affected by

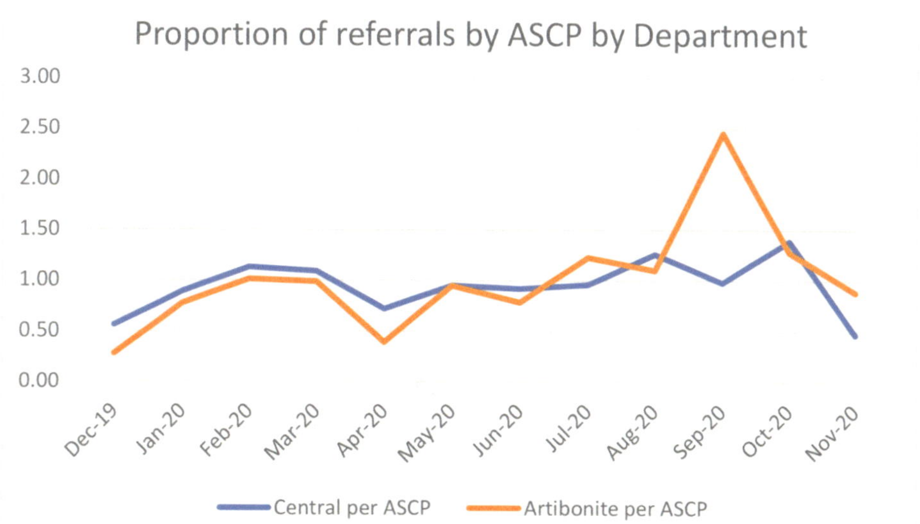

Figure 2.
Referral trends by Department.

the COVID-19 pandemic. Referral peaks reflect the easing of COVID restrictions around movement. At these times, people moved freely from different areas within the country and across the border from the Dominican Republic. Dips in referrals are related to increased COVID restrictions, including social distancing guidelines, mask wearing, and limits to gathering at assembly posts and hospital waiting rooms.

3.2 How did the referral strengthening intervention affect referral processes?

We qualitatively assessed what the referral process looked like before and after the introduction of the triplicate referral form and associated trainings. Our pre-implementation assessment showed that the referral process involved an ASCP providing a verbal or simple referral slip to the patient. The referral slip included the name, phone number of the ASCP, and patient information. Facilities were not notified of referrals. ASCPs stated that they never or rarely received counter-referral slips after referrals were completed. ASCPs were not notified if patients completed their referrals; however, ASCPs recorded the date of referral in their notebooks, and often followed up 4–5 days later to see if the patient completed the referral.

> *'The referral is usually done informally; the patient is told to go to a health center, no documentation, whatsoever... The Department's "referral" form ...[though]... printed and distributed at departmental level, is rarely available in the field, at least, not on a regular basis. Community workers therefore simply tell the patient to" go to a health facility and tell the nurse that you have such a problem"."*
>
> – National Policymaker

After the implementation of the triplicate referral form, ASCPs commented that the new forms are detailed and helpful for assessing if people are in urgent need of care, since there are limited resources at health centers. They mentioned receiving training on how to fill out the forms and found the forms easy to use. ASCPs generally did not have any additional recommendations for the forms. Similar to our pre-intervention assessment, ASCPs confirmed that they typically follow up by phone or in-person a few days after they make referrals, and people usually received the intended services. ASCPs commented that triplicate referral forms allow other members of the medical community to better serve their patients. One ASCP describes their modified process for referral:

> *"When I make a referral to a Health Center, the referral form guides me. It includes the place to write the date, the service [referral type], the place to take the service - the nearest hospital or dispensary. I write the name, signature, date of birth, gender. After that, there is a place that says why you refer the person who has signs like big headache or shortness of breath. As an ASCP, I put my code, name and phone number in case of needed follow-up."*
>
> – ASCP, Central, Mirebalais

While consistent across setting, ASCPs and ASCP supervisors describe how the referral process has changed and been made easier after implementing the triplicate referral form.

> *"It has rendered the process easier. At one time, we did not have a form, we would use a sheet of paper from a notebook or pad. When the patient showed up at the hospital,*

the staff did not really know what to do with the sheet of paper or they would drop it somewhere, it could have been written by anyone. Now it is more structured, formal, and the hospital staff receive the patients."

– ASCP, Central, Mirebalais

"It [referral process] changed in that it gives you more motivation, because now it is a reference form that represents a registry. So when making the referral, the remaining source [copy] allows us to verify the referral was well done. [Previously it]… was a small sheet that was given and the person went with it, there was no source [copy] left. We can follow up on the referrals as supervisors."

– ASCP Supervisor, Artibonite, PRA

3.3 What factors affected implementation of the intervention?

Supervisors and ASCPs describe the importance of supportive supervision as critical to ASCP's work, including the use of the triplicate form. Specifically, the value of supervision arises in technical support, training, and correcting ASPC's behaviors and practices as needed on the job. Monthly group supervision on various topics including referral, allows for ASCPs to work out challenges with the referral process and allows for upward and downward communication between the department and central MSPP through to ASCP supervisors and ASCPs. Our sample's ASCPs and supervisors describe supervisory meetings as opportunities for receiving encouragement by supervisors and peers.

"There are changes [over the last year]… My supervisor is always present, he is always on time, he is a supervisor that I love very much. When I have concerns… he tells me to look how he does it, gives me strength, and says, 'Let me see.' Sometimes he tells me, 'it's not this, come let's go on.' He always encourages me."

– ASCP, Artibonite, PRA

Supervision on applying the triplicate referral form was similar across all settings and reportedly helpful from the perspective of most ASCPs and supervisory stakeholders. ASCPs and supervisors noted that supervisors provide support with filling out triplicate referral forms when challenges are encountered.

"He always double-checked if I keep record of the reference forms that I delivered to patients… Sometimes it happens that we remove them both and the supervisor couldn't trace the reference. To prevent this, he always keeps an eye on the reference forms we are using, trying to ensure that we give the first one and keep a copy, to be able to report on the number of references we give."

– ASCP, Artibonite, PRA

Observational notes from monthly meetings showed that despite the usefulness of the triplicate referral form, one complaint voiced by ASCPs included the difficulty in receiving counter referral information from facilities. Often there was lack of information shared by supervisory facility-based staff on patients completing their referrals, a result of fragmented and delayed data-reporting systems.

ASCPs noted that the modeled communication between ASCPs and their supervisors translates into how ASCPs mobilize their clients, underlining the downstream benefits of the ASCP-supervisor relationship. Supervisors also back up and/or accompany ASCPs as needed, particularly in emergencies and when ASCPs experience difficult client refusals. In some cases, supervisors provide corrections personally after a group session to not embarrass or offend ASCPs in front of their peers.

> *"It is a good relationship, everyone knows their role and the hierarchy - as such, no one dominates another, we each have tasks to accomplish. If there is a problem, I may make a recommendation; if something needs my changing, I oblige. I also do the training [monthly meeting] sessions, our relationship is based on our set objective that we work together to attain."*
>
> – Nurse, Artibonite, Verrettes

There are mixed perspectives as to how accessible supervisors are to ASCPs. Most ASCPs say that supervisors are accessible when you need them and are often close to the field, however, a few describe limited accessibility in situations of political turmoil and roadblocks. ASCPs and ASCP supervisors alike describe the importance of having individual phone-based communication, particularly when ASCPs have quick questions or need clarification while in the field. ASCP supervisors also provide in-person on-site visits and/or accompany ASCPs to homes and posts, especially when health workers and communities are in remote areas.

> *"We work together and when there is something that does not work well, I always reach out to tell them [ASCPs] how things should be. I always hold meetings with them based on our activities... I create my calendar based on their calendar and I would go to them to complete the fieldwork."*
>
> – ASCP Supervisor, Artibonite, Verrettes

Financial and non-financial support also affects implementation of the triplicate referral form and ASCPs work. ASCPs describe the need for salary increase given their current salary is not motivating and they suffer increasing expenses due to inflation and sociopolitical insecurity. ASCPs and supervisors also mention the need for additional funds for transportation (e.g. motorbike taxis, buying gas) and phone cards with sufficient minutes to enable them to conduct their duties effectively. Several ASCPs mentioned needing to borrow money to travel long distances work and some expressed frustration with discontinued transportation fee support. In some cases, the association of ASCPs with government and non-governmental organizations led to a veiled financial stability of ASCPs at the community level.

> *"As a health worker you have a family to care for, you have responsibilities. People think that you work for this giant organization...[and] come to you for money all the time, and there are times you are only able to buy only a loaf of bread... I brought 2 packets of crackers, I did not even get a chance to eat them, I gave them to 2 children who were asking me for money."*
>
> - ASCP, Central, Mirebalais

Though ASCPs maintained access to the triplicate referral form, they expressed limited access to other necessary materials and vaccines to conduct their duties – particularly when it comes to community distribution activities. Some mentioned an inability to give people relevant medications. Supervisors mention similar concerns about materials – supervisors put in many requisitions but claim they have not received items to distribute to ASCPs such as vitamin A pills, iodine pills, folate, vaccines, and menstrual pads.

> *"The role of the government is to provide us with support... they need to provide us more materials, such as notepads, notebooks, and a manual containing the data we need. Sometimes you think you will work on an activity for 2 hours but then you end up working 8 hours; we tend to write extensively, we need other materials to store our documents, bags, and raincoats also."*
>
> – ASCP, Artibonite, PRA

ASPCs expressed that they would like more training for areas that they are less familiar with, such as new or less common diseases. Observation of monthly meetings showed, for example, that ASCPs had some difficulty referring children for problems other than prevalent malnutrition. Community health nurses similarly expressed that they need more training to take advantage of technology innovations in their work. Some ASCPs mentioned that they would like better healthcare treatment for themselves, because even though they are in the health field, when they are sick, it is difficult for them to get are.

The referral process is not without challenges. ASCPs explained that triplicate referral forms are easier than the previous process, but some non-state hospitals do not accept the forms. They explained that it is easier when they refer people to Zanmi Lasante-supported hospitals where the forms are received. When the triplicate referral forms are not recognized nor received, ASCPs feel ashamed, and in some cases blamed, that their patients are not able to get care. An additional challenge is that facilities are not reliably tracking referrals.

> *"When we make referrals, it is very stressful because sometimes the person spends the whole day in the hospital with the referral in his hand, he never is given an appointment... We even accompany the person even though they [facility staff] do not receive us... The references we provide become of no value to the community."*
>
> – ASCP, Central, Mirebalais

3.4 What factors affect referral completion?

We found consistency in the factors affecting referral completion before and after implementation of the referral strengthening intervention.

Our pre-intervention quantitative assessment examined sociodemographic factors associated with referral completion including gender, age, education, marital status, and religion (tabulated data not shown). Referral completion was significantly associated with were gender and religion. Of 525 respondents who were referred by an ASCP in the last 6 months, men were more likely than women to complete a referral at baseline (62 vs. 49%) as were those with no religion compared to those who were Catholic, Protestant, or other (69 vs. 45%, 20, and 51%, respectively). We also examined several interpersonal factors within the respondent-ASCP interaction including number of visits in the last 6 months, whether or not the ASCP asked questions or gave health information to other family members, service satisfaction, whether or not the information provided by the ASCP was easy to understand, and whether or not the ASCP asked the respondent questions about family members' health. Factors significantly associated with referral completion were whether or not the ASCP asked questions or gave health information to other family members (63 vs. 45%), and whether or not the ASCP asked the respondent questions about family members' health (62 vs. 42%).

Our qualitative pre-intervention assessment showed several factors affected referral completion. First, ASCPs stated that referral institutions are sometimes too far for patients. The cost associated with referral completion are prohibitive for some patients. Some patients do not accept the advice of the ASCPs – for example, some people do not accept that their child is malnourished if the ASCP tells them that this is the case. Some people decide to go to a voodoo priest instead of a health facility, though alternative care seeking emerged less salient at endline.

Following implementation, many of qualitative factors described in the pre-intervention assessment – delayed decision making because of distance, cost, socio-political barriers, and perceived quality – persist. An additional challenge was patients' misunderstandings of the triplicate referral form as it relates to perceived quality of a hospital's responsiveness to a referral. For example, patients believe a referral means they do not have to pay for treatment. Patients think the triplicate referral form means that they are "VIP" and should be treated as such, so they do not want to wait for the doctor.

> *"When we make the referral, the patients always ask us, firstly, to accompany them... secondly, they always complain about not having money for transportation to go to the hospital and that it is difficult to find a service even if they have the referral form."*
>
> – ASCP, Central, Mirebalais

> *"I don't know if this come from the ASCP or if it is a misunderstanding from the patients - patients think that the referral could be used as a pass for everything. A referral doesn't give any right to ["express" care for] the patient -it only indicates that this his problem is identified and the intended service ... Most of the time, [at] the referral institutions, patients with the referral think that they are "VIP" and should be treated as such. They do not want to wait for the doctor... They refuse to pay even their dossier fee... a referral is not a dossier."*
>
> – ASCP Supervisor, Artibonite, PRA

Observational notes from monthly meetings showed that ASCPs raised the more information related to experiences of patients that did not complete referrals. For these patients, the main concerns voiced included wait times at the hospital and the sup-optimal hospital reception, where they felt unwelcome and spoken to in a bad manner.

4. Lessons learned

Implementation of a referral strengthening intervention – a triplicate referral form, supportive training, and monthly troubleshooting meetings – as a part of routine community health programming demonstrates little influence on overarching referral trends, but promising qualitative effects on the referral process for ASCPs and supervisory stakeholders in Haiti. Our piloting shows that despite the persisting challenges to the referral completion at the patient level that further link to the country's extreme poverty and limited emergency and routine relief in the protracted insecurity [12], high quality of supervisory relationships were instrumental in mitigation and reinforced the use of the triplicate referral form. This suggests the value of a streamlined referral form extends beyond the merit of improved community-integrated patient tracking as part of health care monitoring systems, but also to the motivational aspects around individual community health stakeholder goal-setting and achievements.

We glean several lessons around sustaining implementation beyond the project timeline – and in the face of further disaster (e.g. COVID-19 pandemic). First, implementing the intervention demands a nominal cost associated with producing the triplicate referral form and that of personnel to oversee its distribution, collection, and validation. These costs may be reduced if digital tracking were enabled, though such solutions require high preliminary investment and regular updates for failed technology. Second, collaborative development of the triplicate referral form by Zanmi Lasante and the MPSS, enabled its successful integration into on-going referral processes, though further technical assistance and advocacy may be required for its full recognition in non-state hospitals. Third, there is a need to strengthen counter referral processes, including tracking referral completion at the facility level. Communicating care features and monitoring needs back to ASCPs routinely through functional supervisory feedback mechanisms described in this paper can help better follow up with communities over time. Finally, navigating politics to sustain gains in community-integrated referral strengthening is crucial in contexts with shifting and unstable ministerial and policy landscapes. As intervention implementation progressed over time in Haiti, we had to accommodate changes in community health governance and financial investments that re-prioritized aspects of ASCP hiring, training, and retention.

5. Recommendations and conclusions

Community health stakeholders in Haiti find the referral strengthening intervention acceptable – given it can be easily integrated into routine workflows of CHWs, supervisors, and program managers. We recommend integration of the triplicate referral form, training, and follow up meetings as a quality assurance mechanism to strengthen community-facility linkage and equitable communication between supervisors and CHWs. In Haiti, we advocate for scaling the triplicate referral form across the country, as part of the national ASCP curricula; over time transitioning the referral tracking system to a digital platform can be considered. Scaling the form alongside further research is needed, especially around the disaggregation of referral trend effects by distance to a facility and linked trends in referral completion. Globally, particularly in similar fragile humanitarian settings where CHWs carry out much of the primary health care service delivery, we suggest adapting the triplicate referral form as a promising job-aid and data-reporting tool.

Acknowledgements

We want to thank all who contributed to this work, particularly Sarah Kennedy, Smisha Agarwal and Ralph Ternier, for their roles during the early phases of design and implementation. We also thank Guerline Bayas, a member of the Haitian Ministry of Health, for her support of the study.

Funding statement

This study was supported by the Bill & Melinda Gates Foundation [OPP1174594].

Author details

Alain Casseus[1*], Kenia Vissieres[1], Tracy L. McClair[2], Chery Maurice Jr[1], Charlotte Warren[3] and Pooja Sripad[2]

1 Zanmi Lasante, Port-au-Prince, Haiti

2 Independent Contributor, Washington, USA

3 Population Council, Washington, USA

*Address all correspondence to: acasseus@pih.org

References

[1] Agarwal S, Sripad P, Johnson C, Kirk K, Bellows B, Ana J, et al. A conceptual framework for measuring community health workforce performance within primary health care systems. Human Resources for Health. 2019;**17**(1):1-20

[2] Kok MC, Dieleman M, Taegtmeyer M, Broerse JEW, Kane SS, Ormel H, et al. Which intervention design factors influence performance of community health workers in low- and middle-income countries? A systematic review. Health Policy Plan. 2015;**30**(9):1207-1227

[3] Nigussie Z, Zemicheal N, Tiruneh G, Bayou Y, Teklu G, Kibret E, et al. Using mHealth to improve timeliness and quality of maternal and newborn health in the primary health care system in Ethiopia. Global Health: Science and Practice. 2021;**9**(3):668-681

[4] Lal S, Ndyomugenyi R, Paintain L, Alexander ND, Hansen KS, Magnussen P, et al. Community health workers adherence to referral guidelines: Evidence from studies introducing RDTs in two malaria transmission settings in Uganda. Malaria Journal. 2016;**15**(1):1-13

[5] Kok MC, Kane SS, Tulloch O, Ormel H, Theobald S, Dieleman M, et al. How does context influence performance of community health workers in low- and middle-income countries? Evidence from the literature. Health Research Policy and Systems. 2015;**13**(1):1-14

[6] Atun R, De Andrade LOM, Almeida G, Cotlear D, Dmytraczenko T, Frenz P, et al. Health-system reform and universal health coverage in Latin America. Lancet. 2015;**385**(9974):1230-1247

[7] Zeng W, Cros M, Wright KD, Shepard DS. Impact of performance-based financing on primary health care services in Haiti. Health Policy and Planning. 2013;**28**(6):596-605

[8] Cavagnero EDV, Cros MJ, Dunworth AJ, Sjoblom MC, America L, Caribbean DD. Better Spending, Better Care: A Look at Haiti's Health Financing: Summary Report. Washington DC: The World Bank Group, ed; 2017

[9] Sripad P, Casseus A, Kennedy S, Isaac B, Vissieres K, Warren CE, et al. "Eternally restarting" or "a branch line of continuity"? Exploring consequences of external shocks on community health systems in Haiti. Journal of Global Health. 2021;**11**:07004

[10] Jerome & Ivers. Community Health Workers in Health Systems Strengthening: A qualitative evaluation from rural Haiti. AIDS. 2010;**24**(Suppl 1):1-9

[11] Project FH, Lasante Z. Assessing the performance of community health workers in Haiti: Key findings from a mixed-methods study. Reproductive Health [Internet]. 2021;(October 2019:1-4. Available from: https://knowledgecommons.popcouncil.org/departments_sbsr-rh/1383

[12] Leaning J, Guha-Sapir D. Natural disasters, armed conflict, and public health. The New England Journal of Medicine. 2013;**369**(19):1836-1842

Chapter 2

Perspective Chapter: Integrating Traditional Healers into the National Health Care System – A Review and Reflection

Bamdev Subedi

Abstract

This paper reviews and reflects on the policy efforts to integrate traditional healers in Nepal. Most people in rural Nepal rely on traditional healers for their primary health care needs, not only because health facilities in rural areas are poorly functioning but also because these healers meet various health care needs. The kind of traditional medicine provided by traditional healers (such as herbalists, bone setters, faith healers, and traditional midwives) is much more accessible to them than the practitioners of biomedicine and scholarly traditional medicine (such as Ayurveda, Unani, and Homeopathy). However, traditional healers have not been recognized as legitimate practitioners. Policy initiatives are needed to facilitate recognition, accreditation, or licensing of traditional healers so that they can be integrated into the formal structure of the health care system. Nepal's recent initiative of registration of traditional healers is an important policy effort in this direction.

Keywords: integration, traditional healers, primary health care, traditional medicine, Nepal

1. Introduction

Traditional medicine is widely used and the world today sees its relevance for health and well-being [1]. The issue of integration of traditional healers into the national health care system got prominence around the time of Alma-Ata Conference in Primary Health Care in 1978 [2–5]. The Alma-Ata Declaration not only highlighted the wide existence of traditional healers including traditional birth attendants but also the importance of engaging them in the formal health system to meet primary health care needs. The Declaration stated that

> *"With the support of the formal health system, these indigenous practitioners can become important allies in organizing efforts to improve the health of the community. Some communities may select them as community health workers. Therefore, it is worthwhile exploring the possibilities of engaging them in primary health care and training them accordingly" [6].*

Following the recommendation of the Alma-Ata Declaration, many nation-states explored the possibilities of integrating them. Those traditional healers who were practicing scholarly traditional medicine (such as Ayurveda, Unani, and Homeopathy) or qualified in any stream of these systems were recognized as practitioners and integrated into the formal health care system. Those traditional healers (who were practicing "folk", "popular," or "indigenous" traditional medicine) largely remained outside the state's purview and regulation. Only 36 countries have regulated "indigenous traditional medicine providers" that include "traditional healers, bone setters, herbalists, and traditional birth attendants" [7].

Though the integration of traditional medicine into the general public health system has been recognized as a "pressing need" [8], no such laudable efforts were made in bringing traditional healers into the fold of the formal health system. Scholars have recognized the important role traditional healers play in primary health care and often they are described as "the principal health care providers", "primary source of health care", "first point of contact", "first treatment of choice", etc. and appreciated for their healing prowess and herbal knowledge. The contribution of traditional healers in primary health care has been highlighted and scholars argue for their inclusion in the formal health care system [9]. Despite all this, the integration of traditional healers remains to be an unfinished dream in many nation-states.

The scholarly emphasis seems much on traditional medicine, medicinal practices, and medicinal herbs rather than the traditional healers who practice medicine and who have the knowledge of using herbs as medicine. This is something that recognizes the value of medicinal herbs but not the traditional healers who have been using them. This is something that tends to recognize the knowledge but not the (original) knowledge holder.

In many developing countries, health facilities are largely concentrated in urban areas [10] and rural populations are poorly served by the formal healthcare system. Traditional healers are providing at least some form of health care to the rural populations who are underserved by the formal healthcare system [11]. Even in urban areas, formal healthcare services are expensive, and traditional healers work as an affordable substitute. The kind of traditional medicine provided by traditional healers (such as herbalists, faith/spiritual healers, bone setters, and traditional midwives) is much more accessible to them than practitioners of biomedicine and scholarly traditional medicine. Moreover, some traditional healers address the different healthcare needs that patients cannot avail from formal healthcare providers.

Traditional healers, in many settings, lack legitimacy and are practicing informally. The issue of traditional healers' legitimacy has drawn the attention of scholars and activists. In this context, this chapter looks into Nepal's efforts to integrate these healers based on the literature, policy documents, periodic plans, and programs. However, some of the descriptive information about the healers are backed by my field experience [12–14]. The chapter begins with a short note on the health care system of Nepal, looks into the difference between scholarly and popular traditional medicine, and then describes the volume and types of traditional healers and then examines their place in the policy documents and periodic plans. The last part of the paper reviews the recent development of registration standards for traditional healers, reflects on challenges and opportunities, quality concerns, and how government can support traditional healers to provide quality traditional medicine services, and emphasizes the need for the policy initiatives as concluding remarks.

2. Health care system of Nepal

Healthcare services are provided by both public and private facilities. The public sector provides health services from 201 public hospitals, 189 primary health care centers (PHCC), and 3,794 health posts (HP), and the private sector provides from 2082 facilities [15]. After entering into the federal system of government in 2017, Nepal has three levels of government (a federal, seven provincial, and 753 local) and the local level governments' role has become very important in the delivery of health care services. The local government plays an important role in the administration of PHCC and HP and the provision of services to local communities [16].

Traditional medicine services are also provided by both public and private health facilities. Public facilities include a total of 382 Ayurveda facilities (2 Ayurveda hospitals, 14 Zonal Ayurveda Dispensaries, 61 District Ayurveda Health Centers, and 305 Ayurveda Dispensaries), 1 Homeopathy hospital and an Unani dispensary [17]. Several private facilities (hospitals, clinics, and pharmacies) provide Ayurveda, Homeopathy, Sowa-Rigpa, and Naturopathy services.

Nepal is ranked 143 (out of 192 countries) on the Human development index [18] and 98 (out of 163) on the SDG index [19]. Nepal has relatively low health expenditure (around 5% of GDP) and high out-of-pocket spending (around 57% of the total health expenditure) [20] and only 21.35% of the population has been covered by the national health insurance program [21]. People have to pay from their own pockets for traditional medicine services because traditional medicine facilities are yet to be included in the list of service provider institutions.

Nepal has high poverty headcount ratio (32.8% at $3.20/day), high maternal (186/100,000 live births) and under-5 mortality rates (28/1000 live births), and high prevalence of stunting (31.5%) and wasting (12.0%) in under-5 children, and low life expectancy at birth (70.9 years) and low subjective wellbeing score (4.4 in the scale of 0–10, worst-best) [19].

The total population of Nepal is 29.1 million, according to the 2021 census. There are a total of 2,67,891 registered human resources for health (including 28,477 medical doctors, dentists, and specialists; 96,430 nurses and auxiliary nurse midwives; 77,605 health assistants and auxiliary health workers; 14,720 pharmacists, 790 Ayurveda physicians, and 4281 Ayurveda practitioners; 71 Naturopathy and Yoga practitioners, 174 Acupuncture practitioners, and 228 Homeopathy and Unani practitioners) [22]. The Sowa-Rigpa practitioners have not been registered yet but it is likely that they will be registered soon.

The doctor-to-population ratio (0.9 physicians/1000 population) and nurse-to-population ratio (2.1 nurses/1000 population) in Nepal are far less than the SDG index threshold of 4.45 physicians, nurses, and midwives per 1000 population [23]. The concentration of the health workforce in urban areas resulted in an unequal distribution of human resources for health. Although traditional healers are widespread in rural areas, they remain an untapped resource. Traditional healers hold the possibility to contribute to achieving SDG 3, which is about "ensuring healthy lives and promoting well-being for all at all ages." Moreover, their service is in line with the spirit of universal health coverage in the sense that people can access traditional healer's services at their doorstep whenever they need, without financial hardship [24].

3. Traditional medicine: scholarly and popular

Following Dunn [25], traditional medicine can be divided into two groups: (i) Scholarly traditional medicines which are distributed over a relatively large area such as Ayurveda, Unani, and traditional Chinese medicine, and (ii) popular traditional medicines, also known as "folk" medicine, are the local or small-scale medicine rooted in the ethnocultural traditions. Scholarly traditional medicines represent the textual tradition and are codified and institutionalized whereas popular traditional medicines represent oral tradition and largely remain in non-codified and noninstitutionalized forms.

The practitioners of scholarly traditional medicine in Nepal hold academic degrees and are registered with Nepal Ayurveda Medical Council (NAMC) or Nepal Health Professional Council (NHPC). Traditional healers lack such degrees and certificates and practice without getting registered. To date, only 19 traditional healers have been registered with NAMC. This means all the healers, except those registered with NAMC, are practicing without being registered. NAMC is the autonomous body to regulate Ayurveda medicine, practitioners, courses, institutions, and traditional healers in Nepal.

Traditional healers in Nepal do not have a formal status. They are not institutionally trained, accredited, or licensed. The current legal framework does not recognize them as legitimate health practitioners. It is important to bring traditional healers into the regulatory framework in order to ensure the safety and efficacy of their practices. The healers have also felt pressure to be registered to serve as valid practitioners and get needful support from the state [26]. Scholars have continuously pointed to the need for the registration of traditional healers. There is an ongoing policy debate to recognize their knowledge and integrate their practices into the formal health care system.

4. The types of traditional healers

Though traditional healers form a major source of health care for many people, they are not a homogeneous category. Various types of traditional healers are catering to people's health care needs. In this chapter, the term "traditional healers" has been used to refer to herbal healers, bone setters, traditional midwives, massagers, faith healers, or any such practitioners who are experienced enough and recognized as healers by the community people. These healers are the informal providers who are not trained in academic institutions but provide health care services based on traditional knowledge and experience. They hold knowledge of medicinal herbs, healing mantras, traditional midwifery, and massage and are consulted for physical, psychosocial, and emotional health problems. They learn the healing knowledge as a family tradition or work under their gurus, the senior traditional healers. Some of them have expanded their knowledge through long-term practice and self-study. They represent the oral tradition and treat patients with herbal remedies and/or healing mantras, based on lineage inheritance of knowledge and experience. Despite the expansion of healthcare services throughout Nepal, a large number of people take recourse to these healers [27]. These healers command the trust of the community in which they live. The healers and patients share the same culture and worldview. In the villages, they are treated with respect and are consulted for a range of physical, emotional, spiritual, and psychosocial problems.

Traditional healers are invariably described as folk healers, indigenous healers, native healers, or indigenous traditional medicine providers. There is no Nepali equivalent term to refer to traditional healers [28]. They are known by different names in different communities. These healers can be categorized into three broad groups:

4.1 Herbal healers

Herbal healers are informal providers who exclusively rely on medicinal plants for the treatment of different health problems. Though they are also known as *vaidya* (informal Ayurveda practitioner), *amchi* (informal Sowa-Rigpa practitioner), and *hakim* (informal Unani practitioner) but are not qualified from academic institutions. They follow textual tradition by learning privately in the family or with the *guru* and, therefore, hold no certificates or degrees. There are other categories of herbal healers who do not follow textual tradition but hold the knowledge and know-how of medicinal herbs and deal with specific health problems such as jaundice or bone fracture. These healers use medicinal plants and plant parts, mineral substances, and animal products as medicine. Some of them also purchase manufactured herbal medicine and dispense them keeping a margin of profit. The herbal healers are consulted for physical illnesses and injuries. Some specialist traditional healers are consulted for specific illness problems such as bone fractures, snake bites, jaundice, stomach pain, and joint pain.

4.2 Faith/spiritual healers

Faith/spiritual healers use nonmaterial means for diagnosis, prevention, and treatment, invoking unseen/spiritual forces. Some of them may combine healing mantras with herbal medicines. They are known as *dhami-jhankri* (shamans), *jannne-manchhe* (those who know herbal and faith healing), *jhar-phuke* (healers who sweep down or blow out evil spirits), *mata* (a woman healer possessed by Goddess), *jyotish* (an astrologer who foretells star and suggest rituals like *grah-shanti*), *pundit, pujari, lama, gubhaju, or guruwa* (who do faith healing and priestly work). Faith/spiritual healers largely follow the ritual methods of treatment. They are consulted for the illnesses, which are locally understood and explained such as *daraune* (frightening), *jhaskine* (startling), *nidra nalagne* (sleeplessness), *chhatpati hune* (restlessness), and similar other illnesses of emotional, spiritual, and psychosocial nature [12].

4.3 Traditional midwives

Traditional midwives are known as *sudeni*, who assist in homebirth and provide postnatal care and massage. Traditional midwives also use medicinal herbs and oils, treated with ingredients such as fenugreek, for massage.

5. The size of traditional healers

Traditional healers are found in every village and town in Nepal. Scholars and planners often quote a study [29] that had estimated the number of traditional faith healers to be around four to eight hundred thousand. The number also shows that faith healing is the most widely prevalent tradition in Nepal [30]. The number got an entry in the Ninth Five Year Plan [31], which stated: "to encourage about 800,000 traditional healers *(dhami, jhankri, lama, and vaidya)* to provide health services." Till today, no such study has been done to estimate their precise number and types. However, a common understanding is that the number of traditional healers is dwindling, as the young generation is not interested in taking up the profession of traditional healing. In recent times, formal healthcare services are being expanded. Health awareness is increasing and faith healing is fading. There are instances of faith healers who have left their long-standing faith-healing professions. Similarly, traditional midwives' role has been shrunk with the promotion of institutional deliveries [13]. However, herbal healers have retained their relevance, and even today, traditional healers have a robust presence in Nepal, especially in rural areas. They outnumber the medical practitioners and "85% of the rural population turns to traditional healers as their first point of care" [28].

6. Traditional healers in policy and periodic plans

Ayurveda Medical Council Act 1988 allowed registration for those traditional healers who were 50 years and above and practicing herb-based Ayurveda medicine as a family tradition for the last three generations and [32]. The Section 5.1.1B of the Act states that "In the case of a person who is Fifty years of age, and having obtained recommendation from the concerned District Office with the certification of experiences being involved in the Ayurveda medical science since three generations, such person may carry on Ayurveda medical profession by obtaining permission under separate provisions as specified by the Council within one year from the date of commencement of this Act." The Act also barred the unregistered traditional healers to practice as this was made punishable offense with "a fine not exceeding 3000 rupees or with imprisonment for a term not exceeding six months or with both." This provision was criticized as "ridiculous and humiliating" [33]. Indeed, this provision was restrictive for those who were below 50 years of age and even for the eligible healers it was just a one-time opportunity to get registered. This may be the reason why there are only 19 traditional healers registered with the NAMC. The Act illegitimated many traditional healers but they kept practicing without getting registered. Rather, they continued to advocate for their rights and recognition. The scholars and activists also argued in favor of traditional healing/healers and questioned the government's reluctance, inaction, and skepticism (see **Box 1** below). The issue of registration and integration invited much debate and discussion among scholars, activists, planners, and policymakers.

"The government cannot remain silent about those who are providing health care to the people in one way or another. Either it [government] should say that there is no use of traditional healer's service, with strong reason; otherwise, it should investigate and open a way to legalize traditional healing"—Shantalal Mulmi, RECPHEC

"The knowledge received from their forefathers, the treatment method of preparing medicine at home from naturally obtained herbs and other things is the original method of Nepal and it is the responsibility of the state to build it and properly manage it"—Dr. Sarita Shrestha

"Such treatment methods which are used for the sake of service rather than financial gain are cheap and accessible as well as being close to the way of life should be mainstreamed"—Madhubajra Bajracharya

"Therefore, in order to register the traditional healers, the government should take an initiation to formulate plan and policies focusing on traditional healers" [26].

"Traditional healing deserves its due share in government budgetary allocation" [28] .

"The roles and responsibilities of traditional healers must be identified and clearly defined" [34].

Box 1. *Activists and scholars speaking in favor of traditional healers.*

6.1 Healers in the periodic plans

An examination of national policies and planning documents reveal inconsistent and insignificant efforts to recognize and integrate healers. In 1998, Nepal Human Development Report [35] wrote, "Traditional healing received little direct support from the state, but in the last 15 years there have been efforts to integrate it with the public health system. But such efforts were peripheral and lukewarm." This shows that there was only a half-hearted effort to integrate traditional healers. Though some of the periodic plans emphasized traditional healers' training. For example, the Sixth Five Year Plan [36] had a program to provide training to traditional healers (such as *vaidya* and *jhankri*) and then the Eighth FYP [37] also repeated to provide training to traditional healers including birth attendants and mobilize them. The Ninth FYP [31] specified the number of healers and planned to encourage them to provide health care services. Subsequent periodic plans did not mention traditional healers but repeated government's commitment to protect and expand Ayurveda and other alternative systems. Thus, in the planning documents, traditional healers sometimes got a mention and sometimes did not. Nevertheless, traditional healers' training remained one of the regular activities of DOAA and at times NGOs also included traditional healers' training in their programs. The training events were mostly intended to increase knowledge of the formal treatment processes and seek referral support rather than to enhance their knowledge and skills in traditional healing (for example, see [38–40]).

6.2 Healers in the health policy

National Health Policy 1991 emphasized the participation of women volunteers and birth attendants (Sudeni). National Ayurveda Health Policy 1996 also emphasized the training of traditional healers and the protection of their knowledge. National Health Policy 2014 continued to repeat "develop, protect, and promote Ayurveda and other complementary medicine." However, the National Health Policy 2019 states that "the existing traditional health care system shall be enlisted, managed, and regulated as per the standard" [41]. This policy provision seems developed from the Nepal Health Sector Strategy [42], which had iterated the government's commitment to the protection and promotion of traditional medicine. The strategy accepted the popularity of traditional practices that are being provided by traditional healers and showed the need to study the effectiveness of this method by bringing them into the mainstream. Similarly, the second long term health plan was to provide traditional healers with appropriate training in health, nutrition, and family planning, and use them in health education activities at the local level [43].

7. Registration standard for traditional healers

After a long debate and series of discussions, the Department of Ayurveda and Alternative Medicine (DOAA) drafted registration standard for traditional treatment providers [44] to facilitate local governments in the registration of traditional healers. The registration standard recognizes traditional healers as *Paramparagat Upacharak*. This Standard has been adopted, approved, and published in the Local Gazette by some municipalities (*Palika*), the local government body. The Standard provides guidance and criteria for the registration of traditional healers. The Standard aims to provide a regulatory framework to ensure the efficacy, safety, and quality of traditional healing; to provide for the management and control over the registration, training, and conduct of practitioners.

The registration standard is based on the provision of Article 22 of the Public Health Service Act, 2018. Article 22 states that it is mandatory to obtain a license to provide health services. Article 22 (3) of the Act states that "In the case of the traditional treatment service, service shall be provided after obtaining approval pursuant to the standards prescribed by the Local Level" [45]. While the practitioners of Ayurveda, Unani, Homeopathy, Yoga, and Naturopathy are registered with the NAMC or NHPC, traditional healers (except those 19 traditional healers) are practicing without being registered. Since the existing legal framework and regulatory body do not recognize them as legitimate health practitioners, the Standard addresses the registration issue, at least for those traditional healers who meet the requirements.

The registration standard defines traditional healers as "those persons who provide treatment at their home based on the knowledge, skills, technology, and experience acquired from their ancestors or *gurukul* traditions, examining the patients looking at the cause, nature, and condition of the disease, and using or processing various herbs, minerals, and animal products available naturally at the local level" [44]. The registration standard also recognizes the three categories of healers: (i) Herbal healers, (ii) Spiritual healers, and (iii) Traditional midwives (*Sudeni*).

7.1 Objectives of the registration standard

The main objective of the registration standard (see **Box 2**) is to bring traditional healers into the regulatory framework. The Standard recognizes those healers who are involved in providing treatment for certain diseases by using certain herbs or sources, those who have acquired healing knowledge through at least 15 years of closeness to ancestors or gurus, and those who have adopted traditional healing as their main occupation. In addition to having a clear knowledge of the cause and symptoms of the disease to be treated, in case of using herbs or materials, the healers should have a genuine knowledge of the place and source along with properties, process, collection method, and time, processing, storage, preservation, supply, and usage. In the case of those who manufacture medicine from herbs and use it, they should properly follow the manufacturing method, use local resources and prepare medicine themselves, and provide health care services.

1. Identify, classify, and collect data on traditional healers and their health and cultural knowledge.
2. Assist in documenting and preserving the knowledge, skills, and technology of traditional healers.
3. Document, validate, protect, promote, develop, and expand the knowledge, skills, and techniques of traditional healers.
4. Determine the eligible and capable traditional healers and delimits their role by classifying them based on their qualification, capacity, and geographical and subject area.
5. Make the registered healers work within the prescribed limits and prepare a basis for discouraging and punishing those who do not comply.
6. Bring uniformity in the standards of traditional healers at the local levels.
7. Protect intellectual property rights.
8. Preserve traditional healers' professions and promote their knowledge, skills, and techniques.
9. Facilitate research studies related to traditional healing.

Box 2. *Objectives of the registration standard for traditional healers.*

7.2 Rights and duties of healers

The Standard defines the functions, duties, and rights of traditional healers. The healers are required to keep records, not only of the method of collection of herbs, the place of collection, and the manufacturing process but also of patients' symptoms, conditions, services provided, and medicines dispensed, including the quantity and dosage. The healers should be able to identify herbs well and prepare medicines at home from such herbs and should have provided treatment services by making medicines from herbs without using the classical or patent medicines manufactured by different companies. The Standard prohibits healers from using classical or patent medicines of various companies, manufactured by using modern technology or knowledge and skills or those readily available in the market. The Standard allows healers to make medicine required for the treatment but forbid them to produce to sell in the market. The Standard does not allow them to advertise their services and products.

The healers are required to contact and coordinate with the Ayurveda dispensary or municipality in case they have specific knowledge, skill, technique, or original manuscript for verification, protection, enrichment, or printing support. Traditional healers who provide health services without being registered will be prosecuted according to prevailing Nepali laws. The Standard gives authority to the municipality to explain the clause of the Standard, to change and modify the schedule of the Standard, and to issue a notice for the registration of the traditional healers.

8. The challenges and opportunities

Traditional healers are not a homogenous category. Integration of diverse forms of traditional healers is a challenge. There are a variety of traditional healers, classified into three groups, and their practices differ considerably. Some practice herb-based medicine, while others mix with shamanistic and spiritualistic practices making it difficult for scientific validation of their practices. Some healers have adopted healing as their main profession and many others continue as a part-time voluntary service. Some do charge for their sustenance and some accept the nominal amount as an offering, yet others do not accept money as they think charging those who are ill is morally wrong. Some are consulted by their extended family members, relatives, and neighbors but some are also consulted by far-away patients. Some follow oral tradition and some follow textual tradition by doing self-study or learning from gurus or senior practitioners. Some healers specialize in herbal treatment, some in midwifery and massage, some in faith healing, shamanism, and magico-religious and spiritual healing. Some others are consulted for specific health conditions such as jaundice, joint pain, and stomach problem. And there is a mismatch of practices, for example, some of the traditional *dhami-jhankri*, they are known for faith healing also possess knowledge of herbs and include herbal treatment along with ritual treatment. The registration standard as it appears is favorable to those healers who practice herbal medicine and restrictive to those who provide faith healing.

Another challenge is that we do not have a good understanding of the number and types of these healers. And, we have no idea about the extent of use of traditional healers by the population, the kind of health care needs these healers address, the number of illness episodes they treat, and the quality of care they provide. There is no such mechanism to collect periodic data on traditional healing and healers' activities. One of the points often gets mentioned is the declining interest in traditional healing and the dwindling number of traditional healers. The young generation is not interested in taking up their parents' occupation, because healers get neither official appreciation nor any incentives. Traditional healing largely remains an unattractive profession because there is no monetary benefit. Though some healers have started to charge for the services and the medicine they dispense. But a very large number of healers give crude herbs and do not charge or charge nominally or take whatever is given out of happiness.

The young generation lacks knowledge and skills regarding medicinal herbs and traditional healing. The educational system has distracted students away from traditional health knowledge. Most of the healers are elderly, and the young generation is not willing to learn traditional healing (because it takes a long time to learn) and this is leading to the inter-generational loss of health knowledge [12].

Opportunity for integration exists when looked at from two different angles. The first is that ethnic communities form one-third of Nepal's population and the ethnic communities do have their own healing traditions. The UNDRIP recognizes the importance of indigenous knowledge, and indigenous people's "right to their traditional medicines and to maintain their health practices" [46]. Similarly, the ILO Convention (169) states that indigenous people's "traditional preventive care, healing practices, and medicine" shall be taken into account while planning and administering health services. WHO encourages member states to integrate traditional and complementary medicine into health systems "by developing national policies, regulatory frameworks, and strategic plans for T&CM products, practices, and practitioners" [7]. The state policy as enshrined in the Constitution of Nepal is to protect and promote the traditional knowledge and experience of the indigenous people and local communities [47]. These international conventions, WHO strategy, and national constitution also work as background reasons to move towards recognition of traditional healing. Moreover, traditional healers are appreciated for their role in conserving traditional knowledge, biodiversity, and plant resources. Another important opportunity for Nepal is that a large number of traditional healers have been serving informally and struggling for recognition and integration. Moreover, traditional healers have community support and cultural legitimacy to their practice, and many scholars and activists see the potential of popular traditional medicine and traditional healers.

9. The question of quality in traditional healing

One of the questions often asked is the quality of treatment services traditional healers provide. If we accept that the kind of medicine people use should be of sufficient quality, it is reasonable to ask about the quality of medicine and services traditional healers provide. Since traditional healers lack academic training, doubt over their prowess, experience, and wisdom exists. Though some studies have found medicinal herbs that are being used by herbal healers are consistent with the principles of Ayurveda [26], their practices have not been validated scientifically and the risk of inappropriate use of herbs exists. Traditional healing is not free from harmful practices and needs extra attention and effort to discourage harmful practices and promote beneficial practices. Beneficial practices "should be scientifically validated and integrated into the health system" [26]. As Dr. Margaret Chan stated, "traditional medicines, of proven quality, safety, and efficacy, contribute to the goal of ensuring that all people have access to care" [1], the quality question is far more important when it comes to traditional healing. From the equity perspective, traditional healing needs additional attention and effort from the state to increase its quality. Steps should be taken to validate traditional healers' knowledge and practices as well as enhance their knowledge and skills.

Popular traditional medicine is the primary source of care for the socioeconomically poor who live in rural areas, and from the equity perspective, it should get priority [48]. However, governments seem reluctant to make a budgetary allocation to address the issue of quality. Traditional healers can be provided with training and modular courses. The registered healers can be recognized by awarding a certificate of appreciation and/or monetary incentives for their outstanding service. They can be incentivized with training, equipment, seed, and saplings to grow medicinal herbs in their home gardens. They can be facilitated to form their associations at local, provincial, and national levels. These associations can be supported to work as a self-regulatory body of traditional healing. An institution can be established to document traditional healing practices and herbal knowledge to build the capacity of traditional healers and promote research activities. Some of the healers can be selected and mobilized as traditional medicine volunteers or Ayurveda health volunteers like the female community health volunteers. There are many things government can and should do to increase access and to enhance/ensure the quality of popular traditional medicine.

People in Nepal often consult traditional healers before consulting formal practitioners [49]. Traditional healers have been making an important contribution to primary healthcare [40] and for the benefit of the community, these healers need to be recognized and integrated into the formal healthcare systems. Integration of traditional healers into the formal healthcare system is likely to contribute to the health and well-being of rural communities. Popular traditional medicine is struggling with the changing socio-economic, educational, legal, and regulatory requirements. The erosion of traditional health knowledge, the young generation's declining interest in the healing profession, the negative attitude towards traditional practices, and the question of safety, efficacy, and quality are some of the challenges traditional healing faces today. The identification of healers, recognition of their practices, promotion of beneficial practices, registering them as treatment providers, and providing them with necessary support can contribute to the integration process.

10. Concluding remarks

Many nations are struggling with the issues of the integration of traditional healers. Nepal is not an exception. Though scholarly traditions have got official legitimacy and academically qualified traditional medicine practitioners have been authorized to practice, traditional healers, the practitioners of popular traditions, have been struggling to secure a legitimate space in the formal structure of the health care system. The issue of integration of traditional healers is complicated. However, Nepal has at least moved ahead from inaction and skepticism towards a more inclusionary health care system in which traditional healers will have a role to play. The recent development suggests Nepal's approval of the idea of recognizing and integrating traditional healers. However much remains to be done to see traditional healers integrated into the health care system. Nepal's example can be a good one if it moves in the desired direction. Policy initiatives are necessary to address issues of recognition, accreditation, or licensing of traditional healers and to help integrate them into the national healthcare system.

Acknowledgements

I would like to thank anonymous reviewer of this chapter who greatly helped to shape this paper in this form. I have received no funding support from any organization for this research. I thank IntechOpen for a publication fee waiver.

Conflict of interest

I declare no conflict of interest.

Author details

Bamdev Subedi
Medical Anthropologist (Doctorate from Jawaharlal Nehru University, New Delhi), Kathmandu, Nepal

*Address all correspondence to: bamdevsubedi@gmail.com

References

[1] WHO. WHO Traditional Medicine Strategy: 2014-2023. World Health Organization, Geneva [Online]. 2013. Available from: https://www.who.int/publications/i/item/9789241506096 [Accessed: July 08, 2021]

[2] WHO Meeting on the Promotion and Development of Traditional Medicine (1977, Geneva) and World Health Organization. The promotion and development of traditional medicine: report of a WHO meeting [held in Geneva from 28 November to 2 December 1977] [Online]. 1978. Available from: https://apps.who.int/iris/handle/10665/40995

[3] Rubel AJ, Sargent C. Parallel medical systems: papers from a workshop on 'the healing process': introduction. Social Science & Medicine. Part B. 1979;**13**(1):3-6. DOI: 10.1016/0160-7987(79)90013-9

[4] Good CM. Traditional medicine: an agenda for medical geography. Social Science & Medicine 1967 1977;11(14):705-713. DOI: 10.1016/0037-7856(77)90156-1

[5] Newell KW, editor. Health by the People. Geneva: World Health Organization; 1975

[6] WHO and UNICEF. Primary Health Care: Report of the International Conference on Primary Health Care, Alma-Ata, USSR, 6-12 September 1978. World Health Organization, Geneva, 1978

[7] WHO. WHO global report on traditional and complementary medicine 2019. World Health Organization [Online]. 2019. Available: https://www.who.int/publications/i/item/978924151536. [Accessed: March 24, 2022]

[8] World Health Organization. Regional Office for South-East Asia, Traditional medicine in the WHO South-East Asia Region: review of progress 2014-2019. World Health Organization. Regional Office for South-East Asia [Online]. 2020. Available from: https://apps.who.int/iris/handle/10665/340393. [Accessed: December 05, 2022]

[9] Lyngdoh JP. In: Kaushik A, Suchiang A, editors. Contribution of Traditional Medicine Toward Primary Health Care in Meghalaya. In: Narratives and New Voices from India: Cases of Community Development for Social Change. Singapore: Springer Nature; 2022. pp. 203-214. DOI: 10.1007/978-981-19-2496-5_14

[10] Tamang AL, Broom A. The practice and meanings of spiritual healing in Nepal. South Asian History and Culture. 2010;**1**(2):328-340

[11] Priya R, Saxena SA. Status and Role of AYUSH and Local Health Traditions under the National Rural Health Mission. New Delhi: National Health Systems Resource Center; 2010

[12] Subedi B. Socioeconomic disparities in access and utilization of health care services in Nepal. In: Christopher S, editor. Caste, COVID-19, and Inequalities of Care, Acharya SS. Singapore: Springer Nature Singapore; 2022. pp. 355-373. DOI: 10.1007/978-981-16-6917-0_18

[13] Subedi B. Medical pluralism among the tharus of Nepal: legitimacy, hierarchy and state policy. Dhaulagiri Journal of Sociology and Anthropology. 2019;**13**:58-66. DOI: 10.3126/dsaj.v13i0.26197

[14] Subedi B. Whose knowledge counts? a reflection on the field narratives

of indigenous health knowledge and practices. Dhaulagiri Journal of Sociology and Anthropology. 2022;**16**(01):59-69. DOI: 10.3126/dsaj.v16i01.50947

[15] DoHS. Annual Report 2020/21. DoHS, Ministry of Health and Population, Government of Nepal, Kathmandu, Nepal. 2022

[16] Lewis TP, Aryal A, Mehata S, Thapa A, Yousafzai AK, Kruk ME. Best and worst performing health facilities: a positive deviance analysis of perceived drivers of primary care performance in Nepal. Social Science & Medicine. 2022;**309**:115251. DOI: 10.1016/j.socscimed.2022.115251

[17] DoHS. Annual Report 2019/20. DoHS, Ministry of Health and Population, Government of Nepal, Kathmandu, Nepal. 2021

[18] UNDP. Human Development Report 2021-22: Uncertain times, unsettled lives: shaping our future in a transforming world. 2022. Available from: https://hdr.undp.org/content/human-development-report-2021-2022 [Accessed: January 05, 2023]

[19] Sachs J, Kroll C, Lafortune G, Fuller G, Woelm F. Sustainable Development Report 2022. Cambridge University Press; 2022

[20] MoHP. Nepal National Health Accounts 2017/18. Ministry of Health and Population (MoHP), Kathmandu, 2022

[21] Health Insurance Board. Health Insurance Board policy and program for the financial year 2022/23 [Swasthya Bima Bord 2079/80 BS ko Niti tatha Karyakram]. Health Insurance Board, Government of Nepal [Online]. 2022. Available from: https://hib.gov.np/en/detail/b-b-aa. [Accessed: January 06, 2023]

[22] MoHP. Nepal's National Strategy for Human Resources for Health 2021-2030 [Nepalko Swasthya Janashakti Sambandhi Rananiti 2076/77-2078/88 BS]. Ministry of Health and Population (MoHP), Kathmandu, Nepal. 2022

[23] WHO. Global Strategy on Human Resources for Health: Workforce 2030. Geneva: World Health Organization; 2016

[24] Bode M, Hariramamurthi G. Integrating folk healers in india's public health: acceptance, legitimacy and emancipation. eJournal of Indian Medicine. 2014;7:1-20

[25] Dunn F. Traditional Asian medicine and cosmopolitan medicine as adaptive system. In: Leslie C, editor. Asian Medical System: A Comparative Study. Berkeley: University of California Press; 1976. pp. 133-158

[26] Aryal K, Dhimal M, Pandey A, Pandey A, Dhungana R, Khaniya B. Knowledge Diversity and Healing Practices of Traditional Medicine in Nepal. Kathmandu: Nepal Health Research Council; 2016

[27] Patel B et al. An assessment of local use pattern and traditional knowledge on medicinal and aromatic plants in Kapilvastu district Nepal. The Healer. 2021;**2**(1):17-41. DOI: https://doi.org/10.51649/healer.54

[28] Pham TV, Koirala R, Kohrt BA. Satisfaction in the soul: common factors theory applied to traditional healers in rural Nepal. Ethos Berkeley Calif. 2020;**48**(1):93-128. DOI: 10.1111/etho.12263

[29] Shrestha R, Lediard M. Faith Healers: A Force for Change. Kathmandu: Educational Interprises; 1980

[30] Subedi MS. Healer choice in medically pluralistic cultural settings: an overview of Nepali Medical Pluralism. Occasional Papers in Sociology and Anthropology. 2003;**8**:128-158

[31] NPC. Ninth Five Year Plan (1996/97-2000/01). National Planning Commission, Government of Nepal. 1997

[32] The Ayurveda Medical Council (First Amendment) Act, 1999 [Online]. 1999. Available from: https://lawcommission.gov.np/en/?p=16371. [Accessed: December 08, 2022]

[33] Bajracharya MB. Traditional ayurveda, the indigenous knowledge and health practice in Nepal. Education and Development. 2006;**22**(Special issue):90-97

[34] Phuyal N. Indigenous people of Nepal and their healing practices. Education and Development. 2006;**22**:69-74

[35] NESAC. Nepal Human Development Report, 1998. Nepal South Asia Center (NESAC), Kathmandu, 1998

[36] NPC. Sixth Five Year Plan (1980-1985). National Planning Commission, Government of Nepal. 1980

[37] NPC. Eighth Five Year Plan (1992/93-1996/97). National Planning Commission, Government of Nepal. 1993

[38] Sharma A, Ross J. Nepal: integrating traditional and modern health services in the remote area of Bashkharka. International Journal of Nursing Studies. 1990;**27**(4):343-353. DOI: 10.1016/0020-7489(90)90093-X

[39] Oswald IH. Are traditional healers the solution to the failures of primary health care in rural Nepal? Social Science & Medicine. 1983;**17**(5):255-257

[40] Poudyal AK, Jimba M, Murakami I, Silwal RC, Wakai S, Kuratsuji T. A traditional healers' training model in rural Nepal: strengthening their roles in community health. Tropical Medicine & International Health. 2003;**8**(10):956-960. DOI: 10.1046/j.1365-3156.2003.01094.x

[41] MoHP. Raastriya Swasthya Niti 2076 (National Health Policy 2019). Ministry of Health and Population, Government of Nepal, Kathmandu, Nepal. 2019

[42] Ministry of Health. Nepal Health Sector Strategy: Implementation Plan 2016-2021. Ministry of Health, Government of Nepal, Kathmandu, 2017

[43] MoHP. Second Long Term Health Plan 1997-2017: Perspective Plan for Health Sector Development. Ministry of Health and Population, GoN, Kathmandu. 1997

[44] DOAA. Paramparagat Upacharakko Suchikaran Maapdand 2077 BS (Namuna Masyauda) [Registration Standard for Traditional Healers 2020 (Sample Draft)] [Online]. 2020. Available from: https://doaa.gov.np/notices/%e0%a4%aa%e0%a4%b0%e0%a4%ae%e0%a5%8d%e0%a4%aa%e0%a4%b0%e0%a4%be%e0%a4%97%e0%a4%a4-%e0%a4%89%e0%a4%aa%e0%a4%9a%e0%a4%be%e0%a4%b0%e0%a4%95%-e0%a4%95%e0%a5%8b-%e0%a4%b8%e0%a5%82%e0%a4%9a%e0%a4%bf-2/ [Accessed: September 23, 2021]

[45] The Public Health Service Act, 2018 [Online]. 2018. Available from: https://www.lawcommission.gov.np/en/wp-content/uploads/2019/07/The-Public-Health-Service-Act-2075-2018.pdf [Accessed: September 23, 2021]

[46] UN General Assembly. United Nations Declaration on the Rights of Indigenous Peoples: resolution/adopted

by the General Assembly, 2 October 2007, A/RES/61/295. United Nations [Online]. 2007. Available from: https://www.refworld.org/docid/471355a82.html [Accessed: February 26, 2020]

[47] GoN. The Constitution of Nepal 2015. Constitution Assembly Secretariat, Simha Darbar, Kathmandu, 2015

[48] Subedi B, Joshi LR. (Un) popular traditional medicine community perceptions, changing practices, and state policy in Nepal. eSocial Sciences and Humanities. 2018;**1**(2):157-167

[49] Jimba M, Poudyal AK, Wakai S. The need for linking healthcare-seeking behavior and health policy in rural Nepal. The Southeast Asian Journal of Tropical Medicine and Public Health. 2003;**34**(2):462-463

Chapter 3

Implementation of the Posyandu Program and Healthy Living Behavior of Mothers and Children in Sidomulyo Village, Godean District, Sleman Regency, Yogyakarta Special Region

Umar Nain

Abstract

This study aims to: (1) analyze the continuity of healthy behavior of mothers and children even though their involvement in *Posyandu* is low due to poor *Posyandu* services; (2) analyze the healthy behavior of mothers and children in the community that is institutionalized by the community itself, although at the initial level, it was introduced by *Posyandu*. This research uses a descriptive survey approach. The population of this research is 348 mothers who have babies and toddlers, who are the target of the *Posyandu* service program. The number of samples taken was 100 respondents with a simple random sampling technique because the population was homogeneous. Data were obtained through questionnaires, in-depth interviews, and direct observation. The results showed that the low involvement of mothers in Posyandu was not an obstacle for mothers to behave in a healthy manner on an ongoing basis. This is because in the community there are various formal, semiformal, and village institutions that institutionalize healthy living accompanied by the availability of service facilities outside the *Posyandu* that can be used by mothers to meet the needs of a healthy life. The healthy behavior of mothers and children in the family is included in the high category seen from the frequency of mothers providing nutritious food for the family, maintaining food hygiene, boiling water before drinking, providing complete immunizations to their babies, baby clothes and utensils, conducting pregnancy checkups 7–9 times during pregnancy, using modern health care facilities for childbirth, as well as actively participating as an acceptor for independent family planning.

Keywords: Posyandu program, healthy lifestyle, mother and child, healthy behavior, Indonesia health system

1. Introduction

There are still many obstacles in the way of Indonesia's health development and its goal of improving maternal and child health. Still high rates of maternal and child mortality, as well as malnutrition in babies and toddlers, are indicative of these difficulties. The 2012 IDHS maternal mortality rate (MMR) in Indonesia was calculated to be 359 per 100,000 live births due to complications during or immediately after delivery [1, 2].

Deaths among infants (IMR) and young children (under-5 mortality rate, AKBAL) occur at a rate of 32 and 29 per 1000 live births, respectively (www.depkes.go.id). Since 1982, the government of Indonesia has used the primary health care (PHC) plan to pursue health development with the aim of lowering maternal and infant mortality rates. Community health centers (Puskesmas) use a primary health care approach, seeing patients as their first point of contact when they are ill and acting as a referral hub for more advanced medical care [3].

The government established the integrated service post program (Posyandu) in response to geographical challenges, a shortage of medical professionals, and the community health center's expansive service area, all of which made it difficult to provide accessible public health services, especially those focused on mothers and children [4, 5].

Family planning services (KB), maternity and child health (KIA), vaccination, nutrition enhancement, and diarrhea prevention make up Posyandu's basic service package as a health care institution offered by the government to rural communities. Nutrition counseling, family development for toddlers, dengue hemorrhagic fever, child care, food processing, and the promotion of healthy living are only some of the other initiatives carried out *via* counseling [6, 7].

It seems that the strategy of relying on the target population's (mothers and children) visits to the Posyandu to achieve service program coverage has not been successful. Visits to Posyandu by pregnant women, babies, and toddlers, as measured by the Ministry of Health's own data collection methods (1997 report), indicate that Posyandu is still not widely used in the community. Coverage for family planning services is 32.40%, with 8.99% of pregnant women seeing Posyandu, 23.51% of newborns, and 67.51% of toddlers [8].

Because the Posyandu service program places an emphasis on preventative health services, including vaccination, pregnancy checkups, and child weighing, community participation in Posyandu has dwindled. The unpredictability and lack of consideration for the activities of the local community in setting the Posyandu's service schedule is a major factor in the low rate of mother participation. We may, thus, infer that subpar Posyandu services will work against efforts to boost citizen participation in Posyandu.

The success of a development program depends on three factors aligning perfectly: the needs of the beneficiary and the outcomes of the program; the requirements of the program and the actual capabilities of the auxiliary organizations; and the recipients' ability to express needs and the decision-making processes of the auxiliary organizations. If Posyandu is able to tailor its services to the need of the local population, it will play a part in enhancing the community's health, as shown by this research [9].

Affordability, timeliness, and precision in medical care are all indicators of rising service quality. The capacity, outlook, and demeanor of service officers in their dealings with members of the community as service receivers are decisive in ensuring the execution of excellent service. Police personnel may demonstrate courtesy and friendliness in these encounters. Posyandu's decision-making process, as well as the ease with which demands may be communicated, will influence the extent to which the organization can gain public support [10].

The democratic method, which places a great deal of responsibility above the community, and the autocratic approach, which holds that people are fully responsible, work together to ensure that those with the right to act and educate the community are the ones who do so. Since the success of development depends on community engagement and the support of local resources, including labor, finances, and facilities [11], Posyandu will obtain support from the community if it employs a democratic method in decision making.

At the community level, development success may be gauged by how well the Posyandu program has been ingrained into people's daily routines. Institutions in the community and other groups may help with the institutionalization process. The organization is a set of official and informal roles that everyone understands and plays. The institution, however, is understood to be a social standard and pattern of conduct that occurs in order to accomplish certain ends. Meanwhile, various constraints on institutions make patterned behavior a sequence of social connections that occur in communities or groups. Patterned behavior is now a shared feature of our society as a whole [12].

Promoting healthy lifestyles is the ultimate aim of health initiatives, such as Posyandu. There are three types of influences on behavior: (i) predisposition, which includes individual knowledge, attitudes, traditions, and social norms; (ii) enabling factors, which include the accessibility of health service facilities; and (iii) reinforcing factors, which include the attitudes and behaviors of health workers. The high expense of transportation and treatment, as well as the difficulty in accessing medical facilities, are two examples of nonbehavioral issues. There are many different types of healthy lifestyle choices, including those that affect one's physical and mental health, as well as one's approach to food and the environment [13, 14].

The presence of Posyandu, a health service institution, is an indicator that people in rural regions have access to health care resources. Both governmental and grassroots institutions have contributed to shaping modern civilization. Community health centers, sub-health centers, village maternity boarding schools (Polindes), village drug posts, village midwives, and skilled traditional healers are all examples of those who actively participate in delivering health services. Village Community Empowerment Institutions (LPMD), Family Welfare Empowerment (PKK), Dasa Wisma Group, Toddler Family Development Groups, Craftsmen Groups, arisan, and so on all serve to inculcate and encourage villagers to live healthily [15, 16].

Given the above, the study's primary concern is whether or not mothers and children's healthy behavior would persist in the face of their low engagement in the Posyandu as a result of the poor quality of Posyandu services. Second, even if Posyandu was the one who first presented the concept of good parenting to society, how is it being institutionalized by the community itself?

2. Methods

The purpose of this research was not to test hypotheses but to provide a descriptive survey. This study also included in-depth interviews with respondents and many informants to supplement the data collected through questionnaires. Researchers not only conduct in-depth interviews but also actively participate (observer as participant) in Posyandu services in order to observe, comprehend, query, and document all phenomena that emerge throughout the course of a Posyandu service [17]. Sidomulyo Village in Godean District in Sleman Regency in Yogyakarta, a special province, was the site of the study. Firstly, Sidomulyo Village is highly typical for other villages in Godean District due to its relatively homogenous degree of Posyandu development and community features; and secondly, Sidomulyo Village has never been employed as a comparable study site before.

In this study, the population was mothers who had newborns and children under five at the time the research was carried out, with the consideration that they were the focus of the Posyandu service program. There are 348 individuals in all, living in eight different Posyandu (hamlet). Random sampling was used for the sampling process. The sample size collected from the population is 30%, which is carried out proportionately for each Posyandu by lottery. A total of 100 participants were included in the sample. The study variables associated with the issue and the unit under investigation were described by the processing of descriptive statistical data (descriptive statistics). In this research, the mother-child dyad serves as the unit of analysis. So, the mother is the unit of analysis at the individual level, since the child's healthy behavior mirrors the mother's good conduct [18, 19].

3. Results and discussion

3.1 Implementation of the Posyandu service program

Each Posyandu is required to carry out at least five different program packages as part of the implementation of the Posyandu service program. These program packages are collectively referred to as minimum service activity packages. Improving nutrition is one of these five programs, along with mother and child health (MCH), family planning (KB), vaccination, and preventing diarrheal illnesses. The supplemental feeding package (PMT) is also a part of the nutrition improvement program (P2-Diarrhea). It is clear from the findings of the field study conducted in Sidomulyo Village that not every Posyandu is capable of doing each and every one of these basic service activity packages [20].

Participant observations led to the discovery that the types of Posyandu services in Sidomulyo Village that were carried out by 40% consisted of two types of services: nutrition services (20%) and maternal and child health services, particularly services for weighing toddlers (20%). The findings of this discovery were based on the fact that 40% of the village's residents were surveyed. Family planning and diarrhea prevention were not included among the three categories of services that were not provided since they were not implemented. The insufficient nature of the Posyandu service, which places the utmost emphasis on weighing toddlers, gives the impression that Posyandu is primarily a weighing station for children under three years old.

The results of field research can be used to get an idea of what people think of Posyandu as a post for weighing toddlers. The results showed that 85% of respondents stated that it was not suitable, while only 3% stated that it was suitable. This gives the impression that Posyandu is not an appropriate post for weighing toddlers. The number of respondents who claimed that it was suitable was made up of responses from mothers who had toddlers; hence, the most clear need was to manage the health progression of toddlers *via* activities including weighing. Even while the vast majority of respondents (85%) said that they were qualified, they in fact need additional sorts of services, including counseling on family planning, vaccination, extra food (nutrition parks), and counseling on environmental health. According to the findings of the poll, an overwhelming majority of respondents (88%) claimed that the service for the registration desk went well, while just 5% of respondents stated that the service was not smooth. On the other hand, with regard to the second table (weighing), as many as 97% of the respondents claimed that the service was operating well, while just 1% of the respondents stated that it was not operating smoothly.

As for the recording of the findings (table three), the majority of respondents indicated that they were up to date, which is represented by the percentage 90% of respondents who stated that they were current and the percentage 3% of respondents who stated that they were not current. Posyandu gives the appearance of being a toddler weighing station due to the fact that registration, weighing, and the recording of results all go through without a hitch [21].

It was discovered that as many as 38% of respondents stated that it was not operating smoothly for the fourth table (individual counseling/referring), and it was discovered that as many as 38% of respondents stated that it was not operating smoothly for the fifth table (KB-Health services). In the meanwhile, according to the responses of those who were asked about the sufficiency of the Posyandu amenities in Sidomulyo Village, it would seem that the facilities that are enough are mostly those that are administrative in nature. In the meanwhile, essential facilities or equipment, such as cooking utensils, contraception, as well as tables and chairs, are in short supply. Even the respondents themselves expressed their opinion that these amenities were inadequate in some way. As many as 65 respondents indicated that there was an insufficient supply of cooking utensils, as many as 35% of respondents stated that there was an insufficient supply of contraceptives, and as many as 33% of respondents stated that there was also an insufficient supply of table and chair facilities [7].

3.2 Mother and child involvement in Posyandu

The involvement of mothers and children in Posyandu activities can be seen from the frequency of mother and child visits in utilizing the services available at the Posyandu. This can be seen from the variations in the answers of mothers (respondents) to the frequency of visits to Posyandu. The results of the study explained that as many as 57% of respondents stated that the utilization of family planning services at Posyandu was very low; this was related to the quality of family planning services provided. The low quality of family planning services causes mothers to be more inclined to carry out family planning services at the local doctor, midwife, or health center.

For prenatal checks, most of the respondents stated that they were very lacking in utilizing the service, namely 55%. The lack of utilization of this service is not due to the reluctance of Posyandu participants but rather due to inadequate service factors such as the absence of technical staff at the Posyandu (e.g., midwives) to examine mothers, lack of adequate facilities, and infrastructure, for example, a blood pressure measuring device. The lack of quality of antenatal care services has caused most mothers to use the services of doctors, midwives, or Puskesmas as a place to carry out prenatal checks [22].

For immunization services, it was shown that the majority of respondents stated that the quality of immunization services was very poor, namely as much as 50%. This lack of immunization services is mainly caused by the dependence of immunization services on the presence of midwives at the Posyandu who bring vaccines as needed. Because the vaccines are stored at the Puskesmas, and if on Posyandu open days the midwives do not bring the vaccines, the immunization services are abolished [23].

In the case of giving ORS, the majority of respondents also stated that their visit to this type of service was lacking, namely as much as 48%. The low involvement of mothers in this type of ORS service is due to a lack of ORS supplies at the Posyandu. This is also due to the fact that the supply of ORS at Posyandu is highly dependent on distribution from the Puskesmas. The types of Posyandu services that show the high involvement of respondents in utilizing the service are weighing children under five, giving vitamin A for toddlers, and providing additional food.

The involvement of mothers and children in Posyandu activities can also be seen from the participation of mothers in the payment of health fund contributions (IDS). The results of the study explained that 48% of the respondents paid contributions to the health fund (IDS). While mothers who do not make IDS payments are as much as 38%. The amount of health fund contributions (IDS) among Posyandu varies, but field findings show that health fund contributions (IDS) range from IDR 1000.00 to IDR 1500.00 for each mother.

Mothers' involvement in Posyandu activities can also be seen from the frequency with which mothers provide donations/assistance in procuring service facilities needed by Posyandu. The results of the study found that most of the respondents had never contributed to the provision of Posyandu service facilities, namely 62% and there were 22% of respondents who stated that only occasionally, while 16% stated that they often made donations to procure Posyandu service facilities. Forms of donations include money, food, medicines, and vitamins.

The involvement of Posyandu participants in service activities can also be seen from their involvement in discussing Posyandu issues. The results of the field findings revealed that the respondents' answers varied quite a lot in terms of involving these members. As many as 40% of respondents feel that they are always involved in discussing problems in the Posyandu. Meanwhile, another 40% feel that they are only occasionally involved in discussions about the ins and outs of Posyandu service activities. Meanwhile, there were 20% of respondents who said they had never been involved in discussing problems in Posyandu services. This means that the decision-making system has not run democratically so it can affect their involvement in Posyandu.

3.3 Healthy behavior of mother and child

Field data showed that the majority of respondents in this survey lead healthy diets and diet-related lifestyles, with 71% of participants reporting that they regularly serve healthy meals for their families. Rice, tempeh, tofu, pork, fish, eggs, carrots, beans, kale, and fruits, as well as vegetables, milk, and iodized salt, are all eaten to provide for his family's nutritional requirements. Most people already have a good grasp on the value of a healthy diet, therefore it is not commonly questioned whether or not to provide wholesome meals. Most respondents also had incomes above Rp. 750,000.00, which means they are able to afford to regularly serve healthy meals. They will be able to afford enough food to suit their dietary requirements with this sum of money. In contrast, 29% of respondents said they only sometimes supplied healthy meals for their family, and 0% said they never did. It is not that they do not understand the need of maintaining a healthy lifestyle by eating well, but rather that financial constraints at home make it difficult to do so. A mother's involvement in family planning programs is an indicator of her commitment to healthy lifestyle choices, especially those that promote her reproductive health (KB).

The majority of respondents (74%) actively accepted family planning, according to the data from the field. Eleven percent, however, reported being less active, while 15% indicated they did not exercise at all. Most of the respondents at the research sites were now independent family planning participants; that is, they could afford to pay for services from private midwives or practicing physicians, which explains the large number of active family planning acceptors at the study sites.

A mother's propensity to attend prenatal visits is another indicator of her overall health throughout pregnancy. Women who are expecting children are offered prenatal care at regular intervals. During pregnancy, women should see a Puskesmas or midwife at least four times (K1–K4) for checkups (antenatal care). According to the data collected in the field, just 8% of pregnant women went in for between one and three prenatal checkups, while 35% went in for between six and seven and 57% went in for between seven and nine. This indicates that expecting women are well aware of the need of prenatal care. This indicates that the mother is practicing exemplary prenatal hygiene [24].

When it comes to delivering their children, field data indicated that as many as 7% of respondents used a traditional birth attendant, 80% used a midwife, and 13% used a doctor or medical professional in some capacity. Due to the fact that most respondents have given birth with the assistance of a midwife or doctor and just a small number have sought the services of a dukun beranak, it is evident that the mother's healthy behavior is high.

Immunizations against diseases, including diphtheria, pertussis, and tetanus (DPT), hepatitis-B, polio, measles, and Bacillus Calmette Guerin (BCG), are a good indicator of a mother's dedication to keeping her child healthy. Findings from the field showed that almost nine in ten respondents vaccinated their infants and toddlers entirely, with 3% providing just partial vaccinations and 8% reporting that they did not vaccinate at all.

Mothers' healing behavior may be inferred from the lengths they go to in order to treat their children, just as it can be from the measures they take to protect them from illness. When respondents' children were under the age of five and unwell, the majority took them to a midwife (64%), a community health center (64%), or a community health center (80%). Midwives, health centers, and auxiliary health centers are frequently visited by parents who have brought their sick children there because they are reliable, accessible (*via* walking or public transportation), inexpensive (relative to other medical options), and open to people of all socioeconomic backgrounds.

The results of the fieldwork indicated that all respondents boiled their drinking water before ingesting it, which is a healthy practice for families. In addition, research from the field shows that 42% of people who have latrines at home utilize them. Those who fall within this group of respondents understand the significance of maintaining a clean environment and taking measures to eliminate potential health hazards in the comfort of their own homes. However, 13% of respondents reported using a public restroom and 45% reported not having access to a private lavatory in their homes.

The respondents' high socioeconomic status, represented in their education and income levels, is a key factor in the achievement of the aforementioned healthy behavior of mothers and children. Findings from this research show that the vast majority of respondents are well educated, with 43% having completed high school and 7% having completed college or university, and that over half (52%) earn more than IDR 750,000.00 per year. Mothers with higher incomes will have an easier time affording the costs of a healthy lifestyle, and mothers with higher levels of education will be better able to appreciate the significance of maintaining a healthy lifestyle.

4. Conclusion

Subpar service hindered the Posyandu program's rollout. The inability of Posyandu to provide all sorts of services, poor quality service systems, and insufficient service facilities and equipment all contribute to the quality of service that customers get. Because Posyandu only provides weighing services for toddlers and nutrition services, whereas women additionally require prenatal care, vaccination, family planning, and treatment for diarrhea, poor mother participation in Posyandu might be attributed to this mismatch. Posyandu only captures a fraction of the community's mothers and children's healthy behaviors. Most of their knowledge about how to live a healthy life comes from sources other than the Posyandu, such as community health centers, sub health centers, private midwives, and medical professionals. The high levels of education and wealth within the family help to prove this. Even if mothers are not actively participating in Posyandu, this does not prevent them from exhibiting positive health habits in the long run. This is due to the availability of service facilities outside the Posyandu that mothers may utilize to satisfy their daily requirements, as well as the presence of numerous formal, semiformal, and rural institutions that institutionalize healthy living.

But the regularity with which mothers offer nutritious meals for the family, maintain food hygiene, boil drinking water first, give their newborns full vaccines, and bathe their babies twice a day all fall into the "high" category of healthy family behavior, as well as being independent-KB participants, who practice cleanliness in all aspects of their lives (eating, drinking, dressing, and caring for baby equipment), who visit their doctors 7–9 times during pregnancy, who utilize contemporary health service centers for delivery assistance, and who actively engage in these practices.

Since Posyandu is not the only health care facility available to mothers, the healthy behavior of mothers and children will persist even with minimal participation. In rural areas with a high standard of living, residents choose not to employ Posyandu services in favor of more contemporary medical options.

Author details

Umar Nain
Institute of Home Affairs Government, Indonesia

*Address all correspondence to: umarnain1388@ipdn.ac.id

References

[1] Halfon N, Larson K, Lu M, Tullis E, Russ S. Lifecourse health development: Past, present and future. Maternal and Child Health Journal. 2014;**18**(2):344-365

[2] Organization, W. H. World Health Statistics 2016: Monitoring Health for the SDGs Sustainable Development Goals. World Health Organization; 2016

[3] MacDorman MF, Mathews TJ, Mohangoo AD, Zeitlin J. International Comparisons of Infant Mortality and Related Factors. United States and Europe; 2010

[4] Nirwana MD, Utami IH, Utami HN. The cadre of integrated health service post (Posyandu) as an agent in the socialization of cervical Cancer prevention in Malang regency, Indonesia: A cultural approach. Procedia-Social and Behavioral Sciences. 2015;**211**:681-687

[5] Pratono AH, Maharani A. Long- term care in Indonesia: The role of integrated service post for elderly. Journal of Aging and Health. 2018;**30**(10):1556-1573

[6] Apanga PA, Adam MA. Factors influencing the uptake of family planning services in the Talensi District, Ghana. Pan African Medical Journal. 2015;**20**(1):1-9

[7] Gavin L, Moskosky S, Carter M, Curtis K, Glass E, Godfrey E, et al. Providing quality family planning services: Recommendations of CDC and the US Office of population affairs. Morbidity and Mortality Weekly Report. Recommendations and Reports. 2014;**63**(4):1-54

[8] Kadarina TM, & Priambodo R. Preliminary design of internet of things (IoT) application for supporting mother and child health program in Indonesia. 2017 International Conference on Broadband Communication, Wireless Sensors and Powering (BCWSP). 2017. pp. 1-6

[9] Julian R. Is it for donors or locals? The relationship between stakeholder interests and demonstrating results in international development. International Journal of Managing Projects in Business. 2016;**2016**

[10] Syed SB, Leatherman S, Mensah-Abrampah N, Neilson M, Kelley E. Improving the quality of health care across the health system. Bulletin of the World Health Organization. 2018;**96**(12):799

[11] Lunenburg FC. The decision making process. National Forum of Educational Administration & Supervision Journal. 2010;**27**(4)

[12] Fosu AK. Achieving Development Success: Strategies and Lessons from the Developing World. Oxford University Press; 2013

[13] Grembowski D. The Practice of Health Program Evaluation. Sage Publications; 2015

[14] Schell SF, Luke DA, Schooley MW, Elliott MB, Herbers SH, Mueller NB, et al. Public health program capacity for sustainability: A new framework. Implementation Science. 2013;**8**(1):1-9

[15] Abuse S. Mental health services administration. Results. 2013;**2**:13

[16] Bowling A. Research Methods in Health: Investigating Health and Health Services. McGraw-hill Education (UK); 2014

[17] Showkat N, Parveen H. In-depth interview. Quadrant-I (e-text). 2017;**2017**

[18] Acharya AS, Prakash A, Saxena P, Nigam A. Sampling: Why and how of it. Indian Journal of Medical Specialties. 2013;**4**(2):330-333

[19] Emerson RW. Convenience sampling, random sampling, and snowball sampling: How does sampling affect the validity of research? Journal of Visual Impairment & Blindness. 2015;**109**(2):164-168

[20] Closa-Monasterolo R, Gispert-Llaurado M, Canals J, Luque V, Zaragoza-Jordana M, Koletzko B, et al. The effect of postpartum depression and current mental health problems of the mother on child behaviour at eight years. Maternal and Child Health Journal. 2017;**21**(7):1563-1572

[21] Gatto NM, Ventura EE, Cook LT, Gyllenhammer LE, Davis JN. LA sprouts: A garden-based nutrition intervention pilot program influences motivation and preferences for fruits and vegetables in Latino youth. Journal of the Academy of Nutrition and Dietetics. 2012;**112**(6):913-920

[22] Agha S, Tappis H. The timing of antenatal care initiation and the content of care in Sindh, Pakistan. BMC Pregnancy and Childbirth. 2016;**16**(1):1-9

[23] Assija V, Singh A, Sharma V. Coverage and quality of immunization services in rural Chandigarh. Indian Pediatrics. 2012;**49**(7):565-567

[24] Perry GS, Patil SP, Presley-Cantrell LR. Raising awareness of sleep as a healthy behavior. Preventing Chronic Disease. 2013;**10**

Chapter 4

The Kongsi Covid: A Cultural and Religious Belief Approaches for Covid-19, Battling Stigma and Strengthening Family Resilience for Villagers in Padang, Indonesia

Rizanda Machmud, Finny Fitry Yani, Feri Mulyani Hamid, Yuniar Lestari, Irvan Medison, Emilzon Taslim and Bestari Jaka Budiman

Abstract

Background: The stigma of Covid-19 is culturally rooted in health beliefs and practices in Padang-Indonesia. The aim of this intervention project is to develop cultural & religious belief approaches for Covid-19 battling stigma and strengthening family resilience for villagers. Intervention: The Kongsi Covid-19 is community-based preparedness and response strategy preventing the transmission of Covid-19. The sub-village RT/RW is subordinate to the village as a cluster that has supervision directed in the community and requires 10–14 volunteers. All activities are monitored, coordinated, and supervised by the village leader, sub-district, community health centers, and city health offices. Results and Impact: Padang had developed 1,252 Kongsi Coovid-19 covering 100% of sub-villages. More than 3000 people with positive confirmed cases with asymptomatic or mild symptoms, doing self-isolation under Kongsi COVID-19 local monitoring. The government of Padang was awarded the Best rating II due to its policy for preparing strategic planning which includes efforts to deal with the COVID-19 pandemic through the innovations of the Kongsi COVID-19. Conclusions: Kongsi Covid-19 strengthens existing partnerships to reach and engage with wider community networks. It has an active role to resolve the health issue of Covid-19 battling stigma and strengthening family resilience for villagers in Padang-Indonesia.

Keywords: cultural religious approach, empowerment, family resilience, social, Covid-19

1. Introduction

The Covid-19 pandemic has led to cause large-scale morbidity and mortality globally. During the early Covid-19 pandemic, positive numbers of Covid-19 patients in Padang continued to increase every day [1, 2]. The proportion of positive numbers due to Covid-19 increased from 484 cases on June 15, 2020, to 488 cases on June 16, 2020, and on June 17, 2020, to 492 cases [2]. Thus, the city of Padang was designated as a red zone category prone to the transmission of the Corona Disease Virus (Covid-19). Another problem is that the health protocol and self-isolation protocol, which are government programs to control the increase in Covid-19 cases, have not been socialized properly, and what is worrying is the existence of stigma in society, which hinders the control of Covid-19 [1–3]. The Covid-19 pandemic has distanced people from the healthcare system due to excessive fear.

The high number of cases in the Padang requires a new strategy and order to increase this achievement in the New Normal era [3]. In New Normal conditions, according to the Ministry of Internal Affairs No. 440-830 of 2020, in the end, society must live side by side with the threat of the coronavirus, as an effort to restore community life activities and administration of government conditions such as before the occurrence of Covid-19, so that people become productive and safe in carrying out their activities [3, 4]. As for the activities in this New Normal era, what needs to be done is to carry out activities based on the principles of Covid-19, namely wearing a mask when leaving the house, washing hands with soap and running water, and keeping distance [5–7]. The activities of this new order should be community-based. This means that this community-based activity is expected to eliminate the stigma against Covid-19.

Meanwhile, the community is the vanguard that has been forgotten so far; it has more impact and builds social solidarity and mutual cooperation. Community engagement plays a role in maximizing the effectiveness of Covid-19 preparedness and response strategies and preventing transmission at the community level.

The communities, when engaged, are the front line in detecting and managing epidemics. They are the most affected and have the greatest influence in anticipation and preparedness as new diseases emerge or old ones re-emerge [6–8].

By engaging communities in the preparedness and response to Covid-19, the health sector can avoid the emergence of cases that will worsen the pandemic. It can also give the health sector more time to prepare to respond in realistic, relevant, and appropriate ways to the needs and challenges of every population group. Further, community engagement can serve to address and prevent health and gender inequities during the Covid-19 pandemic.

Therefore, we need a community-engaged communication strategy that focuses on Covid-19 messaging in a cultural context that can be a potential channel for responding to the Covid-19 pandemic. Efforts are being made to involve a culture-based community that is already inherent in the Minangkabau community by modifying it to suit the handling and control of Covid-19 in the community. The focus of activities on Covid-19 at this time can be a positive synergy.

2. Rationale: cultural and religious approaches for Covid-19, battling stigma and strengthening family resilience for villagers

Research in another setting has shown the need to address cultural health beliefs about the locus of control in the design and development of programs. In this sense, the word "community participation" is the key word for increasing access to make it easier to detect cases, the socialization process for each stage of the action, as well as community participation in handling Covid-19.

People in West Sumatera are mostly of the Minang tribe and have culturally rooted health beliefs and practices. This activity is based on the sub-village. Every time someone dies in the sub-village, it will be held together in mutual cooperation by the local sub-village residents. It is such as a community bereavement service which is initiated by community in favor to support the loosing family by the neighbourhood where they lived. The community is homogenous and solid. It is called Kongsi Kematian.

Leveraging existing networks and community forums in sub-village. We have modified a strategic approach for addressing the preparedness and response strategies and preventing the transmission of Covid-19 in the community. We modified a community engagement that has been rooted in Minang Kabau devise such as Kongsi Kematian.

It is hoped that this concept can be applied in the preparedness and response strategies and preventing transmission of Covid-19 at the community level, which is called the "Kongsi Covid".

We also had already identified and reviewed Kongsi Covid as the terms of reference for previously established partnerships that could be of value in reaching and engaging solid communities.

Strong existing networks in Padang have established a platform to facilitate discussions among the community about how they can support one another and come up with their own solutions that would be beneficial in Covid-19 promotion and prevention. Kongsi Covid, with the principle of mutual cooperation, removes stigma, increases family resilience, and raises awareness and mental health of the community.

The assignments of the Kongsi Covid are to keep negative cluster areas negative; to monitor clusters, if there are positive people, to become negative; to remove stigma; to raise public awareness; and to work on mental health. The community empowered by the principle of working together means that the concern of promoting and preventing behaviors becomes and is controlled by society itself.

3. The intervention and implementation of the Kongsi Covid

The 'Kongsi Covid-19' concept is a micro lockdown unit in a sub-village, called RT/RW, where the RT/RW sub-villager community serves as a sharing center for food, medicine, and information. Its establishment requires 10–14 volunteers.

Therefore, the RT/RW sub-village is a Covid-19 Consortium Cluster. The clusters as a micro lockdown unit are smaller and more numerous, in fact, minimizing the risk of transmission and making it easier to monitor and evaluate the handling of Covid-19. The role of the sub-village RT/RW in the Kongsi Covid-19 is that of supervision at the community level, no longer at the family nor at the regional government level.

For this reason, for the success of the Kongsi Covid-19, we cannot rely on the role of the health sector alone, but cross-sectoral roles, such as RT/RW, youth organizations, NGOs, the head of village, the head of district, and the presence of academics also play a decisive role. One of the real supports from academics in the success of this partnership is through community empowerment, together with students and lecturers, to improve the management of Covid-19.

We selected Mata Air Village, Padang Selatan District, as the pilot project of the implementation of Kongsi Covid-19. Mata Air has the highest cases among the subdistricts in Padang Selatan District and tends to increase the cases of Covid-19. It has 20 positive cases, 9 people recovered, and 2 people died. The challenge of Mata Air Village is the area that has a dense population, making it easier for Covid-19 transmission to occur [9].

The activity model that will be carried out is as follows: socialization regarding health protocols during the Covid pandemic and the self-isolation protocol.

Collaborating with cross-sectoral partners such as villages, Youth Organizations, NGOs, Head villages, Head sub-district, and Health Offices.

The activity model that will be carried out is as follows: 1. Socialization regarding Health Protocols during the Covid Pandemic and the Self-Isolation Protocol; 2. Collaborating with cross-sectoral partners such as villages, Youth Organizations, NGOs, Head villages, Head sub-district, and Health Offices; 3. Preparing the Establishment of the Kongsi Covid-19 at the sub-village level, and its organizational structure and duties and responsibilities; 4. Make periodic reports that describe conditions in each RT/RW sub-village using the Google form or application; 5. Form socialization by using print media and online media; 6. Create an RT/RW WhatsApp (WA) group for monitoring; 7. Monitoring and evaluating the implementation of the RT/RW Kongsi COVID-19 activities through regular virtual meetings; 8. Creating a Covid Positive community monitoring system; 9. Create a monitoring and reporting system through an application that contains: case identification, reporting of suspected Covid-19, recording of suspected Covid-19, and monitoring of independent isolation that occurs in each sub-village [10, 11].

4. Flow and stages of the implementation of Kongsi Covid-19 activities

The activity indicators are the formation of the RT/RW Kongsi Covid-19; activities of the Covid-19 partnership, discovery of new cases of Covid-19, and self-isolation patients are well monitored (**Figure 1**).

If there are people with symptoms of COVID-19:

1. People contact the call center at 112 or 081112112112.

2. The Department of Health, through surveillance officers, will trace people with close contacts (cases within 2 days; before the case develops symptoms; until 14 days after the case develops symptoms).

3. Contact data include complete personal data, contact category, and date of contact/exposure to the duration of contact.

4. The Department of Health, through surveillance officers/Primary Health Care (PHC), will contact close high-risk contacts and convey:

a. Risk communication against close contact.

b. No need to be hospitalized.

c. Mandatory self-isolation at home for 14 days.

5. Covid-19 specimens will be collected.

6. Periodic monitoring will be done by the health center to evaluate the presence of symptoms for the next 14 days.

7. Primary Health Care (PHC) can provide a certificate in monitoring if necessary.

8. If Covid-19 is not confirmed, then it is considered not a Covid-19 case. Continue to prevent transmission of Covid-19.

9. If Covid-19 is confirmed, continue self-isolation and periodic monitoring by the Primary Health Care (PHC) for up to 14 days.

10. If after 14 days, you are healthy/have no symptoms and the test results after 14 days are negative for Covid-19, you will be declared cured.

11. If within 14 days, the person has symptoms (fever (≥38°C)/cough/flu/sore throat/shortness of breath or acute respiratory infection (ARI)).

12. Immediately contact the nearest Primary Health Care (PHC).

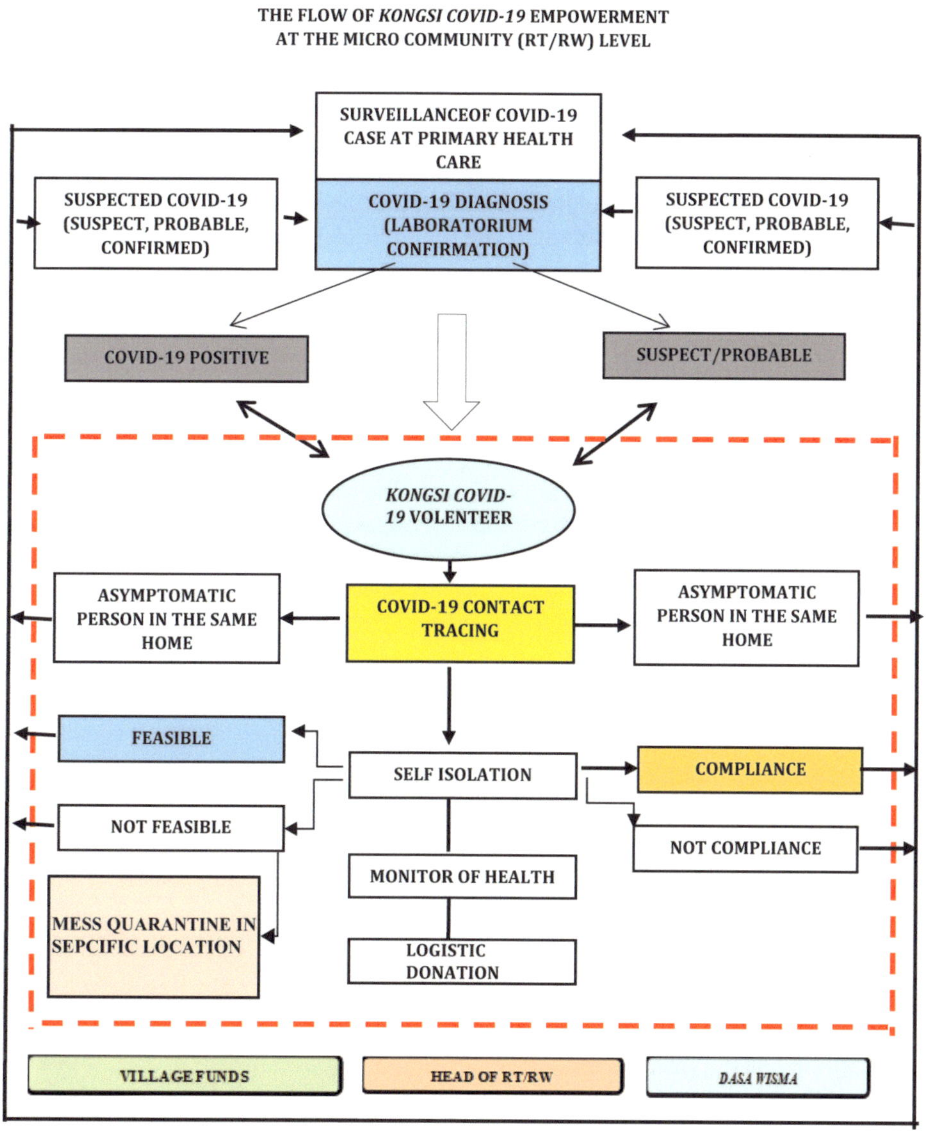

Figure 1.
The flow of Kongsi Covid-19 concept and platform [10, 11].

5. Result

The Kongsi COVID-19 has been developed after all set in Mato Aia Village as a pilot project model. There are 1.252 Kongsi Covid-19 in other sub-villages in Padang. It covers 100% of sub-villages which has an incident of Covid-19. It spreads in all eleven districts in Padang city.

There are more than 3000 people with positive confirmed cases, but with asymptomatic or mild symptoms, doing self-isolation under Kongsi Covid-19 local monitoring. Several of Kongsi Covid-19 societies have quarantine houses that can be used by the local citizen for self-isolation. This Kongsi Covid-19 has collaborated with the health care workers from the health center in managing and reporting the suspected cases and facilitated doing contact tracing to persons who have had contact with the confirmed cases.

We advocate the stakeholder—the mayor of Padang city—to make a local regulation concerning guidelines for the implementation of Kongsi COVID-19 in Padang city and a guideline book with ISBN.

The innovation of the Kongsi Covid-19 has been rewarded by the national government for the success in preparing quality planning in order to achieve better regional development. The award from the Ministry of National Development Planning-Bappenas was handed over virtually at the National Development Conference, which was opened directly by the President of the Republic of Indonesia Joko Widodo, in Jakarta, Tuesday (4/5/2021).

The city of Padang was awarded the Best rating II in the city category, because from a planning perspective, it has a policy for preparing strategic planning, which includes efforts to deal with the Covid-19 pandemic through the innovations of the Kongsi Covid-19.

The villagers in Padang City developed deep relationships within the community and organizations to work together to address Covid-19 issues. It promotes and prevents behaviors to decrease morbidity and mortality due to Covid-19. The principle of mutual cooperation removes the stigma and raises awareness, strengthening the family resilience and mental health of the community. It has established a platform to facilitate discussions among the community about how they can support one another and come up with their own solutions that would benefit in healthcare and treatment.

6. Conclusion

A community-engaged communication strategy that focuses on Covid-19 messaging in a cultural context, which is called Kongsi Covid-19, can be a potential channel for responding to the Covid-19 pandemic. Efforts are being made to involve a culture-based community that is already inherent in the Minangkabau community by modifying it to suit the handling and control of Covid-19 in the community. It is a modified activity that has existed for a long time in the city of Padang, where this activity is based at the sub-village level.

Kongsi Covid-19 is a local community-based social restriction that is more sustainable or supportive because it requires constant vigilance. This intervention in the community made the front line in preventing Covid-19.

Kongsi Covid in the Mato Air Village, Padang Selatan District, became a pilot model, which was followed massively in other villages in the city of Padang. It has been held jointly in cooperation with local sub-village residents to help eliminate stigma in society and raise awareness and community mental health and family resilience.

Acknowledgements

Thank you to our Dean Faculty of Medicine Andalas University give us full support on Kongsi Covid project. And especially to our collages Irvan Medison MD, Dr. Emilzon Taslim, MD have a huge contribution to the implementation.

Conflict of interest

The authors declare no conflict of interest.

Notes/thanks/other declarations

Thank you to our Major of Padang City Mahyeldi Ansharullaah, District Health Office of Padang Feri Mulyani Hamid, MD, M.Biomed, head sub-district of Padang Selatan, and head of sub-villages, head of Primary Health Cares in Padang and community where Kongsi Covid implemented, with all collaboration that made Kongsi Covid had a national level reward.

Author details

Rizanda Machmud[1*], Finny Fitry Yani[2], Feri Mulyani Hamid[3], Yuniar Lestari[1], Irvan Medison[4], Emilzon Taslim[5] and Bestari Jaka Budiman[6]

1 Department of Public Health/Community Medicine Medical Faculty of Universitas Andalas, Padang, Indonesia

2 Department of Child Health, Dr. M. Djamil General Hospital, Padang, Indonesia

3 Padang City Health District, Padang, Indonesia

4 Department of Pulmonologist, Dr. M. Djamil General Hospital, Padang, Indonesia

5 Department of Anesthesia, Dr. M. Djamil General Hospital, Padang, Indonesia

6 Department of Ear Nose Throat-Head Neck Surgery, Dr. M. Djamil General Hospital, Padang, Indonesia

*Address all correspondence to: rizandamachmud@med.unand.ac.id

References

[1] Online News. Kasus COVID-19 Sumbar Kian Landai, Kini Peringkat 15 Setelah Sempat Nomor 8 Nasional [Internet]. 2020. Available from: https://langgam.id/kasusCOVID-19-sumbar-kian-landai-kiniperingkat15setelahsempatnomor-8-nasional/ [Accessed: June 17, 2020]

[2] Padang Departement of Health. Situasi dan Perkembangan COVID-19 [Internet]. 2020. Available from: http://corona.padang.go.id/ [Accessed: June 17, 2020]

[3] Ministry of the Internal Affairs Repubkic of Indonesia. Keputusan Menteri Dalam Negeri No 440 – 830 Tahun 2020 tentang Pedoman Tatanan Normal Baru Produktif dan Aman Corona Virus Disease 2019 Bagi Aparatur Sipil Negara di Lingkungan Kementerian Dalam Negeri dan Pemerintah Daerah. Kepmendagri, Jakarta; 2020

[4] Directorate General of Disease Prevention and Control. Pedoman Pencegahan Dan Pengendalian Coronavirus Disease (COVID-19). Jakarta: Ministry of Health Republic of Indonesia Directorate General of Disease Prevention and Control; 2020

[5] World Health Organization. Naming the Coronavirus Disease (COVID-19) and the Virus that Causes it [Internet]. Geneva: World Health Organization; 2020. Available from: https://www.who.int/emergencies/diseases/novelcoronavirus2019/technicalguidance/naming-the-coronavirusdisease-(COVID-2019)-and-the-virus-thatcauses-it

[6] World Health Organization. Coronavirus Disease 2019 (COVID-19) Situation Report-70 [Internet]. WHO; 2020. Available from: https://www.who.int/docs/defaultsource/coronaviruse/situationreports/20200330sitrep70-COVID-9.pdf?sfvrsn=7e0fe3f8_2

[7] Fotterl Q. Here's How Here's How the Mysterious Coronavirus has Spread Around the World so Rapidly.[Internet]. 2020. Available from: https://www.marketwatch.com/story/howthemysterious-coronavirus-fromchinahasspread-so-quickly-2020-01-21

[8] Ministry of the Health Republic of Indonesia. Situasi dan Perkembangan COVID-19 [Internet]. 2020. Available from: http://corona.padang.go.id/ [Accessed: June 16, 2020]

[9] Provincial Government of West Sumatra. Situasi dan Perkembangan COVID-19 [Internet]. 2020. Available from: http://corona.padang.go.id/ [Accessed: June 16, 2020]

[10] Minisitry of Villages. Development of Disadvantaged Regions, and the Transmigration Republic of Indonesia. Protokol Relawan Desa Lawan COVID-19. Kemen Desa, PDT, dan Transmigrasi RI, Jakarta; 2020

[11] Provincial Government of DKI Jakarta. Pedoman RT/RW dalam Menanggulangi Penyebaran COVID-19. Kementerian Kesehatan RI Direktorat Jenderal Kesehatan Masyarakat Direktorat Promosi Kesehatan dan Pemberdayaan, Masyarakat. Jakarta; 2020

Chapter 5

Poverty and Disease Burden: Reflection on the Rural Community Health Services of the 'Natives' in the Former Northern Transvaal of South Africa, 1930s–1980s

William Maepa

Abstract

The twentieth-century period in South Africa was characterised by social-, political- and economic disparity between blacks and whites. Poor socio-economic conditions of blacks resulted in subjection to tuberculosis and other poverty-related diseases. This study explores rural exposure to diseases due to segregationist and subsequent state of racial disparity in all spheres of live. Focus is particularly thrown at incidents of malaria and tuberculosis in the rural communities of the Transvaal. This study also considers efforts forged by government in an attempt to abate and arrest the spread of these and other epidemics through rudimentary health services. The study relies on the use of published sources, archival materials and data collected through interviews. It is the position of this study that the escalated incidence of these diseases had immense impact on the lives of the rural than urban population. Other related pandemics, such as HIV-AIDS and COVID-19 will be explored. Lastly, the study will argue that evidence of ill health and death continued to surface irrespective of invented vaccines and other related medications.

Keywords: rudimentary, black/African healthcare, preventative primary healthcare, rural-urban migration, South Africa/Transvaal, unequal health, disease burden

1. Introduction

The chronic prevalence of pandemics has been a toxic threat to the lives of South Africans and the world in general. Over many decades after the establishment of the union government, the killer diseases such as malaria, tuberculosis, HIV-AIDS and lately COVID–19 had been a 'headache' to the Department of Health and the World Health Organisation, respectively. It was upon these challenges that blacks found themselves vulnerable due to their state of poverty and other socio-economic defects. The Northern Transvaal, which included the so-called 'native areas or reserves' and later the 1960s ethnic-based homelands of Lebowa, Venda and Gazankulu, became victims of disease diffusions. At times these conditions compelled many young and adult to migrate to the white farms and mining towns where poor living conditions, marginalisation, poor wages and ultimate disease infections were common. The deterioration of health of the blacks compelled the state to come up with measures to deal with the diseases through the establishment of native health, which was followed by popularisation of the concepts such as preventative, progressive and community-based primary health care. The killer diseases such as HIV-AIDS and COVID-19, which erupted in the early 1980s and early 2020s, respectively also continued to inflict ill health and death among the blacks in the country.

2. Malaria in the transvaal and its impact on health care provision

Malaria has been a life-threatening disease that affected Africa and other world countries. As a seasonal disease, in South Africa, it starts to appear in October and reaching its peak in January and February. The disease is usually transmitted through a bite by a female mosquito that carries this disease. It targets mostly the humid high-temperature regions of the world. The Lowveld areas of the former northern and eastern Transvaal, with extreme high annual temperature and rainfall, are popularly known to have favourable breeding ground for malaria-carrying mosquitoes. It has generally been noticed that the intensity of this disease decreases from east to west [1] as reflected in **Figure 1** of the map. One can, therefore, also realise that there is a positive correlation between the rate of malaria, temperature and rainfall, with serious risk areas followed by moderate and light risk areas.

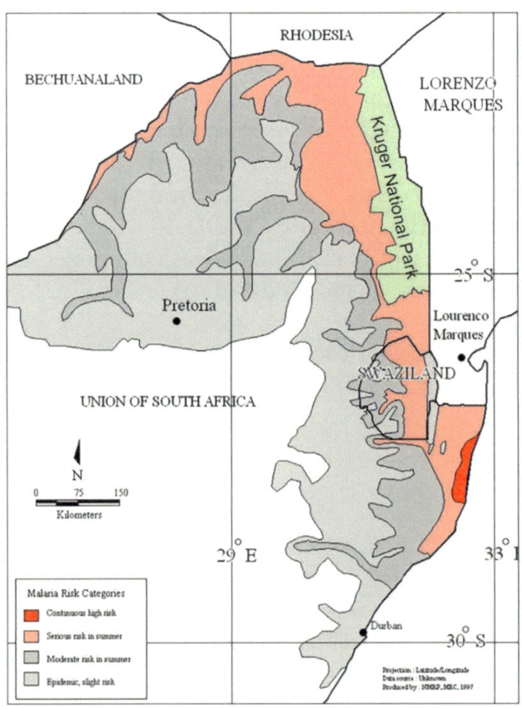

Figure 1.
Malaria risk areas in South Africa, 1938 [1].

The effect of malaria was witnessed during the *Voortrekker* movement to Mozambique when Louis Trichardt, as a leader of the movement, his wife and 20 members were killed between 1837 and 1838 [2]. As a precautionary measure, farmers in the entire area of Transvaal Lowveld considered choosing the high-lying slopes and dry areas for settlement as they were deemed free from malaria-carrying mosquitoes [3].

It was in the midst of the growing malaria challenges that the state saw it fit to come up with workable measures to control and prevent the disease. *Gambiae* and *Funestus* were the mosquitoes typologies that were causing malaria in the area. The Department of Public Health was assigned to carry out this duty through the efforts of N.H Swellengrabel. Meanwhile, malaria continued to worsen in the Lowveld area of the Transvaal, Swellengrabel recommended the establishment of a malaria station in Tzaneen. His influence led to building of the station in 1932 by the South African Institute of Medical Research (SAIMR) under the leadership of De Meillon and Annecke, to carry out research and control of the disease. This effort encouraged the establishment of another station in Eshowe, Natal, in 1934 [2]. Annecke recommended the spraying of indoors and roof surfaces using Quinine Hydrochloride to the Tzaneen Malaria Station in 1939 to control the disease [4, 5]. Traditional leaders were visited and supplied with quinine for distribution to Thabina and the entire Lowveld region [3]. The utilisation of native commissioners through effective depot system was considered critical through constant supervision in the affected areas (**Figure 2**) [7].

Meanwhile, malaria showed an upward trend in the 1940s and 1960s, and the state continued to resort to other additional measures. Educating the communities through the engagement of Tzaneen malaria station staff was crucial as lecturing was presented to black school teachers in the districts of Waterberg, Potgietersrus and Groblersdal [8]. This effort was supplemented by the recommendations of the Tzaneen magistrate, who saw the need for the control malaria depots in Tzaneen and the surrounding countryside [7]. Other areas included Mphahlele's location in the Pietersburg district, municipalities of Potgietersrus, Naboomspruit, Nylstroom and Warmbaths [9]. Towards the end of the Second World War, Annecke endorsed the use of *dichlorodiphenyltrichloroethane* (DDT), which was recommended internationally as effective in the control and prevention of malaria. The reported cases were also dealt with at Giyani area of the Letaba District, the Shingwedzi area of the Letaba District and the Shingwedzi area of the Sibasa District [7].

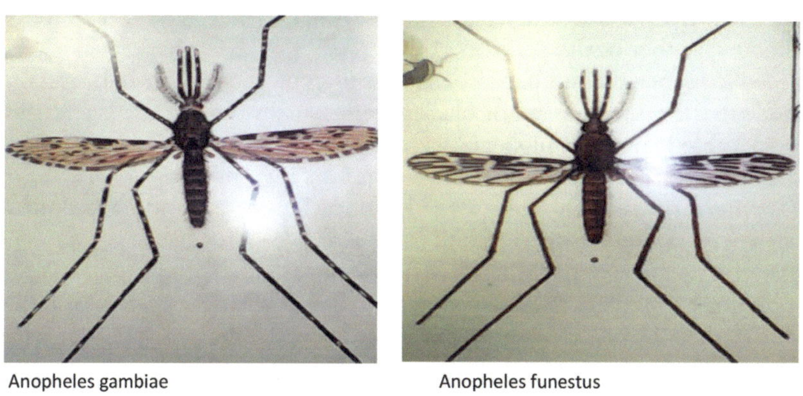

Figure 2.
The two malaria transmitter mosquitoes in southern Africa [6].

When DDT was banned in 1970, followed by its complete replacement in the mid-1980s, the disease once more reflected an upward trend. The banning was influenced by the poisonous impact of this insecticide to the biotic and abiotic environment. Although the public concern was justified, the malaria trends started to increase again, reaching the highest peaks between 1996 and 2015 [10]. Since millions of people throughout the world, including South Africa are currently at risk of contracting this disease, the National Department of Health considered it as a matter of urgency. Its impact as a barrier on social and economic development in the country compelled the state to prioritise meaningful measures to prevent its escalation.

3. Tuberculosis and health services

Tuberculosis (TB), which is caused by a virus called mycobacterium tuberculosis, was unknown to South African blacks until the arrival of whites of European descent in the nineteenth century [11]. People with tuberculosis can be detected by symptoms, such as excessive coughing, physical or body weakness, weight loss, shortness of breath and continuous stress. The discoveries of minerals during the early 1800 in the TVL had a significant impact on the rural-urban migration by the impoverished blacks. As such, blacks became targets of this disease [1]. Researchers such as Shula Marks and Neil Anderson associate poverty and racial discrimination with the high rate of tuberculosis in the rural areas.

In the industrial towns and cities like in the Witwatersrand, the black migrants found themselves vulnerable to the tuberculosis infections caused by unfavourable living conditions. These migrants could easily spread it to their rural environments where health services were poor and inadequate. The soaring ill health and mortality appealed to those in power as well as the employers in the domestic, mining and industrial environments to remedy the situation. They feared the dwindling of labour force and ultimate negative impact on the country's economy. One of the measures initiated by the state was the National Health Service Commission during the early 1940s, which recommended the increase of hospital nurses, doctors, beds and health education for the rural black communities [12]. Apart from the state's request for local authorities to increase hospital beds as a way of overcoming the challenges, immunisation through vaccination was considered the most effective preventative measure. The efforts to combat tuberculosis were made easier when the radiological services were improved with several authorities and mission hospitals having acquired X-Ray units suitable for other health services [13].

The need to increase a number of beds for tuberculosis patients in hospitals coincided with the acute increase of black population during the 1950s and 1960s. Statistics in **Table 1** show the highest incidence of tuberculosis for *Bantu* (blacks) as compared to whites, coloureds and Asiatics in all six regions in 1964 [14].

The Northern Transvaal homelands of Lebowa, Transvaaal and Gazankulu continued to experience increasing reported cases of tuberculosis in the 1970s, with the north-eastern Transvaal in the Mhala district of Gazankulu recording the highest trend. Attempts by the state to deal with this challenge led to the testing of tuberculosis in primary schools including those formerly owned by the missionaries, with subsequent immunisation through vaccinations and distribution of tuberculosis tablets [14]. The forced removal of blacks by the state and subsequent inception of homelands or Bantustans, rural-urban migration, overpopulation, unemployment, poverty and ill health mitigated infection rate. The homelands became breeding grounds for TB and

Region	Whites	Bantu	Coloureds	Asiatics	Total
Eastern Cape	74	3684	5	18	3781
Western Cape	118	2601	2593	—	5312
Natal	16	5047	76	245	5535
Northern Transvaal	—	2709	—	—	2709
Southern Transvaal	50	5408	—	—	5458
O.f.S	38	1487	12	—	1537
TOTAL	447	20,936	2686	263	24,332

Table 1.
South African tuberculosis infected patients in 1964.

other poverty-related diseases. For example, in the Transkei homeland tuberculosis notification growth was at the rate of 489 per 100,000 in 1975 [1].

Alarming notification of tuberculosis encouraged meaningful efforts of educational researches through conferences and symposiums by various institutions of high learning. Attempts at dealing with the challenges of increasing infections in the homelands and developing countries were highlighted during the symposium held at the then University of the North (now the University of Limpopo) on 28–29 October 1976. Pulmonary tuberculosis, which is the tuberculosis of the lungs, was singled out as still by far the most common threatening disease in the homelands [15]. A wide range of recommendations was initiated based on the idea of primary health care approach, with emphasis on preventative and community-oriented care. The reported findings of the health officials from the Pietersburg Regional Directorate of Health Service on the 1978/79 after Lebowa hospitals, such as Knobel, Mogalakwena and Kgapane, were visited revealed increasing notifications. Similar findings were reported from other homelands from the findings by the Medical Research Council during the early 1980s.

Challenges associated with tuberculosis continued to surface in South Africa and worldwide. The disease is currently one of the killer diseases with non-HIV tuberculosis as commonly reported at Waterberg district in 2018. It was here that 1.1 million cases have been estimated [16]. Other districts in Limpopo experienced cases of illnesses and deaths caused by this disease.

4. The relation of disease patterns since 1980

The changing patterns of malaria and tuberculosis continued in the country and elsewhere in the African countries in the 1980s until recent times. The government found itself challenged by these fluctuating incidents of mortality resulting from these diseases. At times the emergence of the new pandemics, such as HIV-AIDS in the early 1980s and COVID–19 in the late 2019 became repeatedly linked to tuberculosis. The Limpopo Province, which embraced previous homelands of Lebowa, Venda and Gazankulu, is largely rural, with high rate of poverty and unemployment.

The first cases of HIV/AIDS were reported in South Africa during the early 1980s and evoked mixed perceptions as many people believed that it only affected European and American homosexuals. As a result, the public did not take enough precautions in the earlier stages. Similarly, the government believed that it was easy to control the homosexuals as they were handful and easy to contain. As for the HIV/AIDS in the black townships and rural communities, lack of sufficient interest by the state was motivated by the racial policy of apartheid. As a result, intervention through preventative measures during the first 5 years after the incidence of the disease was reported was deliberately ignored [17].

The rapid spread of HIV/AIDS can certainly be linked to the migrant labour system and poverty. The long-entrenched labour system had a huge impact on the spread of HIV/AIDS in most rural areas of the former Northern Transvaal, most particularly in the former homeland areas of Lebowa, Venda and Gazankulu and other rural homelands in the country during the 1980s. The tendency of having multiple sexual partners among the blacks, which was deemed culturally acceptable, accelerated the spread of the disease. Most of these migrants established second families in urban areas [18]. This practice also escalated the spread of infections to the entire rural and township black communities, both within South Africa and other neighboring states.

Although the AIDS awareness campaigns were launched for years since the early 1980s, the post-1994 elections in South Africa strengthened the need for the full implementation of community-oriented primary healthcare system. The production of numerous drugs in recent years did not help much to cure the disease completely but contained it as chronic through utilisation of antiretroviral dugs. The scientific discoveries revealed that the disease aggravates in patients with tuberculosis and the two became comorbidities that continued to inflict ill health and death. When COVID-19 emerged towards the end of 2019, focus was shifted, and the disease once more escalated.

The outbreak of COVID-19 created fear and panic in the country, leading to ultimate closure of all public, recreational, private and state institutions, forcing people to stay at home through the 'lock-down' regulations [19]. The challenge with the disease was its rapid rate of infection and death due to the absence of medicine to cure it. The changing structural pattern of this disease made it difficult for health scientists to deal effectively with it as they continued to wrestle to find appropriate vaccine. In Limpopo and other provinces of South Africa, the government initiatives were at times hampered by reluctance of most of the rural populations to comply with precautionary preventative measures and the general attitude of distrust against vaccines during the lockdown alert levels. The controversies surrounding the taking of vaccines and some evidences of government officials' breaking of the lockdown regulations in their gatherings and stealing of personal protective equipment also hampered the government's efforts of effectively dealing with the disease.

Violet Chewe, a Sub-district COVID-19 Coordinator in Mankweng located east of Polokwane and surrounding rural areas, noted that most of the patients diagnosed positive with excessive sickness were found to have other diseases, such as sugar diabetes, tuberculosis, HIV-AIDS, excessive flu and other related communicable diseases. She further stressed that common challenges were experienced during the tracing of people with this disease as most of rural people were in denial as well as being afraid of victimisation and hatred from other members of the communities. She indicated that these conditions were common to other districts of Limpopo Province and countrywide [20].

As for the role played by the traditional healers in the treatment of this disease, Nani Ramalepe, who is one of the well-known traditional healers in the rural area of Tickyline outside Tzaneen confessed that she successfully treated many patients who had similar symptoms of COVID-19 by using plant-based traditional medicines [21]. It is indeed clear that apart from the current reliance on vaccines, which at times raised controversial issues, more scientific research to improve the available vaccines and effective involvement of traditional healers should be encouraged.

5. Conclusion

Certainly, over the years Malaria, tuberculosis, HIV-AIDS and COVID-19 as communicable diseases, continued to pose health challenges to the rural areas and nationwide, forcing the governmental and non-governmental organisations to implement various measures based on the precepts of primary health care. However, with the period following the inception of democratic South Africa in 1994, the whole efforts were at times hampered, among others by lack of effective administration, insufficient medications, ever-increasing black population, laxity and corruption. The rural blacks continued to suffer as most of them could not easily access the quality and expensive health services offered by private health institutions. It is despite the intervention measures from the Department of Health that health challenges continued to threaten the lives of the South Africans, most particularly poverty-stricken black population in the rural areas as it happened with its recent aftermath of COVID-19 pandemic. Although the recent the level of infections showed a significant decline in the late 1921, forcing the government to lift the National State of Disaster on 05 April 2022, COVID-19 has joined malaria, tuberculosis and HIV-Aids as a killer diseases. These diseases continued to be a cause for concern for the Department of Health and the World Health Organisation because of their fluctuating patterns.

Author details

William Maepa
University of Pretoria (UP), Pretoria, South Africa

*Address all correspondence to: maepawilly@webmail.co.za

References

[1] Van Rensburg HCF et al. Health Care in South Africa: Structure and Dynamics. Pretoria: Academica; 31 August 1992

[2] Coetzee M et al. Malaria in South Africa: 110 of learning to control the disease. South African Medical Journal. October 2013;**103**(10)

[3] Kruger P. Face-to-Face Interview on Migrant Work and Immunization during the Period Under Study. Polokwane, South Africa: Malaria Control Directorate, Limpopo Provincial Department of Health; 24 March 2016

[4] South African National Archives, GES, Box 2659 File37/56b, Department of Public Health, Malaria, Tzaneen, South Africa. 15 July 1939

[5] South African National Archives, GES, Box 2659 File45/26, Malaria Distribution of Sale of Medicines and Materials, Malaria, Tzaneen, South Africa. 2 December 1939

[6] Gear JHS et al. Malaria in Southern Africa. Johannesburg: University of Witwatersrand; 1989

[7] South African National Archives, GES, Box 2659 File45/26, Malaria Distribution of Sale of Medicines and Materials, Malaria, Tzaneen, South Africa. 27 November 1939

[8] South African National Archives, GES, Box 2659 File45/26, Malaria Distribution of Sale of Medicines and Materials, Malaria, Tzaneen, South Africa. 01 August 1939

[9] Limpop Provincial Archives, Medical and Preventative Services, Tuberculosis Consultative Report. July 1978/June 1979

[10] Mabunda QE. Malaria Trends in Limpopo Province: Presentation of MRC Malaria Conference, South Africa. August 2015

[11] De Beer C. The South African Disease: Apartheid Health and Health Services. Johannesburg: Southern African Research Service; 1984

[12] Packard RM. White Plaque, Black Labor: Tuberculosis and Political Economy of Health and Disease in South Africa. University of California Press; 1989

[13] Annual Report of the Department of Health, Year ended 31 December 1959. Government Printer, Pretoria 28/1962

[14] Wilson F, Ramphele M. Uprooting Poverty: The South African Challenge. USA: David Philip; 1989

[15] Grous J. Physical Factors which Influence Health : International Symposium on Health Services for Developing Community. South Africa: University of the North; 28 and 29 October 1976

[16] Ramaliba TM et al. Tuberculosis risk factors in Lephalale Local Manucipality of Limpopo Province. South African Family Practice. 2017;**59**(5)

[17] Grunglingh L. Government response to HIV-AIDS in South Africa as reported in the Media, 1983-1994. South African Historical Journal. 2001;**45**(127)

[18] Coovadia et al. The Health and Health of South Africa: Health in South Africa. 5 September 2009;**374**(9692):817-834. Available from: www.thelancet.com

[19] Mercer A, Chinchen G. Available from: https://neuroemploy.com/2022/10/09/benefits-of-covid-19-tot-the-workplace

[20] Chewe MV. Face-to-face interview about the link between COVID-19 and other communicative diseases. 2022

[21] Ramalepe N. Face-to-Face Interview about the Contribution of Traditional Healers in the Treatment of COVID-19. Tickyline Village, Tzaneen, Limpopo Province of South Africa. 8 January 2021

Section 2

Reducing Inequities in Access to Health and Social Services

Chapter 6

Perspective Chapter: Health Facilities and Services in Rural Sierra Leone – Implication for Longevity and Well Being of Her Citizenry

Roland Suluku, Abu Macavoray, Moinina Nelphenson Kallon and Joseph A. Buntin-Graden

Abstract

Sierra Leoneans face multiple barriers to accessing health facilities and services in rural communities leading to morbidity and mortality. The objective of this paper is to identify some of these challenges and proffer possible solutions to mitigate morbidity and mortality in rural communities and prolong the lives of their citizenry. The lack of money, the use of cheaper traditional medicines versus expensive medicines at health centers, lack of confidence in health workers, and transportation access to reach health facilities are barriers to accessing health facilities and services by rural community people. The above barriers outline was obtained through thirty years of interaction, discussion, and observations with people and health workers in rural communities. Possible solutions include the provision of free health care, ambulances to ease transportation, the integration of traditional medicine into the national health system, and the encouragement of rural community people to engage in multiple cropping every year. The above solutions and many others will encourage the citizenry in rural communities to attend health facilities and services in the country's rural towns and villages.

Keywords: rural, health, well-being, citizenry, long-life

1. Introduction

Sierra Leone had limited health facilities in rural communities before the rebel war in 1991. This was partly due to low health expenditures by the government due to the reduced tax collection base of the country. In 2001, the African government agreed to allocate 15% of its annual income to health known as the Abuja declaration [1]. However, most countries have not achieved this African objective due to low gross domestic product, low tax collection, and low budget allocation to the health sector as a result of many competing priorities [2]. However, health requires intensive capital investment, as it increases labor efficiency and productivity, increases income, and improves the standard of living of her citizenry [3]. Current health expenditure by the government of Sierra Leone in 2019 was 8.75%, and out-of-pocket expenditure was US$25.47 [4]. This is far well below the WHO recommended US 30–40 per person needed to cover essential health care in low-income countries [5]. Low-income countries currently spend US$8.00–US$129 per capita compared to US$4000.00 for high-income countries However, many countries in Africa have not been able to meet the Abuja declaration, except Botswana, Rwanda, and Zambia [6], while Equatorial guinea who has not achieved toe the Abuja declaration, but has high health per capita [7].

Rural communities' health infrastructures were destroyed, and only 86% of district headquarters health facilities remained functional during the eleven-year-old civil war. In 2003, the government rehabilitated and made 631 available peripheral health units (PHU) across the country [8]. Most communities' peripheral health facilities were 5 miles apart, so distance will not limit people from seeking medical attention. However, the major bottleneck is the need for more trained and qualified health personnel to operate these health facilities in rural communities. United Nations reported that only 38% of nurses and 25% of medical doctors work in health facilities in rural communities [9]. Five of the fourteen districts lacked access to primary health services after the civil war. The government reintegrated ex-combatants who were treating rebels and civilians as vaccinators. The strategy increased the number of health workforce but limited progress in the health sector due to a need for a clear political vision. Despite this improvement in the country's health facilities, most of the population residing in rural communities could not afford the cost, which also contributed to the high maternal mortality rate of 1800/100,000 in 2002 [8].

In 2010, the government introduced free healthcare to increase access to health facilities and services for pregnant and breastfeeding women and young children [10]; at this time, most births in rural communities were done by traditional birth attendants. The government engaged conventional birth attendants and trained them to work with health workers, thereby increasing attendance at health facilities. By-laws were formulated to discourage home birth but to encourage the use of health facilities. The objective was to reduce maternal morbidity and mortality [11].

Free health care and funding performance-based increased coordination in the health system and brought a paradigm shift in the health sector in the country [12]. The government also introduced performance-based financing as a way of motivating health workers. Compounding the situation further was the high death rate of health personnel, which eroded patients' convenience in attending these facilities and accessing the service [13, 14].

In July 2015, the President of Sierra Leone launched the Ebola Health Recovery Plan to attain a resilient sustainable health system to reduce maternal and child mortality and morbidity [4]. However, the presidential recovery initiative was for 24 months, with a critical focus on IDSR, strengthening IPC, Community engagement, enhancing Human Resources for Health, and Improving Management for Health and a Resilient Health System. The government needed help translating this novel initiative into an effective maternal health system. It was, therefore, the plan of the Ministry of Health and Sanitation to design an appropriate and effective program that is economically, socially, and culturally acceptable to the rural population of Sierra Leone.

The WHO designed the External Joint Evaluation to address the health challenges and build a sustainable, resilient health system to reduce maternal morbidity and mortality. Moreover, the Ministry of Health and Sanitation, with international partners and the One Health secretariat, prioritizes zoonotic diseases to improve the health situation in the country. Aside from these strides, people in rural communities face numerous challenges in accessing these health facilities and services.

2. Challenges and constraints in accessing health facilities and services in rural communities

The primary source of income in rural communities is agriculture and mining contributing to employment and gross domestic product [15, 16]. In time past, people in rural communities were engaged in all-year-round income generation. They harvest and sell coffee, cocoa, and piassava from October to January in the southern and eastern provinces. Ginger was harvested and sold from January to march, orange from February to May, and rice was harvested from June to November. Other assorted crops planted and sold include cassava, benne, yam, groundnut, maize, millet, sweet potato, and other multiple crops cultivated on the rice farm [17]. During the dry season in some communities, there are several water catchments and rivers where the women fish and prepare dishes for the evening meals. The men set traps, hunt animals for home consumption, and sell some for emergencies. All these multiple sources of income make it possible for people in rural communities to easily pay medical bills.

Today, massive destruction of the environment through lumbering, charcoal burning, and mining has destroyed the farming environment in rural communities [18] reported that human activities in the environment in which they live have shown a negative impact on the forest ecology in the last 2800 years. Morie Sam [19] confirmed for Sierra Leone that people depend on forest vegetation as a major source of energy. Soils are no longer fertile, yields are low, and the current population is unwilling to farm. Sam and Zhiqiang [20] said, removing the vegetation cover of the forest decreases the forest and soil stability and biosphere and thus impacts the normal environment. Moreover, the massive destruction of the environment has drastically reduced the income of people in rural communities [21]; as such, the majority can no longer afford to pay for basic essential commodities and services. What are the Challenges and constraints of accessing health facilities and services in rural communities?

i. **Lack of money:** most rural people have narrowed their income sources to single or sole cropping or few activities. IFAD [22] reported that the yields of all major crops cultivated in Sierra Leone are significantly lower than most countries in the subregion of West Africa. The government of Sierra Leone estimated that rice yields are 0.97 t/ha far below other countries in the region. The Government attributes the low yields to the unavailability of improved seeds, lack of access to fertilizers, mechanization, crop protection products, weak extension services, and water control in lowlands [22]. Other contributing factors in rural communities are deforestation and charcoal burning, leading to the reduced organic matter in the soil, low fertility, and crop yield, which cannot meet their daily household or domestic needs. About two-thirds of people in rural communities now grow multiple crops to mitigate against crop failure and reduce the risk of cash income failure [23, 24]. Animal rearing is another source of income, but its compounded with numerous disease outbreaks such as PPR, New Castle Disease, Rift valley fever, rabies, and theft. Most animal rearers drop out of animal rearing which decreases their sources of income. The average Sierra Leonean earns less than 1.90 dollars daily. This has led to many deaths and others being unable to access these medical facilities and services.

The lack of money to pay for consultancy services and transportation to reach these facilities has led to the situation where most pregnant women give birth at home. At the same time, others die on the way to these facilities on foot or bikes.

Sometimes, family members are taxed to contribute and pay the medical expenses before a person goes to these facilities. Some members find it challenging to raise their contributions leading to delay or death of the patient.

ii. **Traditional medicine is cheaper than health facilities**: the extended family systems throughout Sierra Leone make information easily accessible to people within their communities. Most people know about traditional herbalists living within their communities, and in some cases, they relate to each other. They see the herbalist and have confidence in them based on their records because it is embedded in their traditions and customs [25]. Payment for such services is based on kinship, which is cheaper and can be paid for when money is available. In some cases, payment is in kind or other forms, making it easier for people to seek medication from an herbalist than from health facilities. Most rural people prefer to give birth through traditional attendants than health facilities because it is relatively cheaper than modern medicine [26].

iii. **Lack of confidence in health workers:** the Ebola outbreak showcased people's unwillingness to attend health facilities in the country for fear of death or contracting Ebola. The government announced that there was no medicine to treat the disease, but at the same time asked people to go to these health facilities for treatment. Tiffany et al. [27], and Sabeti and Salahi [28] reported that the Ebola Virus Disease outbreak in Sierra Leone was fueled by persistent misinformation and conspiracy theories that led to the public health disaster. Most of the people who attended did not return home; as such, people were afraid to seek medical attention through these health facilities; many healthcare workers died, thereby making people run away from these facilities. Sochas et al. [29], and Elston et al. [30] reported that many healthcare staff died, leading to patients' lack of confidence in the healthcare services.

iv. **Lack of medication:** most health facilities in rural communities depend on medicine supplied by the government. People in rural communities cannot afford the cost of these drugs and therefore take to traditional medications. The inability of rural communities to pay for these drugs has caused most pharmacy shelves to go without essential medicines, as reported when Partners in Health entered Koidu health center in 2014. Patients look for places where they can get cheap drugs. A typical example is the traditional birth attendants. These local people get more delivery of babies than the nurses in the health centers because of the cheap cost of delivery services offered to their subjects. The government has to encourage them to work with health facility workers, where they can receive more training to meet international standards.

v. **Lack of transportation fees for vehicles and bikes:** most rural towns and villages in the country are not accessible either by cars, vehicles, or in some cases, motorbikes [31]. Some people trek on foot to access health services in those facilities. Families who lost their strong and abled-bodied relatives during the war stayed in the villages with no one to take them to the medical facilities. Some with strong relatives have to travel with them on a hammock, while others die on the way. With the advent of motorbikes, traveling to health centers has become much easier, as these bikes move faster on bad roads, thereby reducing transportation constraints in rural communities. The disadvantage is the high cost which most people cannot afford in rural communities. The same is true of the ambulance government has introduced in the country.

   Due to the challenging economic status of people in rural communities, providing funds to make use of ambulance services even when available is a major issue. The people not only resort to risky alternatives but also seek spiritual help from traditional herbalists or religious sources. A typical example is in Lumponga village located in Kamajei chiefdom, Moyamba district, the southern province, where a lady suffered for three days before giving birth because of financial constraints. The people have to seek the attention of church members for prayers until the lady gave birth to a bouncing baby boy three days later. So, although the government has provided ambulances, many people, especially in rural communities cannot use them. Alternatively, they also seek the help of traditional herbalists. This is one factor that has increased the use of conventional medicine in these communities.

vi. **Decision-making** as to who should allow the patient to travel: in rural communities of Sierra Leone, the male is the head of the family household. The family head takes all decisions relating to the family. In his absence, all family members will have to wait until the head returns. Aside from being the head of the family, certain decisions require all family members to be present, particularly when it relates to a family member's health. These consultations and waiting for the head to decide denied most people in rural areas access to health facilities. The situation is compounded when the total financial involvement is high. Here the head will tax all members a certain amount of money for them to pay. The amount charged depends not on the amount people get but on what the leader has proposed. In some cases, other family members cannot afford it, leading to the patient's death. As a result, the patient remains suffering for a long time.

vii. **Traditions and customs:** the tradition of some societies limits people from accessing healthcare facilities and services. A named church does not allow its member to go to hospitals when they fall sick. When people in rural communities who are holding high-ranking positions in secret societies fall sick, they are usually taken to their secret society bushes or shrines, where they perform traditional ceremonies on the person. In most cases, the person dies. Such traditional customs refuse their people access to health facilities and services. Some secret societies deny their members access to medical facilities when they fall sick.

viii. **Altitude of health workers:** the attendance at health facilities by rural community people is heavily dependent on the altitude of the health workers.

Some health personnel have good interpersonal relationship with patients, and this encourages patients to attend such health facilities. The patient in such a community informs others of the good attitude of the health staff. The health worker, in turn, receives gifts from the community, such as rice, chickens, fish, yam, palm oil, or whatever agricultural commodity they have. In some cases, because of the bond, rural community people who do not have money pay in kind, and the health worker sells the items received into money, thus increasing access to health facilities and services.

On the other hand, where health workers' relationship with community people is poor, the rural community people run away from these facilities and rely on traditional herbalists for treatment.

ix. **Case study**: during the Ebola outbreak, most sick people ran away from hospitals and medical facilities around the country because the government announced that there were no drugs to cure Ebola. People suspected of or infected with Ebola refused to attend health facilities but instead went to nurses. They had good relationships. My daughter was one such person who received many patients due to her relationship with the communities she worked. In the end, she, too, contracts the virus and dies.

Rural community people believe in friendship and encourage health professional who loves, promotes, and empathizes with their situation.

x. **Lack of bye-laws:** these are effective constitutional instruments, if judiciously used, can increase attendance in rural health facilities. During the Ebola outbreak, all the paramount chiefs formulated by-laws and circulated them in their respective chiefdoms. These were later digested by the chiefdom authorities and became chiefdom by-laws. It was fully implemented, which helped reduce the epidemic in those communities where it was enforced.

In some communities during the Ebola outbreak, people were asked to report to the hospital if they fell sick. Fines were levied against those who refused to report to health facilities.

xi. **Technical and social infrastructure:** the type of health infrastructure built in the rural areas will attract both technical staff and patients to access the facilities. Medical doctors and other highly trained personnel will stay in rural communities if they have the equipment to work with. Many people would like to stay in rural areas if provided with the necessary infrastructure. Such facilities include hospital services, preventive care, and emergency services. At Njala University hospital, a medical doctor resigned because there was no theater to conduct operations on patients.

3. How do we make people in rural communities attend health facilities and access services to prolong their lives

In many low-income countries, several factors prevent people from equal access from attending health facilities which leads to morbidity and mortality. Particularly so in rural communities [32]. Sierra Leone is one such country where medical bills are paid by the individual, lack of skilled medical staff, and services provided are poor and not to the satisfaction of the patient [33]. Compounding the situation further is the concentration of more than half of the medical staff concentration in the capital city leaving the majority of communities at the mercy of mother nature [34]. The government increased access to health facilities by introducing free health care in 2010 to reduce maternal and neonatal mortality by waiving all medical fees for pregnant and breastfeeding women, children under the age of five years, and those who survived the Ebola pandemic. st as a means of reducing [35].

Another method used to increase access to health facilities was the introduction of the ambulance system known as the National Emergency Service. The government aimed to provide a free-of-charge ambulance service coordinated by a center in all 14 districts [36].

Other strategies used to increase attendance or access to health facilities and services include:

3.1 Encourage rural community people to cultivate multiple crops

In Sierra Leone, multiple crops include rice intercropped with cassava, yam, beans, millet, sorghum, benni, garden eggs, bitter balls, pepper, egusi, cucumber, and maize. After harvest, the farmer will sell some of these crops and use the money for multiple purposes including accessing health facilities and services. Planting multiple crops will militate against crop failure. In Sierra Leone, two-thirds of household families cultivate 12 different types of crops on 2 acres of land [37]. Household plan against food security strategy to prevent crop failure and reduces the risk of income shortage over cash income. An increase in crop production will lead to surplus, and excess crops produced will be sold to earn additional income which they will use to pay for medical bills when they attend health facilities, settle domestic issues and emergencies relating to initiation into secret societies, naming ceremonies, school fees, and unresolved problems within the families or neighbors [38]. The lack of income will prevent many people from accessing health facilities and services thereby leading to increased morbidity and mortality.

3.2 Cultivation of permanent crops

Cultivation of permanent crops such as coffee, cacao, cashew, organ, palm trees, rubber plantation, coconut, guava, kola trees, banana, and plantain. These crops were grown by our rural people for development such as the construction of dwelling houses, payment of school fees, initiation into secret societies, hiring of farm labor, settling bush conflicts, and emergencies such as payment for medical bills. Illnesses that require emergency operations cannot be settled with income from rice farming. These permanent crops were like savings banks and have been used for centuries. Today, the young generation does not grow crops but harvests what their parents have grown, and the yield of crops has drastically reduced. This has led to a shortage of income within the families and hence unable access health facilities. Tree crops currently employ 100,000 rural cacao producers in the country [39] with a total acreage of 235,749 ha, with Kailahun cultivating 114.125 ha, Kenema 58,086 ha, Kono 43,23 ha and Bo district 11,715 ha respectively [39]. This has forced the Government of Sierra Leone to develop long-term planning for expansion, modernization, and improved management to increase income and enhance [40].

3.3 Rotational sources of income

As time passed, rural community farmers had all-year-round income from their farming activities in Sierra Leone. They will plan at the end of the year what they intend to achieve the following year. The plan is based on the income they receive from various crops, animals, or activities they undertake as a family.

3.4 Case study

In the South and Eastern provinces of Sierra Leone, families plant coffee, cacao, ginger, orange, and rice. Rice is harvested between September, and November to the end of December. The rice is sold to buy clothing, shoes, and household condiments for the Christmas celebration. Coffee and cacao are harvested from November until the end of February; Ginger is harvested in the month of November to February end, while orange is harvested in the month of March and April. The harvest is sold, and proceeds are used for house construction, sometimes paying school fees, initiation into secret societies, and settling emergency medical bills. In some families, they will keep or set aside some amount of funds for emergencies. When a family member falls sick, money set aside will be used to send the ill person to health facilities, thus increasing access to health facilities and services. The current generation of abled-bodied men no longer follows this pattern of income generation, thereby reducing access to these facilities and services. Sometimes a portion of the proceeds is plowed back into farming and used to buy food during the lean period.

3.5 Rural transportation

Transportation is a significant bottleneck in accessing rural health facilities and services. About one billion people in rural communities are three miles or 2 km away from a regular road [41]. Aside from the availability of good roads, a large segment of the rural population needs help to afford the cost of transportation. Patients die in rural communities or on the way to medical facilities because they cannot afford the cost of paying for bikes, lorries, and taxis. Lack of safe access roads causes devastating effects on communities leading to high infant mortality in isolated communities [42]. Though the government has provided ambulances in all districts, only a few people can afford the cost. Providing transportation at a subsidized price will increase access to these facilities.

3.6 Education of rural organizations

Organizations raising awareness and educating rural communities on healthcare issues should be provided with adequate education on community social, traditional, and cultural norms. Understanding social behavior and traditional and cultural norms will help them to interact and live with people amicably. Such social cohesion will help increase access to health facilities and services because of the level of awareness of their health in the community. Health education will empower people to improve health care, disease prevention, and control [43]. Such knowledge gained will allow people to adopt healthier behaviors to attend health facilities when sick and use the services provided. Empowerment of this nature will not only help the individual but families, communities, and the nation to contribute to the achievement of the millennium development goal.

3.7 Training community health workers' socio-cultural lives in rural communities

Training community health workers on how to live in rural communities will be a step in the right direction. There are reports of healthcare workers, especially nurses using abusive language against and beating patients. In South Africa, patients refused to give birth in a hospital because they were beaten and scolded by nurses and discriminated against Kruger and Schoombee [44]. Understanding rural people's traditions and socio-cultural customs, will them appreciate you, and either party can live harmoniously. Some of the health workers today are from rural communities, but grew up and spend all their time in the cities or district headquarters towns. As such see rural people as inferior and discriminate against them. Dapaah [45] reported that some nurses discriminate and give preferential treatment to those they love. Such behavior scares people away from attending such health facilities because of a lack of respect [46, 47]. On the other hand, community health workers who understand community life put on a good attitude and live in peace with the people. Small and large health centers are most often flocked with people. Regular training on traditional and socio-cultural behavior will improve personal interaction between health workers and community people.

3.8 Increase incentives for professionals working in rural communities

Most people dislike working in rural communities. The provision of incentives will go a long way in retaining health workers. Retaining health workers in such a community will lead to a strong professional relationship between the healthcare giver and patients thereby improving the relationship between people in rural communities [48, 49]. In many parts of the world, the government and the private sector find it extremely difficult to retain health workers in rural communities [50]. It is vital to retain health workers in rural communities to provide health care and develop a professional relationship between the patient and the health worker to improve the health outcomes of the most defenseless population in the country [49].

3.9 Integrating traditional medicine into national health systems

The integration of traditional medicine into the national health care system will not only help people in rural communities but will meet the health care needs of people in developing and developed countries [51, 52]. In Africa, 80% of the population uses traditional medicine as their first line of healthcare [53]. In Ghana, for example, studies conducted on traditional medicine show treatment of different ailments such as diabetes, fever, foot rot, and stroke [54]. Aside from low-income countries, it is widely used in high-income countries such as France, the USA, Austria Canada, and Belgium [54]. Developing policies, by-laws, and regulations for providers and professionals will enhance rural community access to health facilities and assess services in remote communities.

3.10 Outreach or extension of the internship programs of health care students to rural communities

Students studying medicine and other health care professionals will be better able to convince people in rural communities to attend health facilities and access the services available. Rural community people believe and develop confidence in young people who know how to talk to them when sent on such missions. The rural people do admire the health workers and even try to persuade their children to choose such a vocation. The bond between the two parties sometimes becomes so strong that the community people invite the health personnel into their homes. Such a relationship will boost confidence and increase the attendance of the rural people in the health facilities. Training community children to become healthcare professionals will increase attendance at health facilities and the use of health services.

3.11 Improved infrastructure

People in rural communities easily believe and trust the medical personnel and facilities they have in their communities. When the health center is well constructed and capacitated with adequate equipment, drugs, and trained personnel, rural people tend to frequent such facilities because they are assured of getting the needed services. It is a common saying in rural communities that the medical structure is fine when it has well-trained staff, equipment, and drugs In my village, people prefer seeking medical attention at the Masanka health facilities and Segbwema hospital because they have Europeans who know how to talk to patients and treat them well. People often find money to visit these health centers because of their outstanding performance. Once the trust has been established, they create a friendly relationship with the health personnel and frequently visit them when they are sick.

4. Conclusion

Diversification of income sources, improved infrastructure, and basic services, which include transportation facilities, and reduced cost of out-of-pocket medical bills in rural communities will help them access health facilities and services and increase life expectancy among people.

Acknowledgements

Thanks to members of the serology and molecular diagnostic Laboratory staff who join us to collect information during our visits to animal sample collection throughout the country. Special thanks to health personnel for spearing their time during the interview. The team also thanks all the people in rural communities who visited during the sample collection. Special thanks to my wife who took care of the home during my visits to various communities, and Njala university for using their facilities during this write-up. No fund was received for this write-up.

Author details

Roland Suluku[1*], Abu Macavoray[1], Moinina Nelphenson Kallon[1]
and Joseph A. Buntin-Graden[2]

1 School of Agriculture and Food Sciences, Animal Science Department,
Njala University, Sierra Leone

2 Directorate of Health Security and Emergencies, Ministry of Health and Sanitation,
Sierra Leone

*Address all correspondence to: rsuluku@njala.edu.sl

References

[1] Piabuo SM, Tieguhong JC. Health expenditure and economic growth—A review of the literature and an analysis between the economic community for central African states (CEMAC) and selected African countries. Health Economics Review. 2017;**2017**:7. DOI: 10.1186/s13561-017-0159-1

[2] Gatome-Munyua A, Olalere N. Public Financing for Health in Africa: 15% of an Elephant is not 15% of a Chicken. African Union's 2001 Abuja Declaration on Funding National Health Budgets. 2020. Available from: https://www.un.org/africarenewal/magazine/october-2020/public-financing-health-africa-when-15-elephant-not-15-chicken [Accessed: March 23, 2023]

[3] World Health Organization. Make Every Mother and Child Count. The World Health Report 2005. 2005

[4] The World Bank Current Health Expenditure. Sierra Leone. 2023. Available from: https://data.worldbank.org/indicator/SH.XPD.CHEX.GD.ZS?locations=SL&most_recent_value_desc=false [Retrieved: May 21, 2023]

[5] Ali EE. Health care financing in Ethiopia: Implications on access to essential Medicines. Value in Health Regional Issues. 2014;**4**:37-40

[6] Piabuo SM, Tieguhong JC. Health expenditure and economic growth—Review of the literature and an analysis between the economic community for central African states (CEMAC) and selected African countries. Health Economics Review. 2017;**2017**:7. DOI: 10.1186/s13561-017-0159-1

[7] Dye C, Boerma T, Evans D, Harries A, Lienhardt C, McManus J, et al. The world health report. Research for Universal Health Coverage. 2013. Ref # ISBN 9789240690837

[8] National Recovery Strategy. Sierra Leone 2002-2003. 2002

[9] United Nations. Population Facts Department of Economic and Social Affairs Population Division. 2010 No. 2010/2/E/Ref

[10] UNICEF Annual Report. Covering 1 January 2009 through 31 December 2009. 2009

[11] Edoka IP, Stacey NK. Estimating a cost-effectiveness threshold for health care decision-making in South Africa. 2016. DOI: 10.1093/heal/czz152

[12] Bertone M, Witter S. The development of HRH policy in Sierra Leone, 2002-2012 Report on key informant interviews. Center for Disease Control and Prevention. 2014-2016 Ebola Outbreak in West Africa. 2002-2012. Available from: https://www.cdc.gov/vhf/ebola/history/2014-2016-outbreak/index.html [Accessed: January 2022]

[13] Elston JW, Moosa AJ, Moses F, Walker G, Dotta N, Waldman RJ, et al. Impact of the Ebola outbreak on health systems and population health in Sierra Leone. Journal of Public Health (Oxford). 2 Dec 2016;**38**(4):673-678. DOI: 10.1093/pubmed/fdv158. PMID: 28158472

[14] Sochas L, Channon AA, Nam S. Counting indirect crisis-related deaths in the context of a low-resilience health system: The case of maternal and neonatal health during the Ebola epidemic in Sierra Leone. 2017. DOI: 10.1093/heal/czx108

[15] Gboku MLS, Davowa SK, Gassama A. Sierra Leone 2015 population and housing census: Thematic report on agriculture. Statistics Sierra Leone, Freetown, October, 41. 2017. Available from: https://sierraleone.unfpa.org/en/publications/sierra-leone-2015-population-and-housing-census-thematic-report-agriculture

[16] World Bank in Sierra Leone. The World Bank works closely with development partners to support Sierra Leone in fighting poverty, promoting economic development, and improving living standards. 2022. Available from: https://www.worldbank.org/en/country/sierraleone/overview updated October 20, 2022 [Accessed: March 28, 2023]

[17] Amadu FO, Silvert C, Eisenmann C, Mosiman K, Liang R. Sierra Leone Landscape Analysis. 2017. Available from: https://www.g-fras.org/en/component/phocadownload/category/93-reviews-and-assessments.html?download=821:sierra-leone-landscape-analysis

[18] Feurdean Angelica GF, Vanniere B, Tant I, O'Hara RB, Pfeiffer M, Hutchinson SM, et al. Fire has been an important driver of Forest dynamics in the Carpathian Mountain during Holocene. Forest Ecology and Management. 2017;**389**:15-26

[19] Morie Sam AS. Availability, accessibility, and the road map for clean, affordable, effective, and efficient energy for Sierra Leone. A six years analysis from 2006-2011. International Journal of Scientific and Research Publication. 2018;**8**(5):543-553

[20] Sam M, Zhiqiang Z. The trend of forest cover removal: Case study of Tonkolili district, Northern Sierra Leone. Journal of Environment and Earth Science. 2018;**8**(11). ISSN 2224-3216 (Paper) 2225-0948(Online)

[21] Oduntan OO, Soaga JAO, Akinyemi AF, Ojo SO. Human activities pressure and its threat on forest reserves in your division of Ogun state, Nigeria. Journal of Environmental Research and Management. 2013;**4**(5):260-267. Available from: https://www.researchgate.net/publication/353757276_Effects_of_Deforestation_on_Rural_Household_Income_In_Vandeikya_Local_Government_Area_of_Benue_State_Nigeria [Accessed: March 29, 2023]

[22] IFAD. Sierra Leone agriculture value development project design completion report document date: 21-Oct 2018 project No. 1544 west and Central Africa division programmed management department. 2018

[23] Saravia Matus SL, Gomez y Paloma S. Farm viability of (semi) subsistence smallholders in Sierra Leone. African Journal of Agricultural and Resource Economics. 2014;**2014**(9):165-182

[24] Saravia-Matus S, Gomez y Paloma S. Implementation challenges to the National Sustainable Agriculture Development Plan (NSADP) for (semi) subsistence farmers in Sierra Leone. Cahiers Agricultures. 2015;**24**:240-245

[25] Abdullahi AA. Trends and challenges of traditional medicine in Africa. African Journal of Traditional, Complementary, and Alternative Medicines. 2011;**8**(5):115-123. DOI: 10.4314/ajtcam.v8i5s.5

[26] Antwi-Baffour SS, Bello AI, Adjei DN, Mahmood SA, Ayeh-Kumi PF. The place of traditional medicine in the African society: The science, acceptance and support. American Journal of Health Research. 2014;**2**(2):49-54. DOI: 10.11648/j.ajhr.20140202.13

[27] Tiffany A, Dalziel BD, Kagume Njenge H, Johnson G, Nugba Ballah R,

James D, et al. Estimating the number of secondary Ebola cases resulting from an unsafe burial and risk 138 factors for transmission during the West Africa Ebola epidemic. PLoS Neglected Tropical Diseases. 2017;**11**(6):e0005491. DOI: 10.1371/journal.pntd.0005491

[28] Sabeti P, Salahi L. Outbreak Culture: The Ebola Crisis and the Next Epidemic. Cambridge, Massachusetts: Harvard University Press; 2018. 288 p

[29] Sochas L, Channon AA, Nam S. Counting indirect crisis-related deaths in the context of a low-resilience health system: The case of maternal and neonatal health during the Ebola epidemic in Sierra Leone. 2017. DOI: 10.1093/heal/czx108

[30] Elston JW, Cartwright C, Ndumbi P, Wright J. The health impact of the 2014-15 Ebola outbreak. Public Health. Feb 2017;**143**:60-70. DOI: 10.1016/j.puhe.2016.10.020. Epub 2016 Nov 29. PMID: 28159028

[31] Munguambe K, Boene H, Vidler M. et al, Barriers and facilitators to health care seeking behaviors in pregnancy in rural communities of southern Mozambique. Reproductive Health. 2016;**13**(Suppl 1):31. DOI: 10.1186/s12978-016-0141-0.

[32] Strasser R, Kam SM, Regalado SM. Rural health care access and policy in developing countries. Annual Review of Public Health. 2016;**37**:395-412

[33] Human Development Reports. Sierra Leone. 2020. Available from: http://hdr.undp.org/en/countries/profiles/SLE [Accessed: April 1, 2023]

[34] National Health Sector Strategic Plan. Ministry of Health and Sanitation. 2017-2021

[35] Donnelly J. How did Sierra Leone provide free health care? Lancet. 2011;**377**:1393-1396

[36] Ragazzoni L, Caviglia M, Rosi P, Buson R, Pini S, Merlo F, et al. Designing, implementing, and managing a national emergency medical service in Sierra Leone. Prehospital and Disaster Medicine. Feb 2021;**36**(1):115-120. DOI: 10.1017/S1049023X20001442. Epub 2020 Dec 1. PMID: 33256859

[37] Sesay A, Tejan-Kella M, Thompson A. Agricultural Sector, Background Review for the PRSP. Freetown, Sierra Leone: Government of Sierra Leone; 2004

[38] Suluku R et al. Investigate the uses of goats and socioeconomic impact of Peste des Petits ruminant on farmers engaged in diamond Mining in Tongo Field. International Journal of Zoology and Animal Biology. 2022;**5**(6):000415

[39] Sierra Leone Population and Housing Census. Thematic Report on Agriculture. Statistics Sierra Leone. Freetown. 2015:60

[40] Ex-post Evaluation of Agriculture for Development (A4D) Sierra Leone, Final Report. Freetown. 2018:10

[41] Transport & ICT. Measuring Rural Access: Using New Technologies. Washington DC, USA: Transport and ICT Global Practice; 2016

[42] Sustainable Mobility for All. Global Roadmap of Action Toward Sustainable Mobility: Universal Rural Access. Washington, DC, USA: Sustainable Mobility for All; 2019

[43] Sørensen K, Van den Broucke S, Fullam J, Doyle G, Pelikan J, Slonska Z. (HLS-EU) Consortium Health Literacy Project European. Health literacy and

public health: A systematic review and integration of definitions and models. BMC Public Health. 2012;**12**:80

[44] Kruger LM, Schoombee C. The other side of caring: Abuse in a South African maternity ward. Journal of Reproductive and Infant Psychology. 2010;**28**(1):84-101

[45] Dapaah JM. Attitudes and behaviours of health workers and the use of HIV/AIDS Health Care Services. Nursing Research and Practice. 2016;**2016**:5172497. DOI: 10.1155/2016/517249

[46] Umar N, Quaife M, Exley J, Shuaibu A, Hill Z, Marchant T. Toward improving respectful maternity care: A discrete choice experiment with rural women in northeast Nigeria. BMJ Global Health. 2020;**5**(3):e002135

[47] Afulani PA, Kelly AM, Buback L, Asunka J, Kirumbi L, Lyndon A. Providers' perceptions of disrespect and abuse during childbirth: A mixed-methods study in Kenya. Health Policy and Planning. 2020;**35**(5):577-586

[48] Maarsingh OR et al. Continuity of Care in Primary Care and Association with Survival in older people: A 17-year prospective cohort study. The British Journal of General Practice. 2016;**66**(649):e531-e539

[49] Pereira-Gray DJ et al. Continuity of care with doctors—A matter of life and death? A systematic review of continuity of care and mortality. BMJ Open. 2018;**8**(6):e021161

[50] Dolea C. Increasing Access to Health Workers in Remote and Rural Areas through Improved Retention: Global Policy Recommendations. Geneva: World Health Organization; 2010

[51] Hilbers J, Lewis C. Complementary health therapies: Moving towards an integrated health model. Collegian. 2013;**20**(1):51-60

[52] Payyappallimana U. Role of traditional medicine in primary healthcare: An overview of perspectives and challenges. Yokohama Journal of Social Sciences. 2010;**14**(6):724-742

[53] World Health Organization. WHO Traditional Medicine Strategy 2002-2005. Geneva, Switzerland: World Health Organization; 2002

[54] Boadu AA, Asase A. Documentation of herbal medicines used for the treatment and management of human diseases by some communities in southern Ghana. Evidence-based Complementary and Alternative Medicine. 2017;**2017**:3043061

Chapter 7

Pathology Testing at the Point of Patient Care: Transformational Change for Rural Communities

Mark Shephard, Susan Matthews, Corey Markus, Emma de Courcy-Ireland, Lauren Duckworth, Isabelle Haklar, Ellen Kambanaros, Tamika Regnier, April Rivers-Kennedy and Grant White

Abstract

Point-of-care (POC) testing is an innovative and revolutionary *in vitro* diagnostic (IVD) technology that enables the real-time conduct of pathology testing during a patient consultation, facilitating immediate clinical action. When conducted under a quality-assured framework, POC testing is an essential diagnostic tool, and is now well embedded, in primary health care settings in rural communities around the world. POC testing helps bridge the gap in health equity access that exists in geographically isolated rural communities and empowers patients to invest in understanding and improving their own health literacy. Using POC testing networks for chronic, acute and infectious diseases that are currently operating in rural and remote Australia, this chapter explores the operational, clinical and economic benefits that POC testing can deliver, and the lessons learned that have contributed to continuously improved quality of POC testing service delivery. Investment in POC testing and infrastructure by Australian governments, both federal and state, has reaped significant rewards for patients in rural communities. Additionally, translational research in this field has provided insight into how POC testing can be successfully scaled up for broad application in low- and middle-income countries.

Keywords: point-of-care testing, equity of access, patient-centered care, translational research, scalability

1. Introduction

Point-of-care (POC) testing enables pathology testing to be conducted during a patient consultation in a primary care setting and facilitates timely clinical review and action for the patient. POC testing is the fastest growing sector of the pathology industry, with the global POC testing market worth US $45 billion in 2022 and expecting to reach around US $103 billion by 2030, with a compound annual growth rate of 10.9% [1]. As such, POC testing is referred to as a 'disruptive technology' [2], having transformed the way pathology testing is delivered for the care of patients with non-communicable (NCD) and infectious (ID) diseases, particularly in rural and remote primary care settings. This was particularly evident during the COVID-19 pandemic, where nucleic acid amplification, and later rapid antigen POC testing enabled rapid diagnosis and swift public health action and treatment [3]. Patient-centered care, with specimen collection, POC testing and informed treatment taking place during the consultation, is not only convenient and reduces loss to follow-up, but also enables the patient to become empowered and engaged in understanding and improving their own health and health literacy [4].

POC testing networks within remote Australia have demonstrated that when governments have the political will and are prepared to invest in POC testing and required infrastructure then clinical, operational, cultural and economic benefits can be derived for both the patient and healthcare system [5]. This is particularly evident for remote communities and marginalised populations, where access to centralised pathology laboratories is limited and loss to follow-up is high [6].

Following the rapid expansion of POC testing during the pandemic, current global research discussion in the field of POC testing is now focused on building high-quality, sustainable POC testing networks with the capacity to be scaled up to, for example, a national level; scale-up is defined by the World Health Organisation (WHO) as "the deliberate efforts to increase the impact of successfully tested health interventions [such as POC testing] so as to benefit more people and to foster policy and programme development on a lasting basis" [7]. This chapter explores the evolution of POC testing in rural and remote Australia using both qualitative and quantitative translational research, and highlights lessons learned, from established selected, working POC testing networks in this country. Commentary focuses particularly on the key quality and resource elements that must be embedded into POC testing to enable successful field translation, clinical utility and scale-up.

2. Investment by government in funding POC testing networks in Australia

The Flinders University International Centre for Point-of-Care Testing (ICPOCT) is a specialist POC testing network provider that currently supports eight different NCD and ID POC testing models in primary care settings in Australia; five of these networks are managed solely by the Centre and three are managed in partnership with the Kirby Institute, University of New South Wales. A summary of these networks is provided (**Table 1**). All these networks are funded by either the Australian Government Department of Health and Aged Care or State/Territory governments within Australia. Funding is generally provided for a fixed time period, with re-contracting occurring multiple times for many models, providing key performance indicators set by the government are met.

To illustrate how these models have been established and managed and to discuss the continuous quality improvements that have been made towards the goal of optimisation for scale-up, examples will be drawn from three specific models—one with a chronic disease focus (Quality Assurance for Aboriginal and Torres Strait Islander Medical Services [QAAMS] Program), one with acute care testing as

POC testing program	Funder	Year started	POC device	POC test/s performed & time to result	No. of services	No. of operators[@]
QAAMS	Aust. Govt.	1999	Siemens DCA Vantage	HbA1c^ *(6 mins)* Urine ACR# *(7 mins)*	238	3233
NT i-STAT	NT Govt.	2008	Abbott i-STAT	• Sodium, potassium, glucose, Hb˜, urea, creatinine *(2 mins)*	86	2104
				• Cardiac troponin I *(10 mins)*		
				• Blood gases—pH, pO2, pCO2, base excess; lactate *(2 mins)*		
				• PT/INR* *(5 mins)*		
TTANGO (Test, Treat and Go)**	Aust. Govt.	2013	Cepheid GeneXpert	Chlamydia, Gonorrhoea and Trichomonas *(60–90 mins)*	51	795
Enhanced Syphilis Response (ESR)	Aust. Govt.	2018	Abbott Determine™ Syphilis TP	Syphilis *(15 mins)*	112	1043
Syphilis WA	WA Govt.	2020	Abbott Determine™ Syphilis TP	Syphilis *(15 mins)*	44	369
COVID-19**	Aust. Govt.	2020	Cepheid GeneXpert	SARS-CoV-2+ *(45 mins)*	101	733
NT WBC DIFF	NT Govt.	2020	Radiometer HemoCue® WBC DIFF	Total WBC count plus five-part differential *(5 mins)*	20	175
National Hepatitis C**	Aust. Govt.	2021	Cepheid GeneXpert	Hepatitis C *(58 mins)*	48	103

Aust. Govt. = Australian Government, NT Govt. = Northern Territory Government, WA Govt. = Western Australian Government.[@]*Number of new operator certifications to November 30, 2022.*
^Haemoglobin A1c.
#albumin: creatinine ratio.
˜Haemoglobin.
**International Normalised Ratio.*
***POC testing program managed in partnership with the Kirby Institute, University of New South Wales.*
+Severe Acute Respiratory Syndrome Coronavirus 2.

Table 1.
Summary of primary care POC testing networks managed by the ICPOCT (Flinders University) alone, or in collaborative partnership with the Kirby Institute (UNSW).

its core activity (the Northern Territory [NT] Acute Care POC Testing Program) and one concerning infectious disease (the National Enhanced Syphilis Response [ESR] Program). Each of these models operates in rural and remote Australia and supports mainly Aboriginal and Torres Strait Islander peoples living in those geographically isolated areas. The lessons learned from these models have been important for, and have shaped, the development of government policy for POC testing in Australia [8].

3. Evolution of POC testing models: Building blocks underpinning POC testing and associated translational research

3.1 The Quality Assurance for Aboriginal and Torres Strait Islander Medical Services (QAAMS) Program

The Quality Assurance for Aboriginal and Torres Strait Islander Medical Services (QAAMS) Program was Australia's first national POC testing network in the primary care sector. The program emerged from a recommendation from the National Diabetes Strategy in 1998, which supported a trial of the Siemens (then Bayer) DCA 2000 POC testing device for haemoglobin A1c (HbA1c) in Aboriginal and Torres Strait Islander people with established diabetes [9]. Diabetes and associated renal disease were at the time, and continue to be, a major contemporary health problem for Aboriginal and Torres Strait Islander peoples who experience rates of diabetes that are three times the national average and up to 12% in remote areas [10, 11]. In these latter geographically isolated areas, testing through traditional pathology laboratories was characterised by long delays for turnaround of pathology results and high rates of patient loss to follow-up. Through funding provided by the (then) Australian Government's Office for Aboriginal and Torres Strait Islander Health, in partnership with the National Aboriginal Community Controlled Health Organisation (NACCHO)—the peak body representing the health of Aboriginal and Torres Strait Islander communities in Australia—the QAAMS Program began as a pilot in 45 Aboriginal and Torres Strait Islander health services across Australia in 1999; more than 80% of these services were in rural or remote Australia.

Since that time, the program has been scaled up to reach almost 200 health services at 238 testing sites across Australia and is now fully embedded in the mainstream diabetes diagnosis, monitoring and care of Aboriginal and Torres Strait Islander people.

3.1.1 Surveillance of analytical quality

In 1999, POC testing was in its infancy in Australia. The principal focus of the Australian Government in funding QAAMS was to establish that POC testing in primary health care services, which was conducted principally by Aboriginal Health Workers who were trained by ICPOCT scientists, could meet analytical performance standards expected of a pathology laboratory. Aboriginal Health Workers are health professionals of Aboriginal and Torres Strait Islander descent who live in the community and have a qualification in primary health care. The importance of high quality, robust and culturally safe training for POC testing operators and the surveillance of analytical quality became the initial core elements of this pioneering POC testing model.

Analytical quality in QAAMS was assessed by trained operators regularly testing both commercially available quality control (QC) and blinded external quality assurance (EQA, also known as proficiency testing) samples. Both QC and EQA testing processes form part of mandatory medical testing requirements for pathology laboratories accredited to international standards but had never been implemented in an Aboriginal and Torres Strait Islander primary care setting, nor conducted by non-laboratory trained health professionals. In QAAMS, the QC material was supplied by Siemens and the EQA samples were provided by the Royal College of Australasia's Quality Assurance Programs (RCPAQAP), an accredited global EQA provider; the EQA samples for QAAMS POC testing were identical to those tested by 250 Australasian laboratories (employing 21 different analytical methods) in a separate national laboratory based EQA Program provided by the RCPAQAP. This has enabled a direct comparison of the analytical performance for HbA1c (as measured by imprecision, expressed as a coefficient of variation, CV), in the QAAMS Program versus Australasian laboratories. To enable clinically significant changes in serial patient HbA1c measurements to be detected and not be masked by poor-quality test performance, imprecision goals of 3% (desired) and 2% (optimal) have been set by professional bodies and expert panels [12, 13].

Twenty years of data (from 2002 to 2022) is now available on the comparative imprecision for HbA1c testing in QAAMS and laboratories, with 49,169 EQA samples having been tested in QAAMS (**Figure 1**). In a remarkable achievement, imprecision has continued to improve across time and there has been no significant difference in the imprecision for HbA1c testing observed in the QAAMS Program (mean 2.75% SD 0.46) versus Australasian laboratories (mean 2.68% SD 0.39) over this 20-year period ($p = 0.435$ on a two-tailed p test).

A major improvement to the QAAMS quality system involved the development of real-time entry of QC test results (in 2016) and blinded EQA test results (in 2020) by test operators on the QAAMS website (www.qaams.org.au). This initiative has allowed operators to receive immediate feedback on the results of the quality testing performed at their health service. Once a quality result is entered, operators receive an instant message as to whether their test performance (a) meets analytical standards,

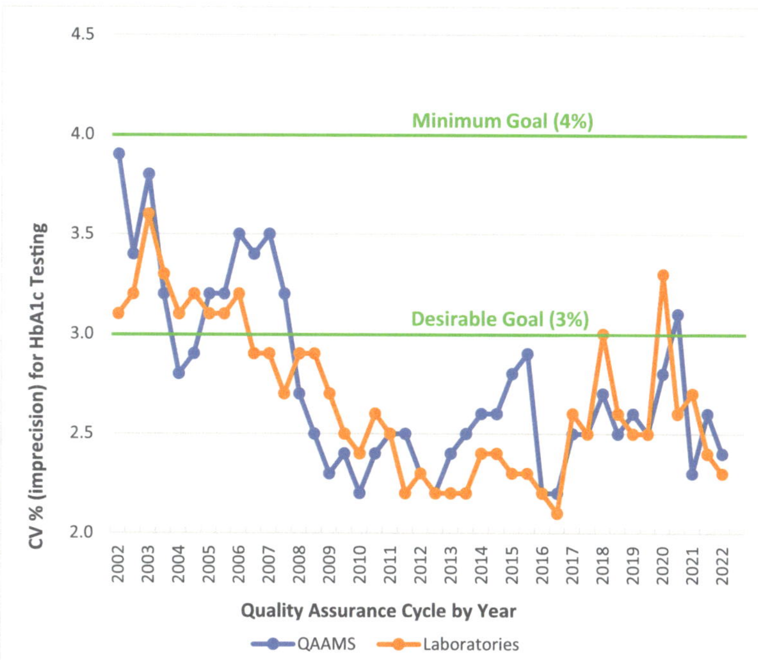

Figure 1.
*Comparative imprecision (median CV%) observed for HbA1c quality assurance testing in QAAMS (by POC testing) and Australasian laboratories (all methods) from 2002 to 2022. *QAAMS sites and Australasian laboratories tested the same EQA material from 2002 to 2020, after which the supplier of EQA material for QAAMS changed (to an Australian-based rather than an international supplier). Three levels of analytical goals for imprecision have generally been recognised for HbA1c testing over the past 20 years—A minimum goal of 4%, a desired goal of 3% and an optimal goal of 2% [12].*

enabling them to continue to test patients, or (b) falls outside acceptable limits for quality, in which case patient testing should be ceased until the reason for poor performance can be identified and rectified through consultation between the operator and the ICPOCT scientific support team.

3.1.2 Training for POC operators

The sound and sustained analytical quality observed in QAAMS is underpinned by a culturally safe training program, which provides flexible modes of training delivery and training resources. Across the 20-year-plus lifespan of QAAMS, variable training formats have been developed and expanded to include face-to-face training for individual services and at regional or annual training workshops; self-directed/self-paced e-learning modules through password-protected access via the QAAMS website; and tele-, video- or now web-conference training sessions (formerly using videocassette, DVD and USB). ICPOCT considers face-to-face training to be the most effective means of training, as it provides an opportunity for operators and training staff to meet and form relationships which then enhance future communication when device troubleshooting, for example, is required. The annual training workshop, which offers attendance support via travel scholarships for remote POC operators from across Australia to meet centrally, is also highly valuable, as it provides a forum for cultural education, operator networking and fosters a sense of inclusion rather than having operators feel they are working in isolation. The training resource package for QAAMS includes a hard copy training manual in full-colour A3 format; a set of posters which provides simple step-by-step visual instructions for operators to conduct patient, QC and EQA testing; training aids on how to interpret patient and quality test results; training videos on the QAAMS website; and a PowerPoint presentation delivered by ICPOCT scientists. Once training is completed, all operators undertake a written and practical competency assessment to formally obtain a competency certificate as a qualified operator in the program. Competency certification lasts for a specified period, currently 2 years, after which a training update and renewal of competency is required. These core learnings from QAAMS training have been invaluable in shaping POC testing policy in Australia [7, 8].

Through this process, a significant workforce for conducting POC testing for chronic disease care has been built in rural and remote Australia, with more than 3200 operators having been trained and/or renewed their competency in the program over 20 years. Further aspects of training will be discussed later in this chapter.

There have been many key time points/significant events that have occurred in the optimisation and scale-up of the QAAMS Program over its lifespan. These will be described in chronological order and provide an insight into how the building blocks of this pioneering POC testing model were established.

3.1.3 Independent evaluation of the program

The program has undergone two independent evaluations—by NACCHO in 2001 and by the Government-commissioned external consultancy company, Campbell Research and Consulting, in 2008. The major impact of the QAAMS Program reported from these evaluations included themes of improved community-based diabetes management, health worker empowerment and appropriate cultural sensitivity (**Table 2**). Continuing evaluation is an important component of a POC testing network and provides an insight into whether the program is fit for clinical purpose,

2002: Evaluation by the National Aboriginal Community Controlled Health Organisation (NACCHO).
"This new point of care technology [the DCA 2000] seems to represent a 'major opportunity' to better care for and manage clients with diabetes and for the clients themselves to better understand its impact on their health." ...
"The machine served as a catalyst for communication to enhance self-management through the speedy return of results and its overall ease of use which led to health workers generally demonstrating a high level of acceptance of this new 'point of care technology'." ...
"A key finding was that nearly two-thirds of services expressed ... [that the DCA] had the effect of raising the esteem of health workers in their community contexts. That is, health worker competence in using this relatively sophisticated piece of technology and the subsequent opportunity this presented for health workers and clients to work together to deal with the multiple effects of diabetes, demonstrated their communities' capacity to take control of the management of [diabetes]." ...
"... a sense of community control was enhanced as a result of the way in which the management of persons with diabetes became more focused within most services."
2008: Campbell, Research and Consulting
"The QAAMS model is firmly rooted in accepted approaches to Aboriginal healthcare. QAAMS has consistently maintained a high level of cultural appropriateness and acceptability ..."
"Aboriginal health professionals and clients alike hold QAAMS in high esteem."
"The program has always been very consultative and culturally sensitive and empowering; those are the things that have made it such a success."
"All sources of evidence suggest that QAAMS is meeting best practice standards in the areas of Indigenous healthcare, diabetes management and Point of Care testing."
"QAAMS is one of the few programs to successfully navigate the cultural complexities and potential pitfalls of chronic disease management in Indigenous communities."

Table 2.
Summary of findings from independent evaluations of QAAMS.

how the program is viewed by its stakeholders, in what areas improvement to the program can be made, and where the program may be failing.

3.1.4 Validation of test performance

Urine ACR POC testing was added to the program in 2003, following the test's approval for use in Australia, demonstration of its clinical use for the detection of microalbuminuria in peer-reviewed international literature, and an independent evaluation of its analytical performance both in the laboratory [14] and the field [15]. Indeed, ICPOCT have maintained the philosophy consistent with best practice that, where possible, laboratory and field evaluations of new POC tests and devices should be conducted before their introduction into a new network [16, 17]. Similar to HbA1c, sound long-term analytical performance has been observed with urine ACR testing in the QAAMS Program [18].

3.1.5 Integration of POC testing into clinical pathways

It is critical that POC testing is not performed in isolation but is integrated formally to improve clinical pathways for the care of patients, who are focus of the program. In QAAMS, POC test frequency was aligned with established Australian clinical guidelines for the use of the tests concerned; for HbA1c, up to four tests per annum are conducted for the management of patients with diabetes while, for urine ACR, tests are performed three- to six-monthly depending on clinical need for those patients with microalbuminuria and annually on patients without microalbuminuria [19, 20]. A new clinical pathway incorporating the use of the HbA1c test for the diagnosis of diabetes was developed and approved by the Australian Government in 2015 [21].

3.1.6 Assessment of clinical effectiveness

The clinical effectiveness of POC testing in facilitating improvements in the glycaemic control of patients with established diabetes was confirmed early in the evolution of the QAAMS Program [22]. Later, a statistically significant reduction in HbA1c of 2.7% was observed in a cohort of 40 diabetes patients across the NT who had access to POC testing in QAAMS for 15 months, while no significant reduction in HbA1c was seen in these patients when laboratory testing was used as part of their care for the 15 months prior to POC testing. In addition, the mean turnaround time for HbA1c test results was 42 hours when laboratory services were used and less than 10 minutes for POC testing, while the mean time for patient follow-up and clinical consultation was 24 days following laboratory testing and less than 15 minutes post the implementation of POC testing [23].

3.1.7 Ensuring POC testing is cost effective

Significantly, in 2002, the QAAMS Program was the first POC testing program outside an accredited laboratory in Australia to be granted a rebate under the Australian Government's Medical Benefits Scheme (MBS). The rebate was approved directly by the Federal Health Minister and enabled services in the QAAMS Program to claim for a POC HbA1c test conducted for the management of established diabetes. (Medicare rebates are usually restricted to medical testing in pathology laboratories accredited to international quality standards by the National Association of Testing Authorities [NATA]). The QAAMS rebate has ensured that the HbA1c POC test is paid for through the national public health system in Australia and not by the health services participating in the network. Subsequently, MBS rebates have also been approved in QAAMS for the ACR test for detection of microalbuminuria in 2006 and for HbA1c for the diagnosis of diabetes in 2015. These rebates have ensured sustainability and growth of the program, as the cost remains neutral for participants. **Figure 2** summarises the numbers of MBS claims for the three item numbers currently available in QAAMS.

Outside of QAAMS, processes for supporting MBS rebates for POC tests remains a significant barrier for the field in Australia and more support and flexibility is required by Governments in this area, particularly if there is a strong clinical need and evidence base to support the clinical, cultural, operational and cost benefits of utilising POC testing in rural and remote environments. The demonstration of the cost benefit of POC testing is now a critical area of research for the field, as predictive cost savings from mathematical modelling for diagnosis and intervention and evidence-based value propositions of diagnostic tests are essential tools for incentivising government investment [24].

3.1.8 Acceptability of POC testing by stakeholder groups

Surveying the views and satisfaction levels of key stakeholder groups such as clinical staff, POC test operators, and patients who are the consumers of the POC service

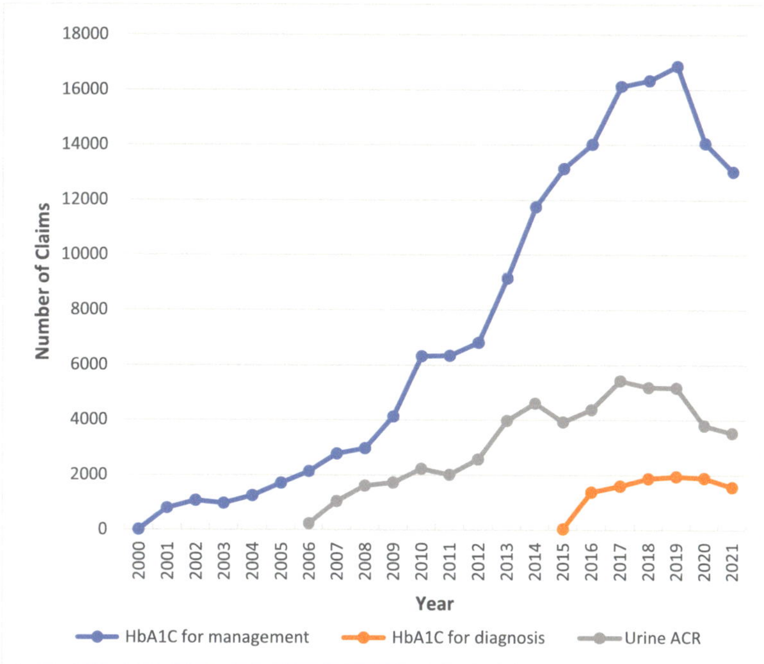

Figure 2.
Total number of MBS items claimed per year by services enrolled in the QAAMS Program—For the HbA1c items for the management of established diabetes and for the diagnosis of diabetes, as well as for the UACR item for microalbuminuria.

is an important component of assessing a model's acceptability, cultural safety and suitability to scale-up.

Surveys has been regularly conducted through the lifespan of QAAMS (as early as 2004 and as recently as 2016) [22, 25]. Ideally, stakeholder satisfaction should be embedded as a core element at the initiation of a new network where, ideally, acceptability can be assessed for example prior to, during and post implementation of a model.

3.1.9 Clinical governance of a network

The governance of the QAAMS Program was initially administered by a small management committee comprising the QAAMS Program Manager and QAAMS Training Coordinator, reporting directly to the Government. However, a more multidisciplinary and inclusive governance structure was implemented in QAAMS in 2006, which included representatives from the following stakeholder groups: RCPA QAP (responsible for EQA support), Medicare Australia (to support services with MBS rebate claims) and Siemens (as an industry representative responsible for logistical supply of devices, cartridges and QC material). A Clinical Support Officer role was also created at this time to provide clinical advice and support to doctors and allied health professionals from participating sites on the appropriate clinical use of the HbA1c and urine ACR tests, as well as interpretation of POC testing results for these analytes. While this was a pioneering appointment in QAAMS at the time, the importance of systematic and integrated clinical governance is now considered paramount for all large-scale POC testing networks in Australia. The clinical governance portfolio can be assigned to a single individual (such as with QAAMS [and the NT POC

Testing network—see next section]) where the Clinical Support Officer is a member of the program's management committee or to a Clinical Advisory Group which act as an advisory panel that sits separate to, and hierarchically above, a management committee. The importance of clinical governance for POC testing networks, with designated and accountable clinical responsibility, is now embedded within the latest *Requirements for POC Testing in Australia* and will become an integral component of future accreditation frameworks for POC testing in this country [8].

3.1.10 Indigenous leadership for QAAMS

In 2006, a QAAMS Indigenous Leadership Team was established. This initiative recognised the ongoing contribution of Aboriginal Health Workers (now also known as Practitioners in some parts of Australia) and their commitment to the success and viability of the program. One representative from each State/Territory of Australia was appointed to the initial leadership team. The Leaders Team act as cultural ambassadors for the program, provide an ongoing Indigenous voice and viewpoint on all aspects of QAAMS, advise on the cultural safety of program's training resource package and, increasingly, participate in training workshops and the development of training resources. The national leader of this group was also appointed to the program's expanded management committee. This initiative has proven one of the most important success stories for the program and continues to the present day, with the group renamed the QAAMS National Leadership Forum in 2021. There is no doubt that any POC testing network that supports the health of Aboriginal and Torres Strait Islander people must include strong Indigenous leadership, co-designed programs, and community engagement.

3.1.11 Connectivity and the electronic capture of POC test results

Most early models of POC testing devices had the capacity to print out a set of POC test results that could be manually placed in a patient's clinical record. However, the importance of connectivity—the capacity to electronically capture POC test results and securely store them in the patient's electronic medical record—has now become an essential post-analytical component of a modern POC testing network.

In the past, connectivity has been a challenge for QAAMS due to issues with individual services' firewalls and different patient management systems used by different groups of health services. Connectivity was first trialled and established in QAAMS in 2010, when a group of 40 new POC testing devices were introduced into the state of Queensland (Qld), following the receipt of a grant from the Queensland government (an initiative approved by the Australian Government at the time). The transition from the Siemens DCA to the Atellica (see Section 3.1.13), which offer improved connectivity functionality combined with the current range of open POC testing middleware solutions available on the market, may enable full connectivity of QAAMS devices to be realised in the future. However, the costs associated with connectivity software implementation, device driver development and licencing for large scale networks remain prohibitive.

For some of our Centre's ID networks, the connectivity system also extends to remote access of the POC device for troubleshooting, real-time POC test dashboard and alert systems, and jurisdictional electronic notification of encrypted positive test results [3].

3.1.12 Scale-up of QAAMS achieved after 11 years

Following the sequential implementation of the building blocks outlined, QAAMS had been systematically scaled up to almost 150 sites by 2010. It had taken the best part of 11 years to achieve what was considered an optimised POC testing chronic disease model. Given QAAMS had been a pioneering, best practice model for POC testing outside the laboratory in Australia and acknowledging the quantitative and qualitative translational research conducted, the quality improvements continually made, and the lessons learned along the journey, this time frame was not unexpected.

However, with an accumulated knowledge of the building blocks required for a POC testing network to be scaled-up, the growth and optimisation of future models (as later outlined) could now be facilitated in shorter time frames.

Before concluding the section on QAAMS, two other aspects deserve brief commentary.

3.1.13 Transitioning to new/updated models of POCT devices

With QAAMS operational across a 23-year period, it was inevitable that changes/upgrades to the POC technology used in the program would occur. For the first 9 years of operation, the Siemens DCA 2000 was used in the program. In 2008, Siemens introduced a newer model known as the DCA Vantage. Fortunately, the method principle did not change, only the external appearance and electronic display features were modified. This facilitated a smooth transition to the new device over the ensuing three-year period, when the existing DCA 2000 devices were systematically exchanged for the Vantage model. Before introducing the Vantage, an independent evaluation of the new device's analytical performance was conducted by ICPOCT scientists. Support from both the industry vendor (where discounted prices were offered in flexible changeover packages) and government (who facilitated the purchase of new devices for nearly half of the enrolled participants) greatly enhanced the transition to the new device. In 2021, Siemens announced the approval of the Atellica® DCA Analyser by the Therapeutics Goods Administration (TGA)—the peak regulatory agency for IVDs, medicines and therapeutics—and availability to the Australian IVD market. A similar transition to the new device has commenced. The method principle has again not changed, albeit there is a reduction in time for result for the HbA1c test from 6 to 4 minutes and progression to a more versatile and smaller device. A further analytical evaluation of this new device has also been completed by ICPOCT scientists. The introduction of both these new devices 13 years apart has necessitated the redevelopment of updated training resource packages, a process which requires co-design and time to complete.

3.1.14 Impact of COVID-19 on test usage in QAAMS

The world has been grappling with the spread of the SARS-CoV-2 virus since late 2019. The COVID-19 pandemic has resulted in severe disruption to the provision of basic health services in many communities, with a focus on isolation of patients with COVID and prioritisation given to the testing for this new disease, especially prior to widespread vaccination. Australia (and QAAMS) have been no exception [26, 27]. As described above, the quality of testing in QAAMS has not been impacted but the number of POC tests performed on diabetes patients has. In the year before the pandemic struck (2019), there were approximately 16,864 MBS claims for HbA1c

POC testing for the management of diabetes. At the end of the first full year of the pandemic (2020), MBS claims for this item had fallen to 14,053 (a decrease of 17%) while, by the end of 2021, only 13,030 tests were conducted (a total reduction in test numbers from pre-pandemic levels of 23%). Similarly, a 32% reduction in MBS claims for ACR testing was seen from 2019 to 2021, while there was a 19% decrease in MBS claims for the HbA1c diagnosis item over the same period.

Across the pandemic, the role of Aboriginal Health Workers changed significantly with a range of other COVID-related tasks preoccupying their role; these included contact tracing; swabbing patients for laboratory COVID testing and/or in some cases conducting molecular-based POC testing for SARS-CoV-2 in remote communities (through the Flinders-Kirby COVID POC Testing network—see **Table 1**); conducting telephone follow-ups and welfare checks; issuing COVID-19 vaccinations (when available), delivering medications, COVID isolation packs and food supplies; promoting COVID-safe health messages and explaining isolation/quarantine requirements. These conflicting roles no doubt contributed to decline in testing rates in remote Indigenous communities.

QAAMS continues to be a landmark and ground-breaking POC testing network in Australia. The fact that QAAMS has operated sustainably for more than 23 years is a testament to the commitment of Government, the National Indigenous Leadership Forum, the QAAMS governance and operational teams, and the Aboriginal and Torres Strait Islander health professionals who deliver the program at the rural and remote coalface.

3.2 The Northern Territory acute care POC testing program

The Northern Territory (NT) of Australia covers an area of 1.3 million square kilometres (km) and represents the third largest state/territory in Australia. It comprises some of the most challenging environments for conducting POC testing in Australia. The landscape is harsh and environmental extremes of soaring temperatures, excessive humidity and tropical monsoonal rains make living and working conditions difficult. Outside of three major towns (Darwin, Katherine and Alice Springs), the vast majority of communities in the Territory are geographically isolated and classified as remote or very remote by the Australian Statistical Geography Standard (ASGS) Remoteness Area Structure [28]. Health services are often spartan, with large road and air distances (often hundreds of kilometres) to reach the nearest regional hospital facilities. Health professional staff (notably remote area nurses) are often transient and overworked. The nature of health care delivery is mainly opportunistic, with multiple daily medical emergencies being a common occurrence among the predominantly Aboriginal and Torres Strait Islander peoples that live in these remote communities.

The NT Acute Care POCT program began in 2008, after the collapse of NT medical retrieval air services meant that pathology tests were unable to be transported to either of the two main pathology laboratories in the Territory. The NT Government investigated POC testing as a possible solution to address the issue and engaged ICPOCT to establish and manage a POCT service, initially in 33 remote health services administered by the Government. The Abbott i-STAT® device was employed due to its capacity to perform a range of acute care tests, notably sodium, potassium, creatinine, glucose, haemoglobin (on a test cartridge known a CHEM8+); blood gases and lactate (CG4+ cartridge), and troponin I. In addition, the i-STAT could test for Prothrombin Time (PT)/International Normalised Ration (INR) on a separate cartridge. The PT/INR test had specific clinical application in the Territory, as Aboriginal and Torres Strait Islander people living in the Territory have one of the highest rates of rheumatic heart disease (RHD) in the world and INR is used routinely to monitor warfarin levels, an anticoagulant used to treat RHD [29]. By placing the i-STAT into a downloading cradle, patient and quality test results can be instantaneously transferred to a central data repository. A more detailed and recent review of the NT POCT program has been published elsewhere [30].

Through lessons learned from the research conducted in QAAMS, the NT program was established using the same core building blocks which had proven successful in QAAMS.

In terms of governance, a NT POC Testing Management Committee was initially established which comprised scientific representatives from ICPOCT (including the chair of the Committee and senior scientist overseeing the program), a clinical support officer (the District Medical Officer for the NT Government's Remote Health Branch), regional POC testing supervisors from Central Australia and the Top End [the northern half of the Territory] (both professional practice nurses), and representatives from the Remote Health Branch's quality and safety committee. Over time, this structure has been modified with more scientific representatives from ICPOCT and a representative from the Aboriginal Medical Services Alliance NT (AMSANT), the peak body representing the Aboriginal community controlled health service sector in the NT, now part of the Committee.

3.2.1 Integration into clinical pathways

Emphasis on clinical aspects of governance has included specified clinical uses for each test measured and the development of NT-based paediatric reference intervals for each test. The integration of POC testing into clinical pathways has been continuously enhanced with POC testing protocols now embedded within the NT Remote Primary Care Manuals, a series of four clinic manuals for primary health care practitioners and allied health professionals in remote and Indigenous health services in central and northern Australia [31].

3.2.2 Growth of the program towards scale-up

The program has undergone rapid growth across the past 14 years. The number of health service enrolled in the program remained between 30 and 35 from 2008 until 2014. However, following the initial success of the program and after a coroner's case found that a patient death may have been avoided if an i-STAT device had been available, the NT Government purchased sufficient i-STAT devices to service every remote NT community in 2015, effectively doubling the size of the program to a total of 72 devices. Since then, and with the support of the NT Government, the program has extended across the NT border into additional remote health services in the Ngaanyatjarra (Ng) Lands, which comprise an approximate 250,000 km^2 area of Western Australia (WA) adjoining the NT and South Australian (SA) borders, bringing the current number of enrolled services to 86 (**Figure 3**).

The total number of operators trained (mainly remote area nurses) has steadily increased across the lifespan of the program to now reach 2104, of which 1340 have undergone at least one competency recertification (**Figure 4**). More than 253,000 POC tests have been performed, rising from just 700 in 2008 to 36,675 in 2021 (**Figure 5**). The CHEM8+ and PT/INR cartridges are the most frequently performed test types (**Figure 6**).

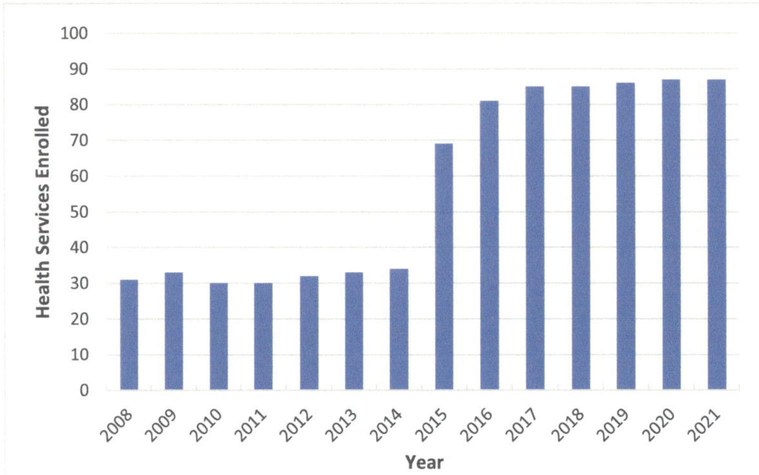

Figure 3.
Number of remote health services enrolled per year in the NT acute care POC testing program using the i-STAT device.

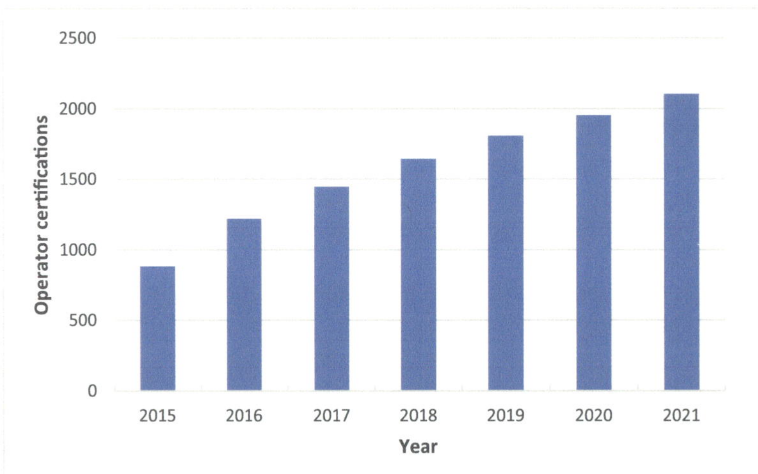

Figure 4.
Cumulative growth in the number of operators trained (new and recertifications) in the NT acute care POC testing program using the i-STAT device.

3.2.3 Analytical quality (and evaluation of test performance)

Quality testing has underpinned the program since its inception. Participation in QC testing has averaged 90% since 2009, and 95% or better for the past 7 years since 2015. The imprecision for QC testing for a representative selection of critical i-STAT analytes–sodium, potassium, creatinine and pH—is shown in **Figure** 7. The average imprecision across the past 6 years for each analyte was: sodium 0.6%, potassium 1.0%, creatinine 3.5% and pH 0.2%, with each analyte meeting or being close to the imprecision goals currently achieved by participants in the RCPAQAP condensed POC testing program, survey 6, 2022 (of 0.5, 1.0, 4.6 and 0.2%, respectively) [30].

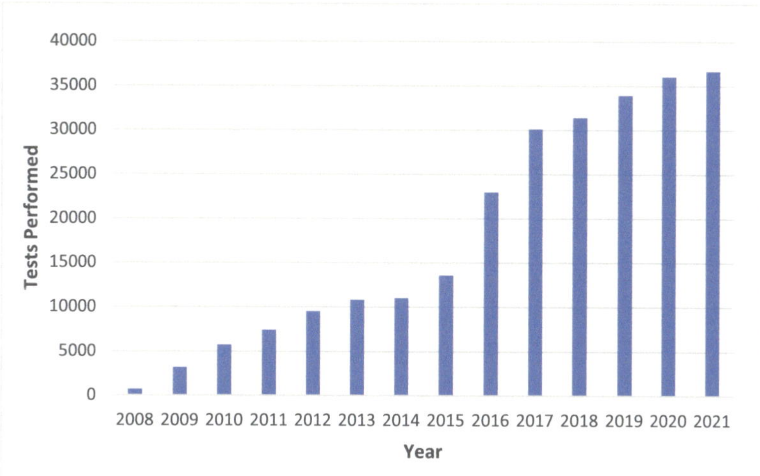

Figure 5.
Total number of tests performed on the i-STAT per annum in the NT acute care POC testing program.

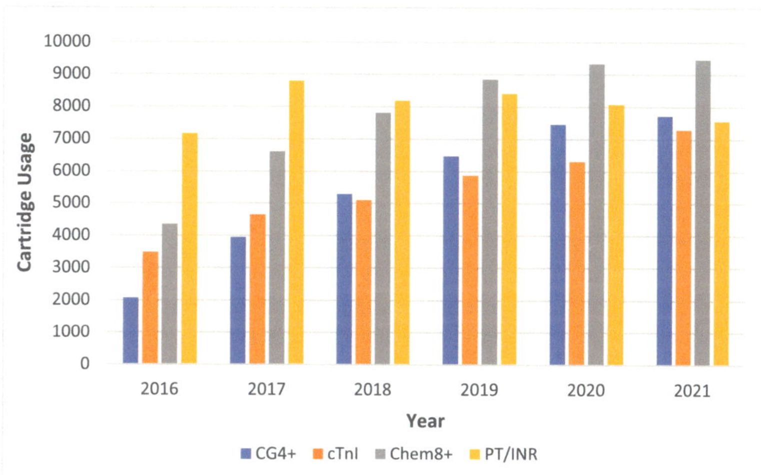

Figure 6.
The number of patient tests performed in the NT acute care POC testing program using i-STAT blood gas (CG4+), cardiac troponin I (cTnI), basic chemistry (CHEM8+), or prothrombin time/international normalised ratio (PT/INR) cartridge types, differentiated by year of test.

This data highlights the remarkably consistent and analytically sound performance of these tests in the hands of remote area POC testing operators.

There have also been continuing evaluations of the analytical performance of the test analytes as part of the broader research and surveillance undertaken across the lifespan of the program [32, 33].

3.2.4 Clinical effectiveness

During the early years of the program, a log of clinical cases where POC testing had resulted in beneficial clinical outcomes was developed. Among these was the case

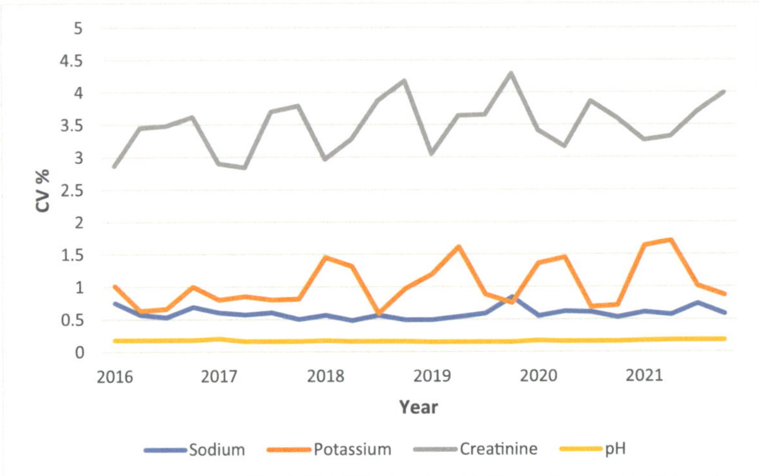

Figure 7.
The average between-site imprecision for selected i-STAT analytes in the NT acute care POC testing program from 2016 to 2021, as assessed by QC testing.

of a 46-year-old male with a history of RHD who had a coronary bypass surgery and was on warfarin to reduce his risk of stroke. In the year prior to the introduction of POCT, the average time between PT/INR tests was 67 days and time in therapeutic range (TTR) was 31% (well below the desired TTR of 60–70%). However, in the year post the introduction of POC testing, the average time between tests was 14 days and his TTR was 74% [29].

In 2015, the ICPOCT was awarded a research grant to investigate the clinical and economic effectiveness of POC testing in the NT. The study investigated 200 patient cases with three acute medical presentations at six remote health services: patients with acute chest pain (n = 147), patients with acute diarrhoea (n = 25) and patients with acute exacerbation of renal failure due to a missed dialysis session (n = 21). POC testing enabled more informed triaging of acutely ill patients requiring evacuation to a tertiary hospital as well as ruling out the need for evacuation for patients who could remain in the community and be stabilised [34].

3.2.5 Cost effectiveness

Perhaps the most compelling evidence for the benefits of acute POC testing came from a cost-benefit analysis that was conducted as part of the 2015 research study. POC testing prevented 60 unnecessary medical retrievals from the cohort of 200 patients. The cost savings for the Northern Territory Government were (AUD) $13.7 million per annum (for chest pain patients), $6.45 million per annum (missed dialysis) and $1.57 million per annum (diarrhoea), translating to an annual total saving of ($21.75 million) for the NT health system [35].

3.2.6 Scale-up complete in 7 years

Applying previous research conducted and lessons learned in QAAMS, the NT acute care POC testing program had been optimised and scaled up to a Territory-wide program in effectively 7 years.

Since 2015, the program has continued to grow in terms of number of services, tests and operators. Despite doubling the size of the program, the robustness and resilience of this optimised model has been sustained, with no diminution of analytical quality (see **Figure** 7). Indeed, in 2021, the NT Acute Care POC Testing program received an Engagement Australia Award in the category of 'outstanding engagement for research impact'.

3.2.7 White blood cell count and differential (WBC DIFF) POC testing network

The success of this program led the NT Government to expand the suite of POC testing devices available to support other acute care presentations by introducing POC testing for white blood cell count (WBC) (including a 5-part differential (DIFF)) on the HemoCue WBC DIFF® device.

An extensive pre-evaluation of both the analytical performance and clinical utility of the WBC DIFF device was initially undertaken. Analytical performance was sound [36], while the clinical effectiveness study demonstrated the WBC DIFF device positively influenced decision making; enhanced patient safety for a range of clinical presentations, including undifferentiated sepsis, appendicitis and meningitis; and produced positive economic benefits (cost savings of approximately $5 million per annum) through reducing numbers of unnecessary aeromedical evacuations [37].

Based on this evidence-based research, the NT Government supported and funded a WBC DIFF network of 20 remote health services in the Top End of the NT in 2020.

Services were prioritised for recruitment by NT Health's Top End Quality and Safety Team, with input from senior District Medical Officers and the Care Flight air service, based on how useful the tests would be for decision-making regarding medical retrieval and which sites would benefit the most from this decision-making capability.

A Primary Health Care Remote Guideline was developed for the clinical use of the device and its operation. This document is an NT Health Policy Guidelines Centre (PGC) Approved and Controlled document.

A workforce of over 175 trained and competent operators has been established, while approximately 1160 WBC DIFF tests have been conducted in just over 2 years (547 in 2021 and 611 to date in 2022).

This albeit smaller POC testing network has been scaled up in a two-year window (having been based on learnings and translational research from the NT Acute Care model). The 20-site program has recently been extended in duration to mid-2024 by the NT Department of Health.

In a more recent development (2021), ICPOCT, in partnership with the NT Government and other researchers, was the lead organisation in a successful Medical Research Future Fund (MRFF) grant awarded by the National Health and Medical Research Council (NHMRC) (Application ID 2016006). This 5-year research grant will investigate whether the availability of a full blood examination (measuring both red and white cell parameters using the HemoScreen [Pixcell Medical] POC device), can further enhance the clinical benefits of conducting acute care POC testing in the Territory, notably for patients with sepsis. The grant will research the analytical quality, clinical, operational, cost and cultural effectiveness of this new technology as well as build an Indigenous workforce competent in using this device before, if successful, making an evidence-based decision to supersede the WBC DIFF device.

3.3 The national Enhanced Syphilis Response program involving POC testing

An outbreak of infectious syphilis (*Treponema pallidum*) has been progressively spreading across Qld, the NT, WA and SA, disproportionately affecting young Aboriginal and Torres Strait Islander peoples predominantly aged between 15 and 29 years [38]. In response to the outbreak, an Australian Government-commissioned working group was established to develop effective community-based strategies to tackle and mitigate the outbreak. The subsequent Enhanced Syphilis Response (ESR) program was established in 2018. Using a co-design approach, NACCHO were engaged to provide advocacy and leadership in the design and delivery of the ESR program, to establish and strengthen partner and stakeholder relationships, to support the enrolment of ACCHOs, to build a 'community of practice', and to increase the uptake of POC testing for syphilis by ACCHOs [38]. The ICPOCT was separately contracted by the Australian Government to establish and deliver a training and quality management system to support safe and accurate syphilis POC testing, as a screening tool, for the ESR program in affected communities. In terms of logistics, NACCHO is responsible for the distribution and stock management of syphilis POC test strips for their participating services. A complimentary program was later initiated by the WA Department of Health in 2020 to expand the reach of syphilis POC testing beyond ACCHOs, and into peri-urban maternal health services and community outreach screening in that state.

3.3.1 The POC test used to screen for syphilis

The Abbott Determine™ Syphilis TP immunochromatographic test strip was chosen as the rapid, screening test of choice for the ESR (and WA) program, as it was (and remains) the only POC test approved by the TGA and has a clinical sensitivity and specificity of at least 96% in a capillary (fingerstick) sample type [39]. The Abbott Determine™ Syphilis TP test detects antibodies to *Treponema pallidum*.

The syphilis screening test is one of simple complexity (being suitable since 2021 as a syphilis self-test) and differs from the moderate complexity POC testing devices used in the QAAMS and NT Programs. The syphilis test provides a qualitative test result ('non-reactive' or 'reactive') rather than a quantitative (numerical) result. Being a manual test (where the operator loads 50 μL of capillary or venous whole blood on to the test strip), electronic capture of test results can only be recorded via digital photographs or imaging software. As such, many participating ACCHOs have created specific clinical items in their patient management systems for the POC syphilis test, with results able to be entered manually. Results can also be incorporated into other general health check data sets that are available for Aboriginal and Torres Strait Islander people in Australia. Nonetheless, these differences between the POC testing technologies used in the three networks outlined in this chapter highlight the broad methodological diversity of POC testing devices and applications which are now available on the global market. Following the advent, wide global usage and eventual definitive case identification of COVID-19 by rapid antigen testing, there is now a broader public awareness, competence and inclusion of lateral flow POC tests for sexually transmitted infections within a self-testing and broader policy environment [40].

A limitation of the Determine™ Syphilis TP test strip is that it is unable to distinguish between an active infection and a past, treated infection, infectious activity or progression of associated complications. Operators are made aware of this limitation as part of their extensive training delivered by ICPOCT scientists for the program.

Patients with 'reactive' POC test results for syphilis antibodies are checked against syphilis registers (available in most jurisdictions) and a serology sample is then sent to the laboratory for confirmation of positivity. The jurisdictional registers and laboratory testing therefore enable services to assess whether an infection is active or not.

In order to respond to the outbreak and build capacity for ACCHO engagement and support, there have been five phases in the rollout of the ESR program since its inception. The first phase commenced in June 2018 in Darwin (NT) and Townsville and Cairns (Qld). The second phase started in October 2018 in the Katherine Region, Nhulunbuy (NT) and the East Kimberley Region (WA). The third phase commenced in April 2019 in West Arnhem Land (NT), Western, Eyre, Far North and Adelaide Regions (SA), and the Pilbara and Western Kimberley Regions (WA). The fourth phase began in May 2020 in Mt. Isa (Qld) and Tennant Creek (NT). A fifth phase commenced in July 2021. In total, 111 services have been engaged in the rollout (**Figure 8**).

3.3.2 Training for syphilis POC testing

The simplicity of the syphilis POC screening test enabled a new model of training to be adopted for the ESR program—that of 'advanced operator training', where local experienced 'POC testing champions' were identified and took part in a higher level of training from the ICPOCT primary training team and were then able to on-train other operators at their health service or surrounding regions. This was particularly advantageous during the initial phases of the COVID-19 pandemic, where face-to-face training sessions delivered by ICPOCT were not possible due to jurisdictional border closures and community lockdowns enforced in many participating services. The use of advanced operators enabled the workforce capacity for syphilis POC testing to be scaled up quicker as part of this emergency response program. Up to November 2022, a total of 872 operators have achieved basic operator certification since the ESR program commenced, while 171 advanced operators (representing 20% of the workforce on the ground) have been certified during this period (**Figure 9**, top). In the WA Syphilis

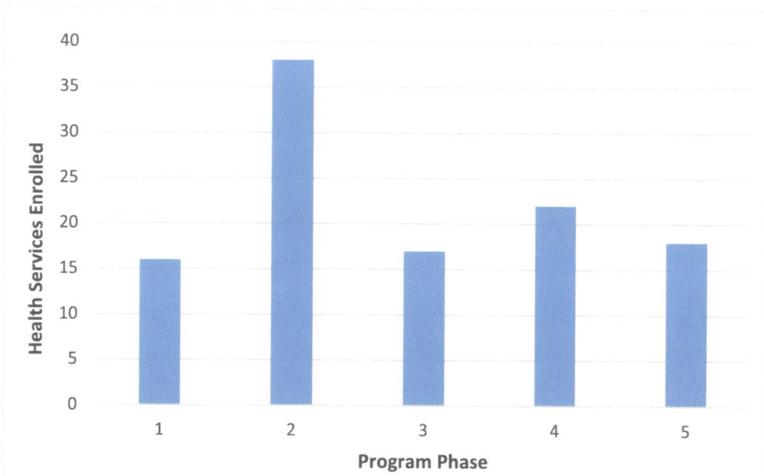

Figure 8.
The number of health services enrolled in the enhanced syphilis POC testing program during the five phases of recruitment from 2018 to 2021.

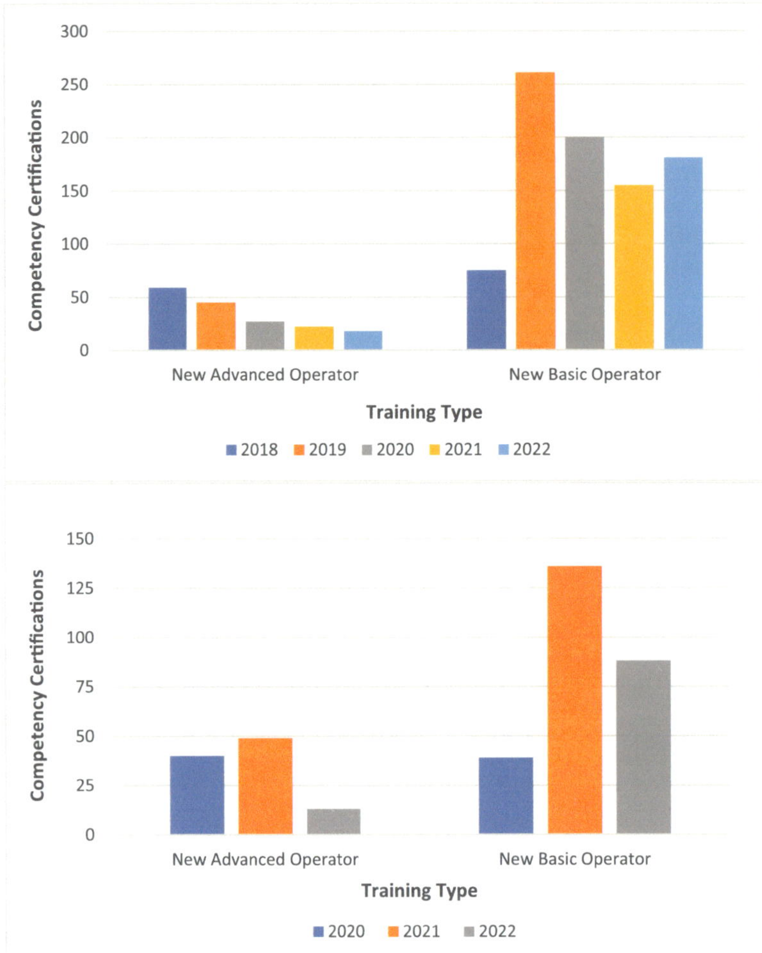

Figure 9.
The number of operators undertaking advanced and basic training in the enhanced syphilis POC testing program (top) and Western Australian syphilis POC testing program (bottom) since the inception of these programs.

program, 263 healthcare staff have obtained basic operator certification, while 106 (39%) have obtained advanced operator certification (**Figure 9**, bottom).

3.3.3 Use of advanced operator training depends on test complexity and patient risk

A critical distinction needs to be made regarding the usefulness of the advanced operator training or 'train-the-trainer' approach. Syphilis POC testing is a relatively simple POC test of low technical complexity (i.e. suitability for a self-test) and relatively low patient risk if analytical performance characteristics are satisfactory. For this type of test, advanced operator training is appropriate, particularly when other forms of training may be limited or rapid scale-up of such a simple test is needed. However, advanced operator training is not appropriate for other POC test methodologies which are more complex and have higher patient and/or operator risk; for example, devices using molecular-based technologies that involve thermal cycling and have associated software packages (both for test ordering and result interpretation). In relation to our ICPOCT networks, the latter category includes tests such as Hepatitis C performed on the GeneXpert device, with the test being classified as Class IV IVD by the TGA, which carries the highest level of patient risk; and the Class III IVD, the SARS-CoV-2 and/or multiplex SARS-CoV-2, Flu A/B and RSV tests, also conducted on the GeneXpert system (in the Australian Government's national respiratory infection program), where operators are required to wear full personal protective equipment and risks of pre-analytical, analytical and post-analytical errors causing false positives or false negatives are high.

3.3.4 What elements of training are not negotiable and which can be consumer driven?

In terms of developing a training framework for POC testing that is compliant with Australian POC testing requirements [8], ICPOCT have identified key elements of POC operator training which are mandatory and thus non-negotiable. These include, but are not limited to, work health and safety requirements which may be specific to the disease type, method or device; clinical governance requirements; competency registers; quality system compliance; and cultural co-design. The only negotiable elements of training are those relating to different modes or formats of training resources and delivery (i.e. allowing advanced operator training), but these should be applied specifically with the POC test and device complexity and thus patient risk at the forefront. Quantitative metrics, including error rates, error types, QC and EQA performance data and comprehensive, embedded qualitative end-user training surveys may be interdependent on training format offered and provide an evidence base for continual quality improvement of POC operator training. Continual quality improvement strategies should be adopted where possible; however, patient safety considerations, international standards and best-practice requirements may not be able to facilitate all end-user training feedback or change requests (**Figure 10**).

3.3.5 Analytical quality of syphilis POC testing

Since late 2018, services enrolled in the ESR program have participated in 17 EQA testing events, with four events per year and two samples tested per event. The EQA material is prepared and distributed by the RCPAQAP (as part of their serology program) and contains both non-reactive and reactive samples with varying concentrations of syphilis antibodies and therefore degrees of reactivity. Concordance with the expected EQA result has averaged 98% (range 93–100%) in the ESR program. For the WA program, which commenced in late 2020, concordance (using the same EQA material and event sequence) has averaged 96% (range 80% during the initial set up of the program to 100%).

Similar to elements of training and competency (described above), assessment of POC test performance via specific requirements for QC and EQA are non-negotiable. Robust quality systems, capable of detecting false negatives or false positives (or quantitative performance at clinically important decision points) underpin POC test result quality and patient safety.

Important to ID POC testing models, where disease prevalence can change from low to high in geographical populations over time, is consideration of the monitoring of QC performance and adoption of individualised QC plans (IQCP) [41]; these plans provide flexibility with changing patient risk (i.e. false negatives and false positives) and permit the customisation of QC plans according to test method and

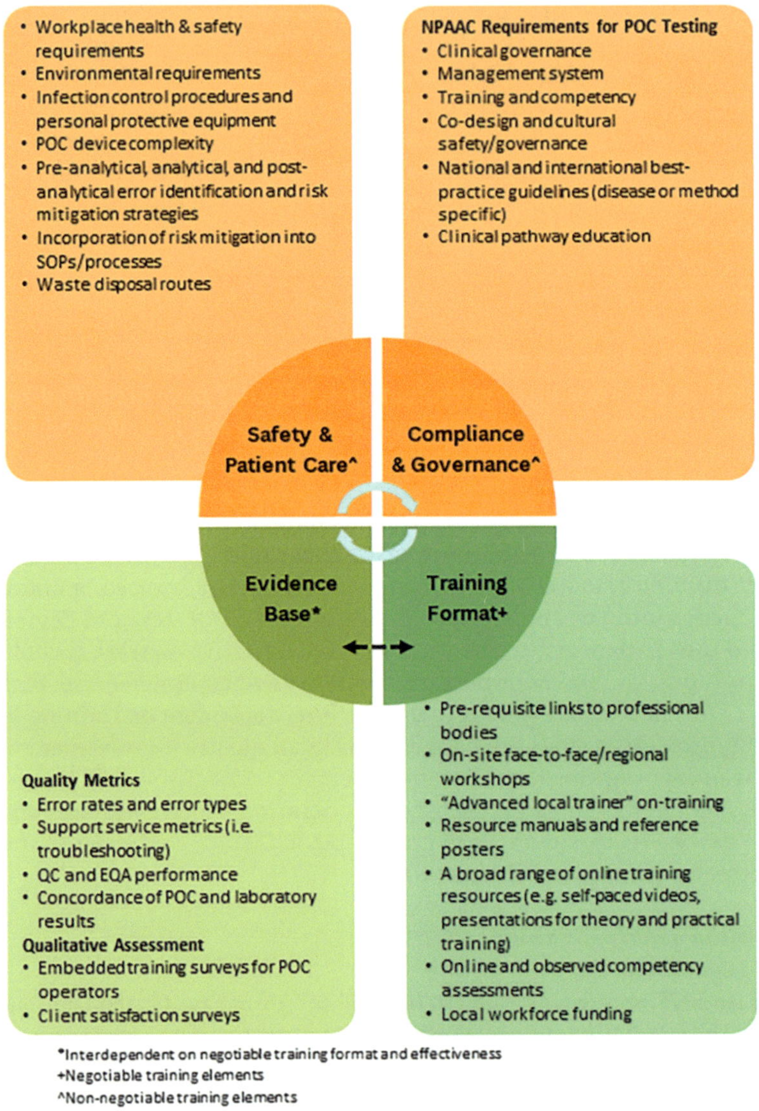

Figure 10.
A framework for the design and continual quality improvement of POC operator training, with elements that should be considered as negotiable, non-negotiable and interdependent.

use, environment, and personnel competency while providing for equivalent quality testing. IQCP could potentially be considered as an additional regulatory option for POC testing in Australia.

3.4 Concluding remarks: implications for POC testing moving forward

Many lessons have been learned from 25 years of implementing POC testing networks in rural and remote Australia. The building blocks to optimise a POC testing network have come together in somewhat of a jigsaw (**Figure 11**) but are now well established following a strong evidence-base of original research and quality improvements carried out along the journey. The optimisation and scale-up of POC

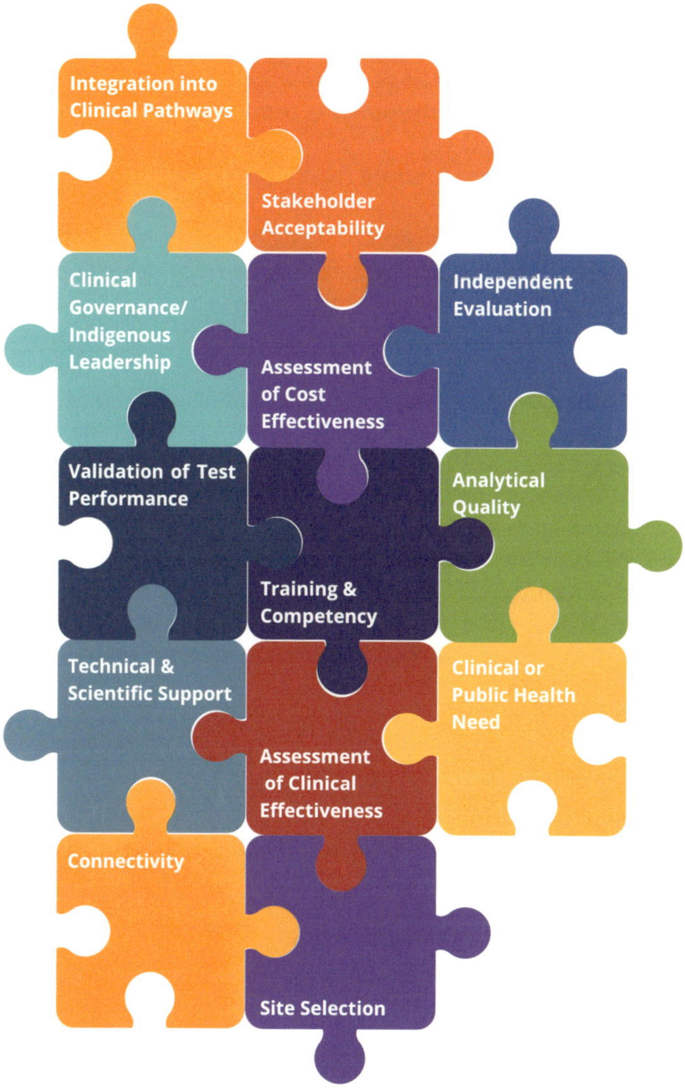
Integration into Clinical Pathways
Stakeholder Acceptability
Clinical Governance/ Indigenous Leadership
Assessment of Cost Effectiveness
Independent Evaluation
Validation of Test Performance
Analytical Quality
Training & Competency
Technical & Scientific Support
Clinical or Public Health Need
Assessment of Clinical Effectiveness
Connectivity
Site Selection

Figure 11.
Building blocks for the development, implementation and ultimate scale-up of a POC testing network—Compiled from lessons learned from ICPOCT experience over nearly 25 years.

testing models remains a 'hot topic' in research conducted around the world in the field [42–44].

Where possible, POC testing scale-up should be accelerated to meet the time frame deemed necessary for the model—depending for example on whether it is a test for NCD versus an ID test that may be required for a disease outbreak or global emergency response. In this regard, ICPOCT remains at the cutting edge of this field through (a) its partnership with the Kirby Institute in an NHMRC-funded Centre for Research Excellence looking at scale-up of POC testing systems (now known as RAPID) and (b) its designation as a World Health Organisation (WHO) Collaborating Centre working *inter alia* on POC testing for sexually transmitted diseases and current gaps in health literacy for NCDs.

There remains considerable blue sky for methodological advancement, technological miniturisation, personalised scope and application of POC testing systems, particularly in rural and remote settings of the world and to service disadvantaged populations. But, as mentioned in the opening remarks for this chapter, success is dependent on policy change and support from governments. Our Australian models have benefitted from continuous funding from governments, albeit with contractual agreements needing to be negotiated repeatedly in time frames as short as 6 months. Ideally, successful models which can demonstrate clinical, operational, economic and cultural benefits as well as sustained analytical quality equivalent to a laboratory, should be underpinned by long-term, integrated funding where possible. This includes ongoing support for the cost of POC testing devices and cartridges; in this regard within Australia, MBS rebates to cover costs of these essential consumables should be in place for models where clinical need is high and laboratory services are lacking. Until recently the QAAMS Program was the only POC testing network with its own rebates. Recently, an MBS item was approved for the performance of POC HbA1c testing in the general practice (family doctor) sector in Australia. The rebate took effect after many years of negotiation with, and repeated submissions to, the main Government authority responsible for approving new rebate items (the Medical Services Advisory Committee, MSAC). When there is an overwhelming evidence-base to support the need for and quality of POC testing, the discipline of POC testing should be expeditiously supported with sustainable funding models.

Acknowledgements

The authors acknowledge and thank the Australian Government Department of Health and Aged Care for their support in funding the QAAMS and ESR POC testing networks. The Northern Territory Government is also acknowledged for funding the NT acute care POC testing program and the WBC DIFF POC testing program, as is the Western Australian Government for supporting the WA Syphilis POC testing network. The authors acknowledge the contribution to these networks of many stakeholders including the National Aboriginal Community Controlled Health Organisation (NACCHO); participating Aboriginal community controlled and government health services; national, jurisdictional and local Aboriginal Community Controlled Health Organisations; national, State and Territory health departments, and other government services; our industry and academic partners; and most importantly, the dedicated health professional staff working as POC testing operators in our networks.

Conflict of interest

The authors have no conflict of interest to declare.

Author details

Mark Shephard*, Susan Matthews, Corey Markus, Emma de Courcy-Ireland, Lauren Duckworth, Isabelle Haklar, Ellen Kambanaros, Tamika Regnier, April Rivers-Kennedy and Grant White
Flinders University International Centre for Point-of-Care Testing, Adelaide, Australia

*Address all correspondence to: mark.shephard@flinders.edu.au

References

[1] Precedence Research, Ottawa, Canada. Healthcare: Point-of-Care Testing Market. Report Code 2270 [Internet]. 2022. Available from: https://www.precedenceresearch.com/point-of-care-testing-market [Accessed: December 7, 2022]

[2] Hayden O, Luppa PB, Min J. Point-of-care testing—New horizons for cross-sectional technologies and decentralized application strategies. Analytical and Bioanalytical Chemistry. 2022;**414**:3161-3163. DOI: 10.1007/s00216-022-03987-8

[3] Hengel B, Causer L, Matthews S, Smith K, Andrewartha K, Badman S, et al. A decentralised point-of-care testing model to address inequities in the COVID-19 response. The Lancet InfectiousDiseases.2020;**21**(7):e183-e190. DOI: 10.1016/S1473-3099(20)30859-8

[4] Shephard M. An introduction to point-of-care testing and its global scope and application. In: Shephard M, editor. A Practical Guide to Global Point-of-Care Testing. Melbourne, Australia: CSIRO Publishing; 2016. pp. 1-14

[5] Spaeth B, Matthews S, Shephard M. Patient-centred point-of-care testing: A life-changing technology for remote health care. In: Onal A, editor. Primary Health Care. United Kingdom: London, UKIntechOpen; 2021. pp. 1-15. DOI: 10.5772/intechopen.100375

[6] Shephard M, Shephard A, Matthews S, Andrewartha K. The benefits and challenges of point-of-care testing in rural and remote primary care settings in Australia. Archives of Pathology and Laboratory Medicine. 2020;**144**(11):1372-1380. DOI: 10.5858/arpa.2020-0105-RA

[7] World Health Organization, editor. Practical Guidance for Scaling up Health Service Innovations. Geneva, Switzerland: World Health Organization; 2009

[8] National Pathology Accreditation Advisory Council (NPAAC). NPAAC Requirements for Point of Care Testing (Second Edition 2021). Australian Government Department of Health. [Internet]. 2021. Available from: https://www1.health.gov.au/internet/main/publishing.nsf/Content/35DE5FC4786CBB33CA257EEB007C7BF2/$File/DT0002469%20-%20NPAAC%20-%20Requirements%20for%20point%20of%20care%20testing%20Second%20edition%202021%20-%2020211215.pdf [Accessed: November 30, 2022]

[9] Colagiuri S, Colagiuri R, Ward J. National Diabetes Strategy and Implementation Plan. Canberra: Diabetes Australia; 1998

[10] Hare MJL, Zhao Y, Guthridge S, Burgess P, Barr ELM, Ellis E, et al. Prevalence and incidence of diabetes among Aboriginal people in remote communities of the Northern Territory, Australia: A retrospective, longitudinal data-linkage study. BMJ Open. 2022;**12**:e059716. DOI: 10.1136/bmjopen-2021-059716

[11] Australian Bureau of Statistics. National Aboriginal and Torres Strait Islander health survey, 2018-19. Ref: 4715.0. Canberra: ABS, [Internet]. 2019. Available from: https://www.abs.gov.au/statistics/people/aboriginal-and-torres-strait-islander-peoples/national-aboriginal-and-torres-strait-islander-health-survey/2018-19 [Accessed: December 1, 2022]

[12] Shephard M. Analytical goals for point-of-care testing used for diabetes

management in Australian health care settings outside the laboratory. Point-of-Care: Journal of Near-Patient Testing and Technology. 2006;**5**:177-185

[13] Liddy AM, Grundy S, Sreenan S, Tormey W. Impact of haemoglobin variants on the use of haemoglobin A1c for the diagnosis and monitoring of diabetes: A contextualised review. Irish Journal of Medical Science. 2022. DOI: 10.1007/s11845-022-02967-2

[14] Shephard MDS, Barratt L, Simpson-Lyttle W. Is the Bayer DCA 2000 acceptable as a screening instrument for the early detection of renal disease? Annals of Clinical Biochemistry. 1999;**36**:393-394

[15] Shephard MDS, Allen GG. Screening for renal disease in a remote Aboriginal community using the Bayer DCA 2000. Australian Journal of Medical Science. 2001;**22**:164-170

[16] Tabrizi S, Unemo M, Golparian D, Twin J, Limnios A, Lahra M, et al. Analytical evaluation of GeneXpert CT/NG, the first genetic point-of-care assay for simultaneous detection of Neisseria gonorrhoeae and chlamydia trachomatis. Journal of Clinical Microbiology. 2013;**51**:1945-1947. DOI: 10.1128/JCM.00806-13

[17] Causer LM, Guy RJ, Tabrizi SN, Whiley DM, Speers DJ, Ward J, et al. Molecular test for chlamydia and gonorrhoea used at point of care in remote primary healthcare settings: A diagnostic test evaluation. Sexually Transmitted Infections. 2018;**94**:340-345. DOI: 10.1136/sextrans-2017-053443

[18] Regnier T, Shephard M, Shephard A, Graham P, DeLeon R, Shepherd S. Results form 16 years of quality surveillance of urine albumin to creatinine ratio testing for a national Indigenous point-of-care testing program. Archives of Pathology and Laboratory Medicine. 2020;**144**:1199-1203. DOI: 10.5858/arpa.2020-0106-OA

[19] Australasian Association of Clinical Biochemists. Pathology Tests Explained. HbA1c [Internet]. 2022. Available from: https://pathologytestsexplained.org.au/learning/test-index/hba1c [Accessed: December 6, 2022]

[20] Kidney Health Australia. Chronic Kidney Disease (CKD) Management in Primary Care (4th edition). Melbourne: Kidney Health Australia; 2020. p. 90. Available from: https://kidney.org.au/uploads/resources/CKD-Management-in-Primary-Care_handbook_2020.1.pdf [Accessed: December 6, 2022]

[21] Australian Indigenous HealthinfoNet. Approval for QAAMS services to use the HbA1c test to diagnose diabetes [Internet]. 2016. Available from: https://healthinfonet.ecu.edu.au/healthinfonet/getContent.php?linkid=320557&title=Approval+for+QAAMS+services+to+use+the+HbA1c+test+to+diagnose+diabetes [Accessed: December 6, 2022]

[22] Shephard M. Clinical and cultural effectiveness of the 'QAAMS' point-of-care testing model for diabetes management in Australian Aboriginal medical services. Clinical Biochemist Reviews. 2006;**27**:161-170

[23] Spaeth BA, Shephard MDS, Schatz S. Point-of-care testing for haemoglobin A1c in remote Australian Indigenous communities improves timeliness of diabetes care. Rural and Remote Health. 2014;**14**:2849. Available from: http://www.rrh.org.au/articles/printviewnew.asp?ArticleID=2849

[24] Price C, John AS, Christenson R, Scharnhorst V, Oellerich M, Jones P, et al. Leveraging the real value of laboratory

medicine with the value proposition. Clinica Chimica Acta. 2016;**462**:183-186. DOI: 10.1016/j.cca.2016.09.006

[25] Shephard M, O'Brien C, Burgoyne A, Croft J, Garlett T, Barancek K, et al. A review of the cultural safety of a national Indigenous point-of-care testing program for diabetes management. Australian Journal of Primary Health. 2016;**22**:368-374. DOI: 10.1071/PY15050

[26] Fekadu G, Bekele F, Tolossa T, Fetensa G, Turi E, Getachew M, et al. Impact of COVID-19 pandemic on chronic diseases care follow-up and current perspectives in low resource settings: A narrative review. International Journal of Physiology and Pathophysiological Pharmacology. 2021;**13**(3):86-93

[27] Parkinson A, Matenge S, Desborough J, Hall Dykgraaf S, Ball L, Wright M, et al. The impact of COVID-19 on chronic disease management in primary care: Lessons for Australia from the international experience. Medical Journal of Australia. 2022;**216**(9):445-448. DOI: 10.5694/mja2.51497

[28] Australian Government Department of Health and Aged Care. Australian Statistical Geography Standard—Remoteness Area [Internet]. 2021. Available from: https://www.health.gov.au/topics/rural-health-workforce/classifications/asgs-ra [Accessed: December 6, 2022]

[29] Spaeth B, Shephard M. Clinical and operational benefits of INR POCT in Indigenous communities in the remote Northern Territory of Australia. Point-of-Care: Journal of Near-Patient Testing and Technology. 2016;**15**:30-34. DOI: 10.1097/POC.0000000000000082

[30] Matthews S, Spaeth B, Duckworth L, Richards J, Prisk E, Auld M, et al. Sustained quality and service delivery in an expanding point-of-care testing network in remote Australian primary care. Archives of Pathology and Laboratory Medicine. 2020;**144**(11):1381-1391. DOI: 10.5858/arpa.2020-0105-RA

[31] Remote Primary Health Care Manuals. Manuals [Internet]. 2022. Available from: https://remotephcmanuals.com.au/ [Accessed: December 6, 2022]

[32] Shephard M, Spaeth B, Mazzachi B, Auld M, Schatz S, Loudon J, et al. Design, implementation and initial assessment of the Northern Territory point-of-care testing program. Australian Journal of Rural Health. 2012;**20**:16-21. DOI: 10.1111/j.1440-1584.2011.01243.x

[33] Shephard M, Spaeth B, Motta L, Shephard A. Chapter 48. Point-of-care testing in Australia: Practical advantages and benefits of community resiliency for improving outcomes. In: Kost G, Curtis C, editors. Global Point-of-Care—Strategies for Disasters, Complex Emergencies, and Public Health Resilience. Washington DC: AACC (American Association of Clinical Chemistry) Press; 2015. pp. 527-535

[34] Spaeth BA, Shephard MDS, Omond R. Clinical application of point-of-care testing in the remote primary health care setting. Quality in Primary Care. 2017;**25**:164-175

[35] Spaeth BA, Kaambwa B, Shephard MDS, Omond R. Economic evaluation of point-of-care testing in the remote primary health care setting of Australia's Northern Territory. ClinicoEconomics and Outcomes Research. 2018;**10**:269-277. DOI: 10.2147/CEOR.S160291

[36] Spaeth B, Shephard M, McCormack B, Sinclair G. Evaluation of HemoCue white

blood cell differential counter at a remote health Centre in Australia's Northern Territory. Pathology. 2015;**47**:91-95. DOI: 10.1097/PAT.0000000000000202

[37] Spaeth B, Shephard M, Kockcinar R, Duckworth L, Ormond R. Impact of point-of-care testing for white blood cell count on triage of patients with infection in the remote Northern Territory of Australia. Pathology. 2019;**51**(5):512-517. DOI: 10.1016/j.pathol.2019.04.003

[38] Equity Economics. Blueprint for the Future: Evaluation of NACCHO's Role under the Enhanced Syphilis Response. A Report prepared for the National Aboriginal Community Controlled Health Organisation (NACCHO). 2021. pp. 2-5

[39] Causer LM, Kaldor JM, Fairley CK, Donovan B, Karapanagiotidis T, Leslie DE, et al. A laboratory-based evaluation of four rapid point-of-care tests for syphilis. PLoS One. 2014;**9**:3. DOI: 10.1371/journal.pone.0091504

[40] Australian Government Department of Health Therapeutics Goods Administration. Chlamydia, gonorrhoea and syphilis IVD self-tests: clinical performance requirements and risk mitigation strategies—Version 1.0 [Internet]. 2021. Available from: https://www.tga.gov.au/sites/default/files/chlamydia-gonorrhoea-and-syphilis-ivd-self-tests.pdf [Accessed: December 6, 2022]

[41] Centres for Medicare & Medicaid Services. Individualized Quality Control Plan (IQCP) [Internet]. 2021. Available from: https://www.cms.gov/Regulations-and-Guidance/Legislation/CLIA/Individualized_Quality_Control_Plan_IQCP [Accessed: December 6, 2022]

[42] Milat AJ, Newson R, King L. Evidence and Evaluation Guidance Series, Population and Public Health Division. Increasing the Scale of Population Health Interventions: A Guide. Sydney: Ministry of Health; 2014

[43] Milat AJ, Newson R, King L, Rissel C, Wolfenden L, Bauman A, et al. A guide to scaling up population health interventions. Public Health Research and Practice. 2016;**26**:1. DOI: 10.17061/phrp2611604

[44] Laferty L, Smith K, Causer L, Andrewartha K, Whiley D, Badman S, et al. Scaling up sexually transmissible infections point-of-care testing in remote Aboriginal and Torres Strait Islander communities: Healthcare workers' perceptions of the barriers and facilitators. Implementation Science Communications. 2021;**2**:127. DOI: 10.1186/s43058-021-00232-8

Chapter 8

The Rural Way: Rural Nurses' Contribution to New Models of Health Care, Reducing Health Disparities – Stories from Practice

Jean Ross, Josie Crawley and Rachel Parmee

Abstract

This chapter reports on a research project that set out to capture the unique stories from rural nurses from Aotearoa, New Zealand. During the past three decades changing socio-political and economic contexts have affected the delivery of health care while rural nurses have responded with new models of practice which has resulted in an emerging rural nurse discourse related and specific to rural New Zealand. Rural nurses have maintained and, in some cases, improved the health care of these rural communities. A total of 26 rural nurse participants shared their stories providing data to explore the structured phenomenon of rural nursing in New Zealand. Personal and human dimensions are illuminated, as the in-depth meaning of the experience is described by each individual storyteller. Interviews were conducted to collect retrospective stories uncovering the participants' rural nurse journey. Revealed are a sense of place and people, involving what nurses' express, as the rural way. A nursing discourse is developed which complements and extends international theories. The rural nurse of New Zealand is imbued with pioneering spirit; entrepreneurial practice shaped by their rural communities highlighting what we suggest is the rural way. Further expansion of the rural way was uncovered with follow up interviews exploring their practice during the COVID-19 pandemic.

Keywords: rural, rural nurse, models of care, reducing health disparities, narrative, COVID-19

1. Introduction

The professional identity of the rural nurse from Aotearoa New Zealand came of age between the 1990s and the early 2000s. This time period is associated with significant changes to the governance, funding and delivery of health care in rural contexts as a result of the global financial crisis of the late 1980s. Changing health care ideologies moved away from a top-down approach to a bottom-up approach reflected in the major health care reforms revealing the adoption of neo-liberal ideology [1]. The National government of the day acknowledged continuing inequalities in health, for

Māori (indigenous population of Aotearoa New Zealand) and Pacific populations was continuing to decline with extensive statistical differences between Māori and non-Māori and equally between urban and rural regions [2]. Changes where needed to address these disparities [2]. The government's aim was to increase efficiency and address these needs while providing healthcare in the most economically and practical ways [3]. The government authorised major health reforms, resulting in changes for the provision of healthcare [1] delivery, funding, governance structures [2, 3] and models of healthcare [4–7].

The establishment of Rural Community Trusts (RCTs) was one outcome of the country's major health-care reforms [8]. RCTs designed and managed their own individual local health services, this model was regarded by the government as innovative and came with associated cost savings. As well as encouraging community involvement in health-care decision-making [8] the RCTs assisted in the development of "by Māori for Māori" iwi providers [9]. The benefits of RCTs became the funding structure that improved and supported community participation, collaboration, and teamwork. Further this ideology was extended and underpinned in the early 2000s by the 'Primary Health Care Strategy' [10] and further laid the foundation in which to position nurses at the foreground of the delivery of Primary Health Care (PHC) and improve nurses' contribution to the delivery of health care. This shift in focus has been beneficial for the advancement of PHC nurses and in particular rural nurses' practice development and contribution to the delivery of sustainable health care.

This original qualitative research aimed to explore rural nurse practice in Aotearoa New Zealand following decades of change leading to the development of new rural health delivery models. The rural nurse participants shared their stories exploring the past, the present and the future experiences leading to a unique rural nursing discourse which complements and extends the international literature from America [11] Canada [12] and Australia [13] in alignment with health beliefs of rural populations and the nuances associated with geographical locations. Traditional discourses aligned with rural nursing practice include personal and professional connections with the rural community; being known in the community; dual relationships; and always being on call; broad scope of practice; jack of all trades, master of none; and a sense of belonging to the geographical location. These discourses are well entrenched within national and international nursing organisations; rural communities; policy development; education, workforce planning and research informing practice.

The occupational title of the 'rural nurse' from Aotearoa New Zealand has been questioned by Ross [14] as to whether this title is an adequate portrayal of their practice and contribution to the delivery of health care? In short, her findings suggest this title does not do justice to their practice and further research into this goal is required. This research seeks to investigate further rural nurses' practice and contribution to health care revealing that rural nurses throughout the latter part of the twentieth century and early part of the twenty-first century were pivotal in pioneering new models of practice; expanding the scope of nursing services available to their rural communities; reducing inequities while maintaining and in some cases improving health. More recently COVID-19 has created new challenges for those rural nurses and rural communities [15]. Follow up interviews in 2020 heightened further demands on rural nurses' practice, further revealing pioneering practice adding to the unique rural nursing discourse.

2. Narrative research: diving into the story

A narrative inquiry approach was the methodology chosen for this research, providing "... a way of understanding and inquiring into experience" [16]. This qualitative research celebrates the power that story has, to explore meaning, make connections, entertain, and build empathy and share experience with others [16, 17]. Haven [18] recognises the power the story has to explore meaning and make connections between the storyteller and the recipients. Stories have provided the data to explore the structured phenomenon of rural nursing in New Zealand—as lived and told by experienced rural nurses.

2.1 Rural nurse participants

Rural Nurses from Aotearoa New Zealand were invited to share their stories. The snowball effect was engaged with revealing a total of 58 expressions of interest, of which 40 rural nurses met the research criteria (rural practice in New Zealand for more than 15 years) and 26 rural nurses were able to commit to the project

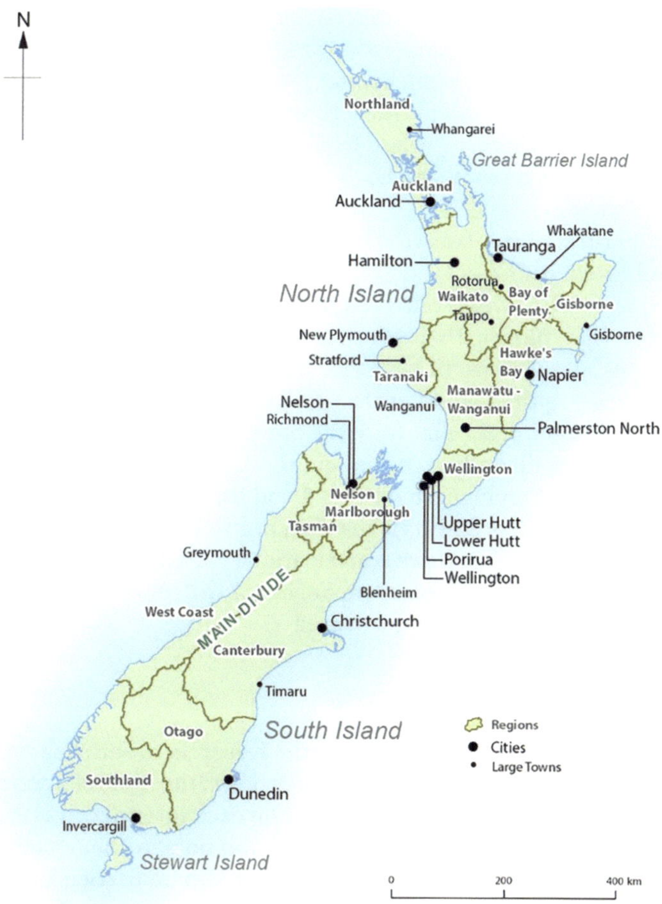

Figure 1.
Map of Aotearoa, New Zealand. Source: Created and published with permission from Chris Garden.

requirements and timeframes. These rural nurses' ages ranged from 40 to 70 years while their demography included nurses of Māori (indigenous population of Aotearoa New Zealand) and European descent, male and female, recently retired and currently employment, representatives from all regions of habited Islands from the far North of the North Island to the far South of the South Island. Island groups (North and South Islands, Great Barrier, Chatham, Pitt and Stewart Island) refer to the Aotearoa New Zealand map in **Figure 1**. Participants for this part of the research project were not identified.

2.2 Data collection

The original research was conducted in 2017/2018 we engaged with semi-structured interviews to collect retrospective stories covering the participants rural nurse stories either face-to-face, SKYPE (video) or telephone. Interviews ranged from 45 to 90 min in length. Interviews were, framed around Clandinin and Connelly's [19] three-dimensional space narrative structure which is a model that examines personal and social interactions across the continuity of time and context, as well as personal and social features experienced by both the researcher, and participant. The framework was shared with all participants before the agreed interviews, however during the interviews began with an open question from the interviewer—"*Tell me about your rural nurse journey*". Each nurse was a primary source, sharing their unique nursing story. Each interview was recorded, transcribed, and sent back to the interviewee (rural nurse) to check validity, or to add key forgotten moments. Each transcript was then returned to the researchers. Each nurse was a primary source, sharing their unique nursing story.

There were 16 rural nurses from the original research project) who agreed to have their stories published in *Stories of nursing in rural Aotearoa: A landscape of care* [20]. These rural nurses in 2020 were contacted by email inviting them to contribute with follow up interviews exploring their practice during the COVID-19 pandemic. Nine of the 16 rural nurses agreed to participate and were interviewed by the first author. This follow up interview enquired whether the COVID-19 pandemic had affected the rural nurses' practice and if so, seek what were the outcome?

The interviews were digitally recorded via zoom meetings, edited to remove identifying features of individuals mentioned and then developed into podcasts and broadcasted on Otago Access Radio (https://oar.org.nz/) before been thematically analysed. Podcasts consist of positive conversations with people from around the world related to COVID-19 is a further expansion of the rural way related to rural nurses from Aotearoa New Zealand uncovered

2.3 Data analysis

Each transcript was read at least twice by the researchers with key repeated concepts identified by commonality across interviews: the umbrella concepts of past, present and future, situation and place. Data from each interview was then coded into themes and subthemes until saturation occurred and no new themes emerged [21]. Researchers could not guarantee absolute confidentiality to participants, as pioneering innovation can be traced back to place and sometimes person. Participants knew personal and community names would be protected, but that emergent themes and specific detail might identify location. We placed safeguards to protect participants by asking all participants to check transcripts, with highlighted areas we thought potentially might be recognisable. Once corrected transcripts were returned, we coded each transcript, removing the participants name, individual participants were identified by code only (by number). A phenomenon of interconnected narratives emerged, showed how stories of the past shape the present and influence discourse All transcripts are kept on a passworded hard drive and will be kept for seven years as per ethical requirements.

Ethical approval was obtained from Otago Polytechnic Research Ethics Committee, Otago Polytechnic, Dunedin, New Zealand in 2017 and extended in 2020 to accommodate further interviews from the original rural nurse participants who consented to have their stories published in a book. Ethical approval also included consultation and engagement from the Office of Kaitohutohu. The Kaitohutohu office at Otago Polytechnic upholds the mana (integrity) of the partnership with the local Māori (indigenous population Aotearoa New Zealand) community, and is consulted during research development, looking at the proposed research from a Māori Kaupapa point of view. Māori are under-represented in the nursing profession, *comprising* only 8% of practising nurses [22] so the inclusion of Māori as part of this research is of the utmost importance to further our understanding and future engagement [23].

We were aware the research was likely to involve Māori as there is a higher number of registered nurses identifying as Māori in the rural practice setting (N = 59; 11.6%) of 6.5% of the overall workforce [24]. Statistics show that 14% of the New Zealand population identify as Māori, with over three quarters of this population living outside the Auckland region, making up a significant part of the rural communities [25] *"Rural nursing is also clearly a valued setting for Māori registered nurses' employment..."* themes from the rural nurses' stories could *"... include reference to tikanga Māori (a Māori concept valuing Māori knowledge into practice), within the context of describing their work"* [23] p. 68.

3. Findings and discussion

Engaging with a thematic analysis has revealed a unique discourse of rural nursing in Aotearoa New Zealand. Rural nurses revealed their innovative practice exposing their contemporary identity of the nurse practising in the rural context. This rural nurse discourse identifies the rural nurse as a pioneer supplying the backbone of health care to the community; an entrepreneurial practitioner expanding the limits of scope of practice to meet community needs. The creative development of tenacious nurses and local communities' embracing responsive solutions and new models of healthcare to accommodate the challenging landscapes and changing socio-political tides, accommodating indigenous provision of health care highlight what we suggest is the rural way, as supported by the following data and discussion.

3.1 The rural way

A description of the rural way incorporates values, attitudes or characteristics that are common in rural indigenous and non-indigenous rural people [23]. These features of rural people or communities were often seen as being different to urban environments, a product of geographic context and isolation from others, encompassing a way of being and a Māori way of being in the rural. Being in the rural revolves around embracing the rural, rural culture, values, beliefs and performing in the rural. For example, resourcefulness (mention is made to #8 fencing wire (**Figure 2**)

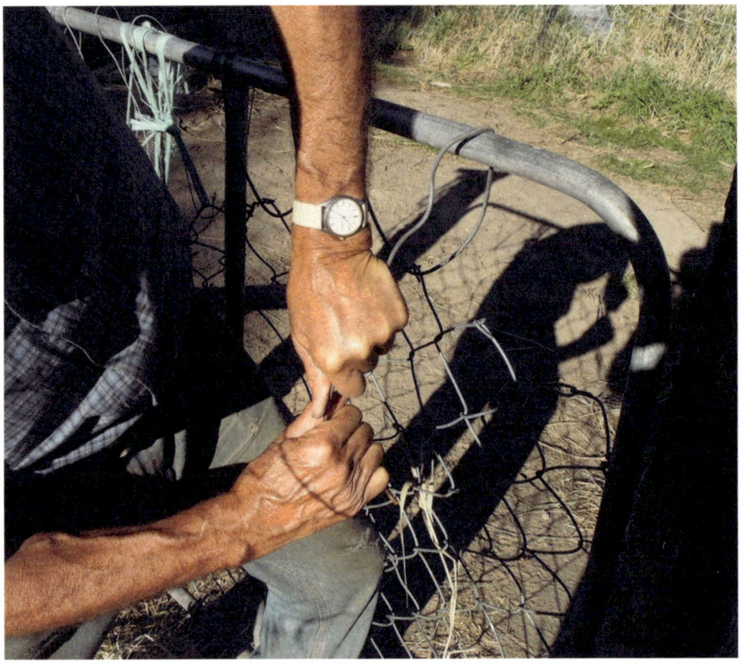

Figure 2.
Dealing to the damage with Number 8 wire. Source: Martin London Photography (published with permission).

a well-known depiction of New Zealanders ability to mend, fix or create solutions to problems by using #8 wire) is made necessary due to being at a distance from many health resources as discussed by the following participants:

> *People are very different in a rural area, I think, than they are in the city. They are very different people; in that they are more community orientated. I think in the city, a lot of people don't even know their neighbours. And in rural areas, they are '#8 wire' people; they manage to fix things that you think 'wow, look at you, look what you managed to do!'. They're quite resourceful. (Storyteller 12)*

> *They've [rural people] got a 'can do' attitude. They care about their neighbours. They're "greenies" in their own right, so they love the environment they live in, and they look after it (believe it or not). They're known for their number 8 wire approach and their ability to diversify when the need arises. (Storyteller 11)*

> *It's about 2 ½ hours. Ambulance, it can be up to 3. And if you've got – obviously - road works, or flooding, we're actually chopped off. We can't get there, and it's only by helicopter. But then, if the weather's no good, the helicopter can't fly anyway. So, we do need to have some sort of independence, and be able to intubate and keep somebody alive until help can come. (Storyteller 16)*

Many (but not all) of the rural nurse participants had been born and bought up in rural communities. The specific rural settings the nurses lived and worked in were often spoken about as part of their own connection with the rural, leading to a sense of place and a sense of belonging (rural knowing) (**Figure 3**). Knowing is associated

DOI: http://dx.doi.org/10.5772/intechopen.109768

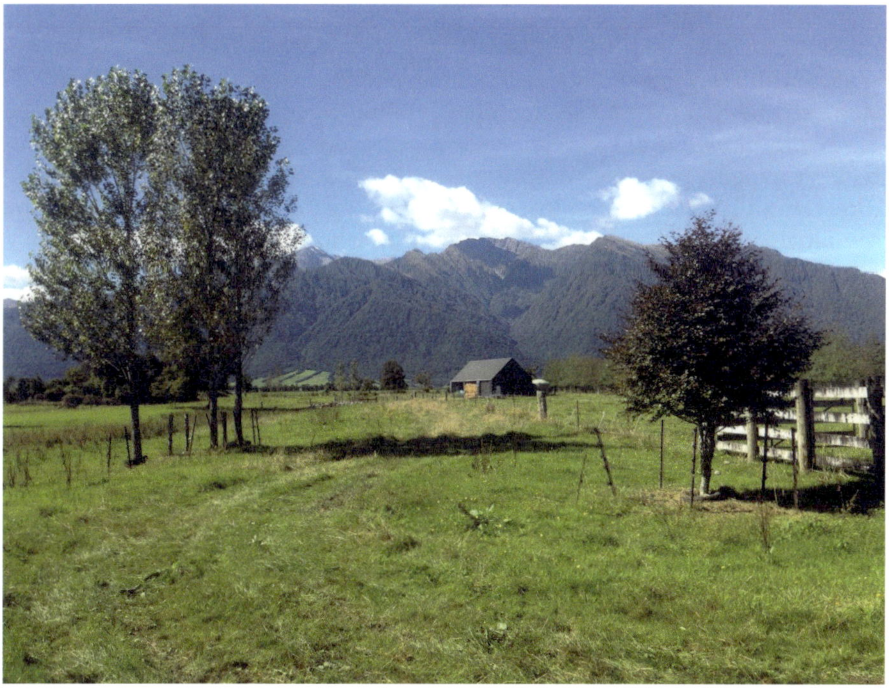

Figure 3.
The hay barn is full on a fine day in Paradise. Source: Martin London Photography (published with permission).

with understanding the rural context, community and the local unique rural community rhythm, which connects the rural nurse to identify with that rural community as revealed by the following storytellers:

> *I live it, dream it. That's massive for me. Space – so, a paddock with some sheep and a hill and a tree and a mountain in the background, for me, is prayer. Literally. Because I love – I love – the rural setting. I love the fact that you're this tiny little town surrounded by this magnificent beauty. (Storyteller 10)*

> *I think this is paradise myself, that's why I wanted to come back, I love the hills, I love the seasons yeah, it's perfect being here I will always stay here. (Storyteller 9)*

> *Living in the rural area, I understand the nature of their farming lifestyle, both dairy and mixed farming, logging, freezing works, the seasonal work like shearing, lambing, tailing, haymaking cropping and all that entails, you know the dangers of tractors quad bikes. I supported the local rugby teams often knowing the players. The families that have been here for a long time, I know them well. (Storyteller 1)*

Despite a love of rural environments, almost all interviewees discussed challenges that they pose. The most cited challenge was isolation due to long distances from other healthcare centres, and weather (and typically a combination of the two). Geographic factors affect healthcare delivery in rural settings but are also cited as a reason why rural nurses require a resilience – they need to be able to provide care and the necessities of life in areas with limited resources, we consider these nurses both pioneers and entrepreneurial practitioners.

3.2 Pioneering practice

Where health services did not exist, nurses employed a pioneering spirit to develop a service that met the client and community needs. They forged new roles, did further training, fundraised for resources, and met challenges with courageous strategies. Changing governance structures meant that nurses were able to shape the direction and delivery of healthcare during the major health care reforms. Rural nurses initiated many practices, whose origins have now been absorbed into contemporary health practice. Like all new practices, changes were scaffolded to make innovation possible. In this case, nurses becoming intravenous-certificated was an important first step to providing local access to chemotherapy. The alternative model required residents to travel 3–5 h, in each direction, to an urban health-care facility (ese rural nurses set out to avoid residents having to travel long distances to acquire treatment in urban contexts) as they progressed with new and never been offered health care services firstly by nurses and secondly in rural regions in the 1990s. This innovative practice was later recognised by the establishment of Nurse Specialists. These approaches to the delivery of healthcare were designed to meet the localised health needs of the community as depicted in the following excerpts:

> *[w]e needed to adapt, which as rural nurses we do very well. So we changed it [the delivery of chemotherapy] to more of a medical day unit and took on doing other transfusions... (Storyteller 16)*

> *So, I pioneered additional services that the nurses could provide for the community, for example cervical smears, which at that time was not the norm for nurses to be offering. (Storyteller 1)*

The rural nurses acknowledge the community role and are encouraged to pioneer and deliver health services in local regions that accommodates the particular nuances related to that community for example, Māori nurses embrace their own identity and have a responsibility to meet the needs of their families or whanau which involves caring for the whole family and not just the individual patient because whanau play a role in a patient's recovery [26].

> *[In establishing operating mobile ear health clinics in rural isolated regions with a high Māori population] We were taking away all the barriers to access, for example, unwarranted cars, unregistered cars, unregistered drivers, petrol in the tank. We were just trying to drop all those barriers so the children could get what they needed without adults putting up the problems that they had, that were getting in the way. (Storyteller 2)*

Rural nurses share on-call (after hours provision of emergency and acute health care) with general practitioners covering 24 h of healthcare at the weekends and during weeknights. One noticeable difference between rural and urban nursing practice has been the expectation that rural nurses would provide an emergency health-care service in the form of Primary Response in Medical Emergencies (PRIME). It is important to acknowledge this in the context of changing models of healthcare and funding and the provision of sustainable healthcare by rural nurses. PRIME is distinct to Aotearoa New Zealand operating only in rural locations and funded by the Ministry of Health and the Accident Compensation Corporation (ACC) and is administered by St. John Ambulance service. PRIME utilises the skills of speciality trained rural GPs and/or rural nurses in areas to support the ambulance service where the response time for assistance would otherwise be significant or where additional medical skills would assist with the patients' condition [27].

... we got a defibrillator and introduced a higher level of care, making the practice more of a casualty outpost rather than just a house with a medical kit in it. (Storyteller 3)

> *[Before PRIME[1]] I found myself stitching people up and putting IVs in without any training... We trained sideways, literally doing our nursing training, our extra training, I trained to Level 4 as an ambulance officer. (Storyteller 3)*

> *...in the local hospital... there were no permanent medical doctors in the hospital and the nurses ran the hospital with the General Practitioners' support... I was a 'jack of all trades' and would do a bit of this and that.*

The RCTs, including nursing services, were driven by the health needs of their communities which, over time, granted rural nurses a strong community involvement while enhancing communities' social capital (as discussed in the excerpts from the rural nurses' stories above). Nurses talked of adapting their practice to accommodate community need to achieve this they needed to be responsive to the community be tentative and pioneer new approaches and models of practice. In the long run, all these trusts ensured the feasibility of community health services, having been redesigned to perform this function [8]. The trusts generally employed all local healthcare staff including the general practitioner and rural nurses. These new employment arrangements gave the RCTs significant advantage the local health professionals were in a strong position to work collaboratively, maintaining effective teamwork and sharing skill base as a result, which benefitted the community.

Many of these aspects of rural nursing show a pioneering spirit, several of these historical practices are now incorporated into community nursing as routine everyday practice. Rural nurses have very autonomous roles, with high levels of responsibility. This both expands nursing skills to the edge of scope of practice, but also sometimes restricts what intervention is possible. Nurses often spoke of "being it", "the only", very different from team nursing in an urban hospital setting as highlighted by the following rural nurses:

> *It really came home to me one night that I was it. ... In the rural setting, I guess, those of us who do work here realise we often have to step up to the challenge... It is a different culture, an unspoken knowing that you will work together to do the best, whatever it takes. (Storyteller 9)*

> *We've had to be quite resourceful in what we do and how we work. We rely on a lot of nurses stepping up into different specialties [like Rural Nurse Specialist, Nurse Practitioners, Clinical Nurse Specialists] because it's very difficult to retain doctors in a lot of those areas... It's an exciting place for a nurse to work. You get to work truly to the top of your scope of practice. (Storyteller 11)*

> *...rural nurses [need to be] recognised for the skill set that they have, because I believe it is different, it's so different. But that we can support them so that they can do it*

[1] PRIME relates to Primary Response in Medical Emergencies and is unique to New Zealand rural practice. Both nurses and doctors working in a solo capacity are skilled in emergency community management.

knowing that they're going to be backed up, knowing that they're not going to fall into working outside of scope. All those things that are very, very difficult when you are on an Island on your own... (Storyteller 10)

Islands provide their own special geographic constraints. Islands are considered as distinct places. Islands are different from the mainland areas especially when they are situated the furthest away from adjacent mainland communities [28]. Islands are surrounded by water; connected/disconnected; isolated; habituated; uninhabited, while having similarities with others or differences and experience their own challenges [29]. Challenges may pertain to the island's own climate which have a direct bearing on island and rural culture and economy. This brings demands on the services and supply industries and can also impact on resources as dis-economy of scale is experienced living on an island because of small community populations that raises costs of living including transport, production of electricity and the moving of goods onto the island all come with a cost (**Figure 4**) [30]. And further consideration of rural peoples' resilience, independence and self-sufficiency relates to rural Island life as highlighted in the following excerpts:

Internationally they say that there is something different – or set apart about people who choose to live remotely... There is a need for the people to be self-sufficient, independent and resilient to enjoy or, in fact, survive island life. (Storyteller 6)

Islands are bound by geographical constraints - distance and boundaries. An island is defined as a piece of land surrounded by water – often also by isolation – by detachment or surrounded in some way.... A good example being in poor weather you just can't get a seriously sick patient off the Island as the helicopter cannot land whereas on the mainland there may be other options. (Storyteller 6)

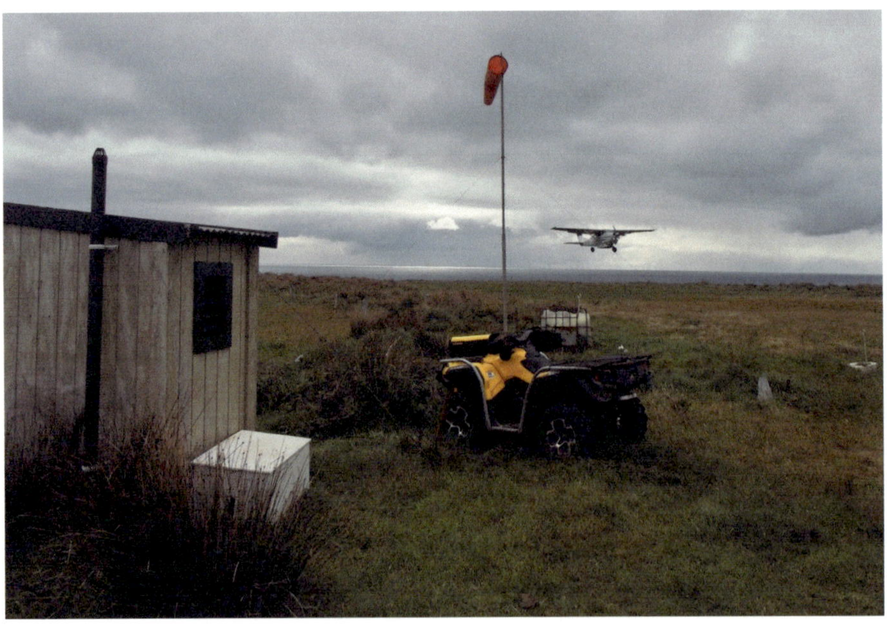

Figure 4.
Terminal building and taxi at Pitt Island airstrip. Source: Martin London Photography (published with permission).

> *...when I realised my father was having a heart attack that night, it was 10 o'clock at night, and the first thing I did was – rather than think 'well, is he going to survive' – I looked out the window to see what the weather was like. You couldn't have a plane because it was dark, so were we going to be able to get a boat to get him off the Island? (Storyteller 10)*

> *We're very vulnerable to commercial decisions here because we rely on businesses that have ferries and planes, and if they change their practices, that can change things overnight for what we do here. (Storyteller 3)*

We further identified several themes that rural nurses' practice typically possesses for example innovation and adaptability while working autonomously but in collaboration with the residents and team members aligned with the rural community which we have identified as the rural nurse as entrepreneurial practitioners.

3.3 Entrepreneurial practitioners

Rural healthcare professionals are usually in reciprocal relationships with the community they serve. They see the community itself as inherent to their practice, and for some nurses, to their sense of self and for Māori nurses this sense of self relates strongly with knowing their communities and whanua contributes to a sense of belonging, provides insight, and helps to establish therapeutic relationships [23]. Many of the rural nurses expressed that they were highly supported and valued by their community. This support is not only due to good will and established relationships, although that is undoubtedly a part of it. Due to matters of geographic isolation and resource scarcity, community support is often a requirement if the community is to have operating healthcare services:

> *I feel supported by the community as I nurse. The proof of that is when there's an emergency. It is common that the locals will stop and assist. Someone might offer to carry my heavy packs into the bush, others will rush off to find family members of the injured. And afterwards some may phone me up saying, 'oh, I realise that you were up really late last night, can I blah blah blah for you?' (Storyteller 6)*

Sense of place is important to both the nurse, and to the patient. Relationships and empowering clients to make their own choices about location are seen as important to the rural nursing role, while recognising the increased risks isolation entails. An often-discussed aspect of rural nursing was enabling people to maintain their independence; to remain in their home or the local community whilst receiving care:

> *And I think a lot of times, when people talk about encouraging people in palliative care to die or saying that people want to die at home, I think 'community' is what they mean. 'Home' doesn't necessarily always mean the house where they lived. But it means where they're comfortable, where their community is, where their support is... (Storyteller 7)*

> *So, yes, I think we provide a magnificent service, I really do. An essential service. We keep people out of hospital or bring them home much earlier. (Storyteller 12)*

Rural nurses show ingenuity in the face of scarce resources, often working in isolation with high responsibility and autonomy. Despite the increased likelihood of working by oneself in a rural context, the interviewees recognise that working with other healthcare professionals is vital to ensuring the best outcomes for patients, but often collegial relationships are at distance:

> *I work in partnership and collaboration with the General Practitioners, I support them, just as they support me. They trust my ability allowing me to manage their patients. There is real teamwork here. (Storyteller 1)*

Although pre-established connections cause challenges with maintaining professional boundaries it can be of benefit to patients in that these relationships can be useful in a therapeutic sense, but also in that health care practitioners feel accountable to the community:

> *... sometimes when you know them [a patient who cannot be saved], you're dealing with your own grief. It's nothing like the grief of the family, obviously, but you're still dealing with your own grief. And then you think – it's the old beat up story – 'did I manage to...', 'was there anything else I could have done', or 'did I not do...'. And as I said, you've got nobody to bounce those ideas off because you're there on your own. ... You're there, until somebody else turns up. (Storyteller 8)*

Understanding the community, and its needs are necessary to be able to forge creative ways to provide services that are accessible and appropriate. Nurses often have a pre-established connection with patients or can quickly form one, sometimes patients are family or friends, working in partnership over long periods of time has numerous advantages for the provision of patient-centred health care linking health requirements and needs and building a sense of connectedness and fulfilment for the nurse. These links create additional complexities, but also opportunities for additional support. Working in partnership with the patient/client is seen as vital, requiring a connectedness to the community. In rural nursing, nurses often get to see the difference they make through continuity of care. Rural nurses describe great satisfaction from seeing their skills being valued by their clients and are professionally invested in the change they help engender with clients:

> *..you tell them to go to so-and-so because they will be able to fix it for you, whether that's home help or something. I'm very aware what's available in the community (Storyteller 13)*

> *If I nurse somebody who comes from [community name removed]..., you know there's issues around distance, you know there is an issue around the limit of health services in their home area, what their shopping and other services are like. You actually really do understand some of the challenges for people, and that makes a big difference. (Storyteller 5)*

> *... you watch people grow. Especially young mums with babies that are struggling... And then you watch them flourish and they get it all together. And you watch the children flourish and go to school, and then you see them in school. It's kind of nice. (Storyteller 8)*

3.4 Entrepreneurial practice the nurse practitioner

The rural nurses we interviewed revealed the practice models they adopted in response to funding changes. Firstly, nurses had the opportunity to purchase and govern general practices, which were traditionally owned and operated solely by GPs – those with a medical background. Nurse Practitioner training was seen by nearly all respondents as the extra training that legitimised what nurses had to do anyway in rural settings, but previously through indirect routes. However – it was generally felt that their work was not understood, appreciated, or valued by those outside of the rural setting:

> *By doing my Nurse Practitioner training, I could then offer this broader, rounder service. I could finish the consult by signing the script, ordering more medication, or – more importantly than the medication – ordering an x-ray, working out which bloods were needed and why. So, investigations were bigger for me in becoming a Nurse Practitioner than prescribing was. Prescribing was the added plus.*
>
> *(Storyteller 10)*

> *Nurse Practitioner was that I felt that it was really helpful to have the ability not just to prescribe, but to actually be able to assess properly; to learn how to assess, diagnose, treat, look for problems and do as much as I can in the areas preventing people from having to come up to tertiary care. (Storyteller 7)*

3.5 Entrepreneurial practice responsive to change

A common sentiment among rural nurses was that industry and demographics within rural communities have changed dramatically over time (**Figure 5**). Changes in industry are said to explain the changes in demographics, with more transient workers and immigrant workers unfamiliar with the Aotearoa New Zealand health system and language barriers. This changes the context in which rural nurses operate, as the high degree of interconnectedness in rural communities, while still existing, is somewhat diminished:

> *But in the rural areas, there are now more transient populations. The dairy farm workers in the [place name removed] area alone are from 10 different nationalities. Many don't speak English. So you have a language barrier, communication barrier, expectations [that do not align with how the New Zealand health system works]. (Storyteller 1)*

> *After starting this job for a couple of years, I could have driven right through my area and named every house, every child, every person. I don't even bother trying these days. (Storyteller 8)*

> *It was very obvious when working in Public Health especially in the school situations as the migrant workers [from diary conversions] brought with them their own social issues previously not seen in the established communities. (Storyteller 14)*

> *I would say we sometimes end up with quite a lot of transient people because they come and get a job and then there's trouble with getting accommodation and stuff, and they have to move on... (Storyteller 9)*

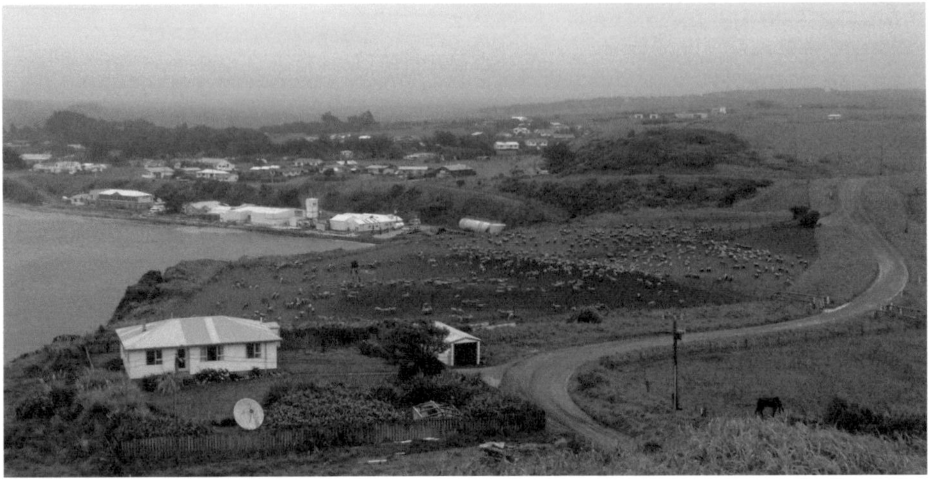

Figure 5.
Chatham Island industries: Hotel, fish factory and sheep penned for embarkation. Source: Martin London Photography (published with permission).

Responsive practice has equally been demonstrated as rural nurses responded to the COVID-19 pandemic. These nurses collaborated with health professionals to ensure adequate care for patients was offered but in different innovative ways. We can acknowledge the pioneering spirit associated with rural nursing practice from Aotearoa New Zealand continued in a similar vein as to the changing health care system identified in the larger research project. This often-involved nurses, health workers and more broadly local authority Council taking on responsibilities outside their normal duties to keep communication lines open and work closely together as highlighted in this excerpt:

> *... very early on in the piece realised that patients weren't going to come see us... because of their own fear around contracting COVID in the practice. So, we activated a project called COVWELL, which basically is a COVID wellness... made these phone calls to all our high risks patients. This was about a 7 or 8 minute phone making sure they were well, that they understood, if they needed to go into isolation what that meant and what it looked like, making sure they had support around them... for them to know that actually you are on the end of a telephone if I do get sick...*
>
> *(Rural Nurse, podcast 46).*

Rural nurses enhanced their practice as community educators and effective collaborators with a variety of local colleagues and members of their rural communities, drawing attention to community resilience and the progressive rural nurses' pioneering spirit.

4. Conclusion

The health care system in Aotearoa New Zealand during the 1990s was subjected to major economic and a change to delivery models, especially in rural regions influenced by neo-liberal political philosophy [3]. Rural nurses put a stake in the ground with the aim of responding to these changes and enabling equity – exploring new practice models to ensure that the best levels of healthcare were available. The aim of this chapter has been to report on a research project that set out to capture the unique stories from rural nurses from Aotearoa New Zealand with the aim to make visible their practice. Narrative inquiry has provided a depth of meaning to the rural nurse experience and uncovered the discourse of rural nursing in New Zealand in the twenty-first century adding to the international rural nursing discourse. Narrative inquiry methodology recognises the power that story has, to explore meaning, make connections, entertain, and build empathy and share with others. This methodology has provided a depth of meaning to the rural nurse experience; the data analysis and research findings demonstrate that rural nurses have maintained and, in some cases, improved the health care of these rural communities in Aotearoa New Zealand. This rural nursing discourse identified in this research identifies the rural nurse with pioneering spirit; as an entrepreneurial practitioner involving what nurses' express, as the 'rural way'. From their innovative practice emerged the contemporary identity of the nurse practising in the rural context which has uncovered the discourse of rural nursing in New Zealand in the twenty-first century and amplified rural nurse voices. This pioneering spirit initially identified in the 1990s has continued in a similar vein, during the COVID-19 pandemic into the 2020s. It is now timely to add to the international dialogue a specific New Zealand discussion and discourse.

Acknowledgements

The authors wish to thank the rural nurses who gave up their valuable time to share their stories and agreed for them to be published in *Stories of nursing in rural Aotearoa: A landscape of care*. Sincere thanks are extended to our colleagues Raeleen Thompson and Rachel Parmee for their dedication as they also interviewed rural nurses as part of this research. Further acknowledgment is extended to Otago Polytechnic, Dunedin New Zealand for contestable funding in support of this research between 2016 and 2021.

Conflict of interest

The authors declare they have no conflict of interest.

Author details

Jean Ross*, Josie Crawley and Rachel Parmee
College of Health, Otago Polytechnic, Dunedin, New Zealand

*Address all correspondence to: jean.ross@op.ac.nz

References

[1] Barnett JR, Barnett P. Primary health care in New Zealand: Problems and policy approaches. Social Policy Journal of New Zealand Te Pura Whakaaro. 2004;**21**:49-66

[2] Matherson D, Neuwelt P. New Zealand's journey towards people-centred care. The International Journal of Person-Centred Medicine. 2013;**2**(1):73-79

[3] Barnett JR, Barnett P. Reinventing primary health care: The New Zealand case compared. In: Crooks VA, Andrews GA, editors. Primary Health Care: People, Practice, Place. Farnham, England: Ashgate; 2009. pp. 149-165

[4] Prince R, Kearns R, Craig D. Governmentality, discourse and space in the New Zealand health care system 1991-2003. Health & Place. 2006;**12**:253-266

[5] National Health Committee. Rural Health: Challenges of Distance Opportunities for Innovation. Wellington, New Zealand: National Health Committee; 2010

[6] Dalziel P, Saunders C. Wellbeing Economics: Future Directions for New Zealand. Wellington, New Zealand: Bridget Williams Books Publishing Trust with the G & N Trust; 2014

[7] Carryer J, Halcomb E, Davidson PM. Nursing the answer to primary health care. Collegion. 2015;**22**(2):151-152

[8] Eyre R, Gauld R. Community participation in a rural community health trust: The case of Lawrence, New Zealand. Health Promotion International. 2003;**18**(3):189-197

[9] Gauld R. Revolving Doors: New Zealand's Health Reforms. Wellington, New Zealand: Institute of Policy Studies Victoria University; 2001

[10] Ministry of Health. Primary Health Care Strategy. Wellington, New Zealand: Ministry of Health; 2001

[11] Bushy A. Orientation to Nursing in the Rural Community. Thousand Oaks, California: Sage Publications; 2000

[12] Macleod M, Browne AJ, Leipert B. International Perspective: Issues for nurses in rural and remote Canada. 2008;**6**(2):72-78

[13] Hegney D, Francis K, Mills J. Rural health. In: Frances K, Chapman Y, Davies C, editors. Rural Nursing: The Australian Context. Australia: Cambridge University Press; 2014. pp. 18-33

[14] Ross J. Place Matters to Rural Nurses. Department of Geography: University of Otago, Dunedin, New Zealand; 2016

[15] Ross J, Mann S, Leonard G. Rural nursing during the COVID-19 pandemic: A snapshot of nurses' experiences from Aotearoa New Zealand. Journal of Nursing Practice. 2020;**3**(1):186-192

[16] Clandinin J. Engaging in Narrative Inquiry. New York: Routledge; 2013

[17] Crawley JM. "Once upon a time": A discussion of children's picture books as a narrative education tool for nursing students. The Journal of Nursing Education. 2009;**46**(1):36-39

[18] Haven KF. Storyproof: The Science Behind the Startling Power of the Story. Libraries Unlimited: Westport, Connecticut; 2007

[19] Clandidin J, Connelly M. Narrative Inquiry: Experience and Story in Qualitative Research. San Francisco, CA: Jossey-Boss; 1998

[20] Ross J, Crawley J, editors. Stories of Nursing in Rural Aotearoa: A Landscape of Care. Dunedin, New Zealand: Rural Health Opportunities; 2018

[21] Birks M, Mills J. Grounded Theory: A Practical Guide. 2nd ed. London: Sage; 2015

[22] Nursing Council of New Zealand. The New Zealand Nursing Workforce: A Profile of Nurse Practitioners, Registered Nurses and Enrolled Nurses 2018-2019. Wellington: Te Kaunihera Tapuhi o Aotearoa/Nursing Council of New Zealand; 2019. Available from: https://www.nursingcouncil.org.nz/NCNZ/News

[23] Brooke L, Hogarth K. Māori rural nurses' stories and their connections to communities: A thematic analysis. Scope: Kaupapa Kāi Tahu. 2021;**6**:62-71

[24] Nursing Council of New Zealand. Nursing Council of New Zealand Annual Report 2015. Wellington, New Zealand: Nursing Council of New Zealand. Available from: https://www.parliament.nz/en/pb/papers-presented/current-papers/document/51DBHOH_PAP67663_1/nursing-council-of-new-zealand-annual-report-2015-e18

[25] Statistics New Zealand (2015) New Zealand in Profile: 2015. Wellington: Statistics New Zealand. Available from: http://www.stats.govt.nz/browse_for_stats/snapshots-of-nz/nz-in-profile-2015.aspx [Accessed: March 10, 2015]

[26] Hunter K, Cook C. Cultural and clinical practice realities of Māori nurses in Aotearoa New Zealand: The emotional labour of Indigenous nurses. Nursing Praxis in New Zealand. 2020;**36**(3):7-23. DOI: 10.36951/27034542.2020.011

[27] Ross J, Kemp T, London M, Jones S. Growing Rural Health: Tipu Haere Tuawhenus Hauora: 30 Years of Advocacy and Support in Aotearoa. Dunedin, New Zealand: Hauora Taiwhenua Rural Health Network; 2022

[28] Baum T. The fascination of islands: A tourist perspective. In: Lockhart DG, Drakakis-Smith D, editors. Island Tourism: Trends and Prospects. London: Pinter; 1997. pp. 21-36

[29] Ross J. Editorial. Scope: Health & Wellbeing. 2021;**6**:7-8

[30] Dillon D. Rural contexts-Islands. In: Ross J, editor. Rural Nursing: Aspects of Practice. Dunedin: Rural Health Opportunities; 2008. pp. 19-30

Section 3

The Quality of Service in Rural Settings: A Multifacet Challenge

Chapter 9

Strategies towards Empowering Nurses on the Rational Use of Antiretrovirals in Children Initiated and Managed on Therapy in Rural Primary Healthcare Clinics of South Africa

Linneth Nkateko Mabila, Patrick Hulisani Demana and Tebogo Maria Mothiba

Abstract

HIV has affected the health and welfare of children and undermined the success of child survival in some countries. The introduction of antiretroviral therapy (ART) in managing HIV is one great public health success story. ART has commanded increased survival for people living with HIV (PLHIV). Barriers to achieving ART outcomes in children have been simplifying the prescribing process for non-paediatricians, such as medical doctors and nurses familiar with prescribing ART for adults but involved in treating children, particularly at the primary health care level. And the lack of appropriate antiretroviral formulations for children. The calculation of individualised doses for liquid oral ARVs for children at each clinic visit is considered complicated and time-consuming. ART failure among children seems to be an under-recognised issue, and adherence to treatment guidelines is reported to be a challenge among nurses caring for children and PLWHIV. Rational medicine use is essential to ensure the success of pharmacologic interventions. The attainment of ART goals depends on the effective use ARVs as recommended in guidelines. It is pivotal that nurses be empowered with strategies aimed at promoting the rational use of antiretrovirals.

Keywords: rational antiretroviral therapy use, children, nurses, rural primary healthcare clinics, antiretrovirals, South Africa

1. Introduction

The concept of rational use of medicines is old. It dates to 300 BC when the physician Herophilus said that "*medicines are nothing in themselves but are the very hands*

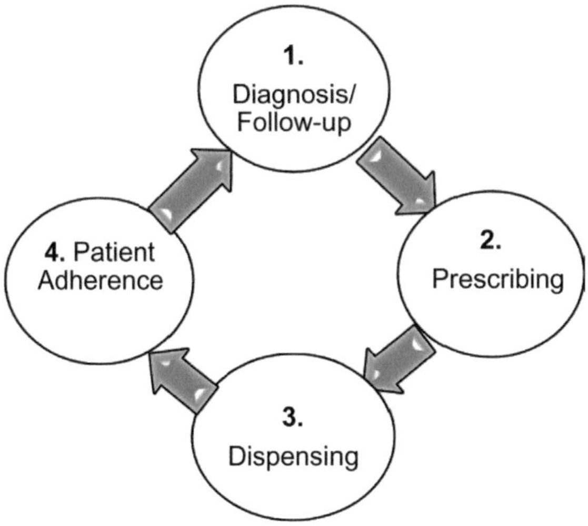

Figure 1.
Medicine use cycle.

of God if employed with reason and prudence" [1]. For many years, the rational use of medicines has been regarded as one of the critical principles of effective and quality health care [2, 3]. In 1985, the World Health Organisation (WHO) convened an expert meeting on the rational use of drugs, from which the rational use of drugs was defined as a contextual picture where "*Patients receive medications appropriate to their clinical needs, in doses that meet their requirements, for an adequate period, and at the lowest cost to them and their community*" [4]. The World Bank also defines the rational use of medical care as two fundamental principles, such as using medicines in accordance with scientific evidence for efficacy, safety, and compliance as well as the cost-effectiveness of the medicines in use within the constraints of a particular health system [4, 5].

Although the World Bank definition considers the financial capacity of medicine use in different countries, the WHO advocates using medicines at the lowest possible cost, regardless of the healthcare system [5]. The WHO and World Bank definitions are primarily based on therapeutic and medical perspectives. Reasonable use of drugs can also be seen from the consumer or patient's point of view. What is considered beneficial from a medical point of view may be regarded as unreasonable by the patient and vice versa [6]. From a medical point of view, improper use of drugs can begin in one of four major stages (**Figure 1**) of the medicines use cycle [2].

Even though half of the patients take almost half of their medicines correctly, half of all medicines are inappropriately used worldwide. The inappropriate use of medicines leads to resistance development, medication therapy problems, and increased medicine and treatment costs [7]. Therefore, both medical and patient perspectives need to be considered to gain a complete understanding of the rational use of drugs.

2. History of antiretroviral therapy in South Africa

When the South African national Antiretroviral Therapy (ART) Program was launched in 2004. It was utterly dependent on the hospital's HIV clinic, where ART services were provided exclusively by medical doctors [8–10]. This means that ART and care at SA at the time were limited to several selected accredited health clinics due to the presence of doctors in these clinics. Most public clinics were run and operated by nurses, so ART services were only seen in hospitals. The doctor then managed the ART program, performed a health examination, and initiated and prescribed treatment for the patient in need. Nurses were not allowed to treat HIV patients or prescribe or administer ART [10]. This practice resulted in the overcrowding of hospital facilities following an increasing demand for HIV care with limited personnel. Consequently, poor management of patients on ART necessitated the decentralisation of services to PHC clinics, rendering nurses essential to managing patients living with HIV [11–14].

Hence, managing the HIV/AIDS pandemic made SA struggle to reply to the troubling impact of HIV/AIDS in conjunction with upholding its democratic mandate to give equitable access to health services progressively. These challenges forced the government to rethink and reorganise its health resources and systems because of the reconsideration of the roles and responsibilities of nurses within the management and care of chronic and complicated diseases [15]. For example, in April 2010, ART was granted a presidential mission stipulating that ART is currently available in all 5500 South African public clinics. It required SA to revise the HIV treatment guidelines in 2010 and request nurses in primary care clinics to enrol for the Nurse-Initiated-and-Managed Antiretroviral Therapy (NIMART) training [16]. The mandate also meant that nurses should be trained to prescribe and treat patients with ART. NIMART has changed the role of HIV treatment and management.

The spread of HIV has led to innovations in the areas of nurse training, job shifts, retention, and practice. This expansion of HIV services was designed to meet the urgent needs of prevention, care, and treatment and embrace the vision of decentralised HIV services to PHCs [15]. Van Damme et al. [17] emphasise that the adoption of ART to reasonable levels, like primary health care, has increased ART access for PLHIV.

Following the implementation of task shifting, it was reported that a total of 2552 public clinics were involved in initiating and caring for patients on ART by April 2011. By March 2015, this number had reached 3591 public clinics [18]. As the numbers grew, training needed to be widened and improved since NIMART required nurses to assess, diagnose, and manage patients with HIV. Nurses, therefore, need to be equipped with skills such as history taking, physical assessment, interpretation of laboratory results, and knowledge about the pharmacological interaction of antiretroviral drugs [19]. The main reason for this integration approach was that in SA, PHC is an identified level of care that reaches most South Africans. Therefore, it is a relevant platform for the ART programme to reach all those in need [20].

Crowley and Stellenberg [21] cautioned that, even though HIV services are a decisive part of PHC, public clinics need to be sufficiently equipped for them to be able to provide quality HIV services to children on ART. This seems to be a global challenge in that Portillo et al. [22] highlight a San Francisco reality that the increasing demand for PHC services and the current healthcare personnel shortage is foreseen to cause compelling reductions in the number of healthcare professionals who are competent to provide HIV care. Moreover, Meyers et al. [23] had foreseen this situation and said that "*there has been a dramatic increase in ART access for HIV-infected children in SSA*". However, the availability of adequate care and treatment programs remains limited. Hence, it is essential to note that the decentralisation of services to rural PHC facilities without the provision of sufficient Human Resources (HR), as well as constant support, could compromise the quality of care provided to patients at this level with long-term repercussions for reaching the National strategic plan (NSP), strategic developmental and global health goals.

Meyers et al. [23] emphasised that essential HIV care, treatment services, and managerial support are vital components for ensuring quality services. Furthermore, they highlight that the provision of ART at the PHC level should be supported with human resources and the implementation process of comprehensive models to decentralise HIV care effectively. In the era of Sustainable Development Goals (SDGs), the UNAIDS set countries the ambitious "90-90-90" target of eradicating global infection with HIV by 2030. This required that by 2020, 90% of people living with HIV would know their status, 90% of whom would be on ART, and 90% of the latter would be virally suppressed [24].

3. HIV care in children and the prevention- of -mother- to- child- transmission

The SA programme for the prevention- of -mother- to- child- transmission (PMTCT) of HIV has, in recent years, achieved noteworthy successes in ensuring good outcomes for pregnant women living with HIV and reducing the risk of vertical HIV transmission to their children [25]. Despite having a persistently high antenatal HIV prevalence of around 30%, South Africa (SA) has made excessive developments in reducing the vertical transmission of HIV in children, especially in their first two months of life, from around 23% in 2003 to about 0.7% in 2019 [26]. Improving ART access during antenatal care has contributed significantly to this success. The integration of ART initiation into Antenatal Care (ANC) is associated with higher levels of ART initiation during pregnancy [27]. Still, it has led to an increase in the relative proportion of vertical transmissions due to breastfeeding in the first six months post-delivery [26].

4. Complexities in the management of children on antiretroviral therapy

The introduction of the NIMART programme in rural clinics brought the emergence of new challenges regarding prescribing and dispensing ART by nurses [28]. The Millennium Development Goals (MDGs) era also confirmed that children living with HIV continue to have less access to HIV services than adults [24]. Issues of ARV tolerability and access to formulations appropriate for children also remain. For instance, the Lopinavir/ritonavir (LPV/r) formulation is very unpleasant to taste. Infants often tend to tolerate it when their taste buds are still undeveloped but spit or vomit it out as the taste buds develop and they grow older [29, 30]. In South Africa, only in 2020 did the LPV/r pellets become available in the state and private sectors. These pellets are developed to overcome challenges with administration and storage experienced with the previously available tablet and syrup formulations for paediatric HIV patients [30, 31].

5. The goal of antiretroviral therapy in children

ART aims at reducing the rate of replication of HIV and breaking its progression into AIDS [32–36]. The use of ART is the basis of clinical interventions that can be used to prevent the transmission and progression of HIV infection in people living with HIV/AIDS. Even though ART does not destroy the virus and cannot cure HIV or AIDS-related illnesses, it significantly reduces the viral load. It slows disease progression, thus increasing the life expectancy and quality of life of PLHIV [37]. Furthermore, when effectively used in children, ART has been shown to improve growth and virologic and immune responses [38–42]. Mortality due to HIV infection in children has meaningfully decreased in the era of effective ART [43, 44]. Quality of life is an essential ART outcome [45] in developing countries that have not been solved yet. The range of HIV/AIDS problems measured by the number of affected children is extensive [46].

6. Challenges with antiretroviral therapy

A noted obstacle towards achieving widespread paediatric ART coverage has been the simplification of the prescribing process for non-paediatricians, including medical doctors and nurses who are more familiar with prescribing ART for adults but also involved in initiating and managing children on ART, particularly in rural primary care levels of South Africa [31]. The calculation of individualised doses for children, especially for liquid oral ARV formulations for infants or young children at each clinic visit using the current weight or body surface area, is also observed to be a complicated and time-consuming process for nurses in resource-limited settings [31, 47]. The development and updating of an integrated weight-based ARV dosing chart for children based on WHO guidelines and adapted for the ARV formulations available in South Africa has contributed to building confidence among prescribing clinicians and pharmacists and helped facilitate children's access to ART [31].

6.1 Adherence to ART in children

The main goal of antiretroviral therapy is to reduce the viral load (VL) in the blood to undetectable levels. Over the decades of ART, various scientists have determined that adhering to this treatment is essential for patients to experience the full benefits of ART, which include the overall and permanent suppression of viral replication, reduced destruction of CD4 cells, the prevention of viral resistance, the promotion of immune reconstitution, and a decreased disease progression. ART improves the prognosis of people living with HIV and reduces HIV-related morbidity and mortality, as well as the development of other opportunistic infections [48–50]. DiMatteo [51] defines this as the extent to which a patient's drug-consuming behaviour aligns with the doctor's recommendations. Although essential, ART compliance is often challenging for people treating ART, especially children. Factors affecting a children's ART compliance include (i) the caregiver, (ii) the child himself, (iii) the prescribed medication or treatment, (iv) socio-economic status, and (v) the provision of services [51–55]. The degree to which patients are compliant with their treatment regimen is an essential determinant of clinical success [56, 57].

There is no generally accepted measure of ART compliance, and each method has various strengths and weaknesses, as well as cost, complexity, accuracy, accuracy, aggression, and bias. Therefore, developing real-time ART adherence monitoring tools can change the development of new preventive strategies to improve adherence. Ultimately, applying these strategies may prove to be the only cost-effective way to reduce morbidity and mortality in individuals and reduce the likelihood of HIV transmission and the emergence of resistance in the community [58].

6.2 Medication errors

Aronson has since 2009 defined medication errors as a failure in the treatment process that leads to or has the potential to harm the patient. Furthermore, he emphasises that medication errors can take place;

i. Whilst deciding which medicine and dosage regimen to use. These are often referred to as prescribing faults, and they encompass irrational, inappropriate, and ineffective prescribing, under-prescribing, as well as over-prescribing,

ii. When writing the prescription (prescription errors),

iii. During manufacturing of the formulation (wrong strength, contaminants, or adulterants, wrong or misleading packaging),

iv. Whilst dispensing the formulation (wrong drug, wrong formulation, and wrong label),

v. During administering or taking medicine (wrong dose, wrong route, wrong frequency, and wrong duration),

vi. Whilst monitoring therapy (failing to alter therapy when required, erroneous alteration).

These errors can be categorised with the help of psychological classifications such as knowledge, rules, behaviour, and memory-based errors. Dosing mistakes can sometimes be serious, but often they are not trivial. However, system failures that lead to minor errors can later lead to fatal errors, so it is essential to identify them. Velo and Minuz [59] predicted that bug reporting should be encouraged by creating an impeccable, non-immunity environment. In addition, prescription mistakes are irrational, inappropriate, and ineffective. There are also recipe spelling mistakes, including the indecipherability of the written recipe. Avoid dosing mistakes in balanced prescribing, that is, the use of drugs adapted to the patient's condition and dosages that optimise the ratio of benefit to harm within the uncertainty associated with therapeutic decisions.

In clinical practice, the separation of prescribing and dispensing activities is considered a *"safety mechanism to ensure an additional independent assessment of the proposed therapy before the patient begins treatment"* [60]. In some settings, such as rural areas with limited health personnel [61], dispensing may be carried out by the prescriber, such as dispensing nurse(s). This is considered *"non-ideal and may promote irrational prescribing, especially if the prescriber stands to gain financially"* [62].

When the prescribing and dispensing functions are separated, proper therapeutic knowledge of the dispensing process is essential to check the prescribing gap and provide the prescriber with necessary recommendations or interventions. Therefore, contact between the prescriber and the patient is important because it can significantly impact the patient's medicine use practice. For example, compliance may improve only if the patient understands the importance of taking the medication, can follow the instructions appropriately, and is aware of the risk of non-compliance [63, 64].

On the other hand, the WHO advocates that *"the rational dispensing principle should be followed to ensure that patients receive adequate information regarding the use of dispensed medicines to achieve the desired benefits. For instance, if dispensing practices such as counting, packaging, and labelling is poorly executed; they are likely to impact the patient's confidence in the dispensed products, and subsequently compliance to therapy"* [65, 66].

7. Healthcare professionals' compliance to treatment guidelines

The appropriate use and monitoring of ARVs have resulted in the enhancement of patient's quality of life [67]. The implementation of task-shifting in South Africa and the decentralisation of ART [68] brought forth noticeable evidence of improved health outcomes, quality of care, and patient satisfaction for PLHIV [69, 70]. In South Africa HIV treatment guidelines, standard treatment guidelines and essential medicine lists are in place as a monitoring and support tool for healthcare professionals to ensure that they appropriately prescribe medicines and can provide good quality care to PLWHIV. There is also a recent (2019) South African National Guideline for the Prevention of Mother-to-Child- Transmission outlining three major strategies for programme improvement. These strategies aim at

1. "*the prevention of primary HIV infection and unintended pregnancies in women of childbearing potential,*

2. *the improvement of maternal viral suppression rates at delivery and in the post-delivery period through potent, well-tolerated antiretroviral regimens, strategic use of maternal viral load monitoring, linking of mothers to post-delivery HIV care, and integration of mother-infant health care, and*

3. *the provision of enhanced prophylaxis to infants of mothers with elevated HIV viral loads in the breastfeeding period, while every effort is made to regain maternal viral suppression*" [26].

Patient safety is a strategic goal and a central value in nursing practice. It is provided through an error-free medication administration which is essential towards achieving positive patient clinical outcomes for patients. In practice, there are therefore a set of guidelines that nurses are required to follow to ensure patient safety. Even though the nurses' adherence to treatment guidelines and factors associated with non-adherence to treatment guidelines among nurses remain under explored [71, 72]. Studies demonstrate a suboptimal adherence to guidelines by all prescribers, and a need for training on the use of these guidelines as well as improved monitoring of compliance at PHC level has been identified [71–73].

8. Strategies for addressing the irrational prescribing of medicines

Generally, the irrational prescribing of medicines is considered a "*disease*" that is difficult to treat even though it is possibly preventable [74]. Therefore, there are several strategies that are aimed at changing patients and prescribing behaviour to encourage the rational prescribing of medicines. These strategies can generally be grouped into targeted or system-oriented approaches [2]. Targeted methods include educational, business, and system-oriented strategies include regulatory and economic interventions [2, 74, 75]. Educational interventions are often aimed at persuading or informative, including printed matter, seminars, or face-to-face contact [76].

Inappropriate medicine management occurs at all levels of the healthcare system, both in hospitals and primary health care. The factors influencing the irrational use of medicines are usually very complex. They are associated with the attitudes of prescribers who are often convinced of the effectiveness of a particular therapy without considering

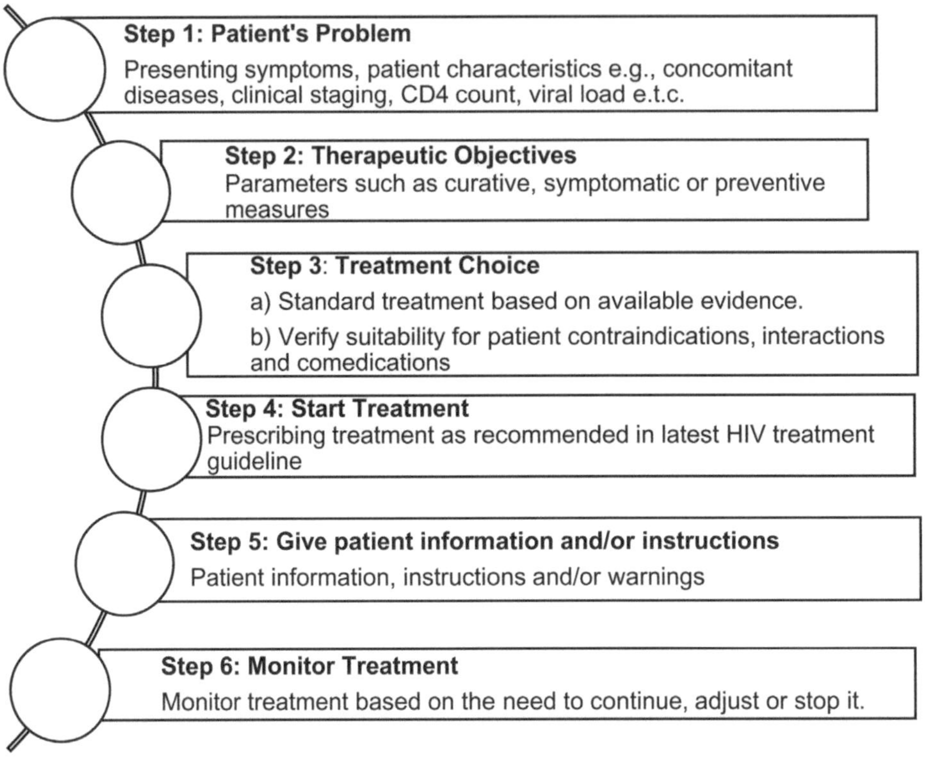

Figure 2.
Rational ARV prescribing cycle (adapted from the WHO-6-step of rational prescribing a guide to good prescribing).

other alternatives, too much staff responsibilities, patient's pressure on the use of a specific drug, lack of knowledge in the field of pharmacoeconomics, and others [77].

According to Wettermark et al. [78] educational interventions can affect the knowledge and awareness of prescribing physicians. Still, their effectiveness in behavioural change remains modest when not combined with other strategies. On the other hand, managerial techniques are specially aimed towards guiding practice. Such managerial interventions that can be hired consist of monitoring, supervision and feedback, the usage of a restrictive drug treatments list, drug utilisation reviews, or the usage of based prescription forms [75]. An example in this case is the "*Swedish Wiselist*". This is the Essential Medicines List (EML), which adheres to only 200 medicines to increase physician familiarity with quality medicines and reduce costs, complemented by regular medical oversight to specialists [79]. Economic strategies, on the other hand, aim to promote positive financial incentives while eliminating the awkward incentives of prescribing physicians [80]. Embrey and Hogerzeil [2, 75] say that economic interventions could include introducing significant changes to the healthcare provider's reimbursement system or banning prescribing drug sales.

In South Africa, to meet the basic constitutional human rights to health care, the new government commissioned a committee that specifically looked at medicine issues, this gave rise to the National Drug Policy (NDP) of 1996. The aim of the NDP is to address deficiencies such as the irrational medicine use, inaccessibility to medicines and cost-ineffectiveness treatment, and inefficient procurement and logistic practices to "ensure an adequate and reliable supply of safe, cost-effective drugs of acceptable quality to all citizens of South Africa, thereby promoting the rational use of drugs by prescribers, dispensers, and consumers". The NDP allowed for the provision of the Provision of the EML guided guided by the Standard Treatment Guidelines (STGs) through the National Essential Drugs Programme [81].

For the intervention to be very effective, it should be targeted at the clinic or prescribers who have the utmost need for improvement, with a particular focus on the identified prescribing behaviours [2, 75]. In some cases, several interventions may often be required to make the necessary changes. Again, it is worth noting that the efforts to promote rational medical care and prescribing should be multifaceted, including the address of aspects of patient and community behaviour [82, 83]. The six steps method of pharmacotherapy education promoted by the WHO (see **Figure 2**) need to be executed in every medical and nursing curriculum "*as part of an integrated learning program which has positive effects on medical students' knowledge of basic and applied pharmacology, pharmacotherapy skills, and satisfaction and confidence in prescribing*." [84].

9. Strategies for promoting the rational use of antiretroviral therapy

Failure of ART in children is an underestimated problem and is not adequately addressed by paediatrics and HIV treatment programs. The failure rate of paediatric ART in facilities with limited resources ranges from 19.3% to over 32%, so a comprehensive analysis of the causes of failure and an approach to addressing impaired adherence to treatment are urgently needed [85, 86].

Studies by Davies et al. [87] and Bunupuradah et al. [88] indicate that a high proportion of virological failures were observed in children in an established HIV primary care environment. These studies also found that the average age at which ART began in this cohort of primarily vertically infected children was 3.4 years, and the need to identify HIV-infected children early is latent. It suggests that you are missing out on the opportunity for a typical diagnosis. In addition, one-third of these children are said to have never achieved virological suppression since they were initiated on treatment. An inadequate system can explain this persistent viremia in the clinic to find a failed child or the lack of clinician knowledge or convenience to manage high viral loads. This is well reflected in the proportion of children (80%) who remained unchanged despite long-term antiretroviral therapy failures. One-fifth of patients aged 10–15 years were not fully disclosed at the start of the study, and this is a known risk factor for ART failure in children [87, 88].

These researchers also emphasise that VL testing in children on ART in resource-constrained environments should be prioritised over monitoring CD4 cell counts to reduce the time it takes for treatment to fail. They also suggest that this facilitates the appropriate conversion of children to secondary ART therapy and minimises immunological disorders. In addition, clinicians need to understand that the most important factor in good paediatric HIV management is achieving reasonable compliance [89]. Furthermore, they point out that easier ways of supporting adherence are very important in frequently visited clinics. This has been shown to significantly improve the quality of patient support that children and their caregivers receive. It is crucial for the nurses to keep in mind that adherence support should not be initiated when a child has a high VL. Very often, proper basic counselling on adherence is not provided until the child fails treatment, so once the child reaches a developmental milestone, proper counselling should be initiated and reassessed at the beginning of ART. Regular and continuous counselling is essential for paediatric patients, as the psychosocial situation of paediatric patients often changes and new barriers to adherence usually arise [90]. Providing paediatric antiretroviral care, particularly at PHC clinics, has distinct obstacles. One of these is a shortage of staff, which includes staff that is comfortable dealing with children [91]. Paediatric ART failure is an under-recognised issue that receives inadequate attention in the field of paediatrics and within HIV treatment programmes. With paediatric ART failure rates ranging from 19.3% to over 32% in resource-limited settings, a comprehensive evaluation of the causes of failure, along with approaches to address barriers to treatment adherence, is urgently needed [90].

In summary, one-third of children aged 0–19 in two HIV clinics with expanded primary care failed to achieve antiretroviral therapy, and 33% did not achieve virus suppression after the initiation of ART. Hence, by addressing the core deficiencies in paediatric HIV care, such as insufficient early diagnosis of HIV-infected children, lack of VL monitoring and clinician comfort in responding to high VLs, and the unstructured and inadequate adherence counselling, we will start to achieve durable VL suppression in children and control this silent epidemic [91]. This will help HIV/AIDS programmes to achieve long-lasting VL suppression within the paediatric HIV population and curb this silent epidemic. An effective response to the challenges of HIV treatment failure in LMICs must include reductions in the cost of second-line agents [92].

The strategies should be comprehensive, evidence-based, and focused on the rational long-term use of ART in children and adolescents [93–95]. Although early mortality and retention in care has been identified by different scholars as early as the year 2002 to be remaining as a significant challenge in HIV programmes, the majority of reports from low- and middle-income countries (LMICs) had in the past decade shown encouraging immunological, virological, and survival outcomes [96–103], with lower than expected reported rates of switching to second-line ART regimens [104, 105], and this was back then attributed to being in part due to actual rates of treatment success, but mainly because of the limited access to both virological monitoring and the unavailability of second-line antiretroviral drugs [105]. In a study by Orrell et al. [106], clinicians were found to be reluctant to switch treatments due to the cost of the regimen, the complexity of the regimen, the inconvenience, and the lack of subsequent treatment options. With the maturation and expansion of the cohort and increased access to virological monitoring and second-line treatment, an increased failure rate of diagnosed treatment and a switch to second-line treatment were expected [107]. This is because the cost of second-line treatment is higher than the cost of first-line treatment. These increases are due to the HIV treatment programs [108–110]. Elliott et al. [111] identified the need for rational ART use in LMICs, which relies heavily on accurately identifying medical malpractices and optimising the timing of the clinician's switch to alternative therapies. In addition, consider various factors such as availability, risk, and benefit substitution to assess the risk of HIV drug resistance and reduced therapeutic efficacy, immunological and clinical progression, and inappropriate early switching of patients. Rivera et al. [112] indicated that HIV resistance develops due to low ARV drug levels because of several factors and variations in drug absorption and metabolism and noncompliance owing to adverse effects or a poor understanding of the importance of the medication. The monitoring of VLs must guide effective treatment [113]. Hence, the recommendation is that the following two conditions are adhered to: Firstly, adequate plasma drug levels must be maintained as results may be inconclusive if adherence is not satisfactory or if the prescribed regimen has not been followed. In addition, the quality of drugs, bioavailability, and drug-drug interactions can affect the outcome. Secondly, the availability of alternative medicines must be assured [113].

10. Adherence to HIV treatment guidelines

The appropriate use and monitoring of ARVs have resulted in the enhancement of patient's quality of life. However, Elliott et al. [111] contend that the complexity of treatment regimens, over and above a multitude of factors such as drug intolerance, poverty, and the level of education of patients, directly influenced the lack of adherence. This also directly influences resistance and treatment failure. Hence, the rational use of ART in LMICs is critically dependent on clinicians' precise detection of treatment failure [111]. The proper use and monitoring of ARV has dramatically improved the patient's quality of life in recent years. However, the complex nature of these therapies, in addition to various factors such as drug resistance, socio-economic status, and the level of patient education, can reduce patient compliance and increase resistance and treatment failure potential. On the other hand, prescribing errors in ART management are said to be common in inpatients [114].

The rational use of ART in LMICs relies heavily on the accurate detection of TF and optimisation of the timing of switching to alternative therapies. Monitoring and switching strategies aim to balance the risk of HIV drug resistance with reduced efficacy of second-line treatment, immunological and clinical progression, and inappropriate early switching. Current and future status of alternative therapies and general medicine availability [111].

There is no well-established link between antiretroviral usage and the development of virological, treatment, and immunological failure, except that virologic failure is highly dependent on the patient's adherence to the prescribed antiretroviral treatment. To the researcher's knowledge, the inappropriate use of ARVs by prescribers is a topic that has never been explored, especially evaluating its impact on the clinical outcomes it might pose to children on ART. When looking at antibiotics as an almost similar class of drugs to ARVs, the literature highlights that the well-established link between antimicrobial usage and the development of resistance emphasises the importance of developing strategies to improve antimicrobial prescribing. It further highlights the possible reasons for inappropriate prescribing: lack of education, misinterpretation of results, prescribing etiquette, and medication errors. These contribute to the increase in morbidity and mortality, the development of antimicrobial resistance, and healthcare costs to such an extent that studies have proven the importance of antimicrobial prescribing [115–117].

Similar to antimicrobials, there is no established nor existing reference for measuring the appropriateness of ART use. [118] highlight that compliance with local, national, and international guidelines as the standard for appropriate therapy is increasingly utilised to reduce subjectivity. Moreover, evaluating compliance to treatment guidelines provides a reproducible method for large-scale evaluations across multiple facilities, especially when sharing similar treatment guidelines such as the consolidated national guidelines for managing HIV/AIDS [119].

The appropriateness of every antiretroviral prescribed can be assessed according to classic criteria established for antimicrobial evaluation by Kunin, Tupasi and Craig [120] (see **Table 1**). Even though this criterion seems outdated, it has since been used and relied upon by many established researchers in appropriate antimicrobial use; for example, researchers such as Dailey et al. [121], Bishara et al. [122] and van Bijnen et al. [123] have all conducted their studies following this criterion depicted in **Table 1**.

Action	Description
Appropriate indication	**Correct choice in presence of one or more of the following):**
Correct choice of antiretroviral drug and correct administration and dosing instructions	1. Tuberculosis 2. Severe malnutrition 3. Neonates <28 days of age 4. Infants weighing <3 kg 5. Hepatitis
Inappropriate indication	**Inappropriate decision** • Selected regimen not suitable for the patient's age • Selected regimen not suitable for the patient's weight **Inappropriate choice** • Different ART needed, than what is prescribed: o unnecessary divergence from HIV/AIDS treatment guidelines o regimen spectrum was overly broad o regimen spectrum was not broad enough **Incorrect use** • Incorrect dose • Incorrect dosing frequency • Incorrect route of administration • Incorrect duration of therapy • Incorrect quantity dispensed **Insufficient information** • No information on whether ART switching was necessary • Insufficient clinical information on whether ART switching was needed **Inappropriate indication** • Inappropriate decision on regimen selection • Inappropriate choice of antiretroviral(s) • Incorrect use of antiretroviral(s)

Table 1.
Criteria for categorising the appropriateness of ART use in children (adapted from Kunin et al. [120]).

11. Good medical record-keeping in HIV/AIDS management

Inaccuracy in prescription writing, poor legibility of handwriting, the use of abbreviations and incomplete prescriptions contribute to the poor keeping of medical records. For example, omitting the total volume of the prescribed syrup or solution or the duration of the prescribed medicine can lead to misinterpretation by healthcare personnel. This can result in medicine dispensing and administration errors [59]. Hence, good nursing practice requires detailed record-keeping that is comprehensive, timely, and accurate. Because, without complete recording, there is no evidence to prove that medical care was offered to the patient [124, 125].

This is supported by the saying in nursing practice that '*what is not recorded has not been done*" [51]. Medication errors are common in general practice and hospitals. Both errors in the act of writing (prescription errors) and prescribing faults due to erroneous medical decisions can result in harm to patients. Any step in the prescribing process can generate errors. Slips, lapses, or mistakes are sources of errors, as in unintended omissions in the transcription of drugs. Faults in dose selection, omitted transcription, and poor handwriting are common. Inadequate knowledge or competence and incomplete information about clinical characteristics and previous treatment of individual patients can result in prescribing faults, including the use of potentially inappropriate medications. An unsafe working environment, complex or undefined procedures, and inadequate communication among healthcare personnel, particularly between doctors and nurses, have been identified as important underlying factors contributing to prescription errors and prescribing faults. Active interventions aimed at reducing prescription errors and prescribing faults are strongly recommended. These should be focused on the education and training of prescribers and the use of online support. The complexity of the prescribing procedure should be reduced by introducing automated systems or uniform prescribing charts to avoid transcription and omission errors. Feedback control systems and immediate review of prescriptions, which can be performed with the assistance of a hospital pharmacist, are also helpful. Audits should be performed periodically [51]. The inappropriate keeping of medical records can influence patient management and the endurance of medical care, leading to inadequate health care [126]. Therefore, the appropriate use of ARVs requires the nurses' understanding of good medical record-keeping and the importance of it in ART management. Patients' clinical records, clinic records, and administrative records are the necessary nursing practice records. Medical records explain all relevant patient details such as the history, clinical findings, diagnostic test results, pre and postoperative care, patient's progress, and pharmacological treatment. If written correctly, notes acquired in these records support a healthcare professional's correctness of treatment [127]. The appropriate keeping of records is important in nursing care in that it provides clear evidence of the care plan, the decisions made, the care delivered, and the information shared with the patient. It is a means of communication with multidisciplinary health team members [124–127].

12. Treatment support systems for the children on ART

The nurses in rural clinics need to facilitate local support systems for the parents and caregivers of children receiving ART, as well as identify local community support groups to support, help, and motivate the parents and caregivers of children receiving ART. Nurses need to remember that children depend solely on caregivers for adherence, treatment administration, and presenting to the clinic for a collection of their antiretroviral treatment. Additionally, caregivers can be their primary parents, guardians, older siblings, aunts, uncles, or grandmothers. As clinicians, you can support the parents/caregivers as they suffer emotional strain in caring for children on ART. Give information about support groups in the community of your facility. The emotional well-being of a parent/caregiver plays a huge role towards the child's adherence to treatment [128–130].

13. Knowledge of the rational and irrational medicine use concept

Promoting the rational use of ARVs will require effective policies and efficient collaboration between health professionals, patients, and the entire communities.

An adequate understanding of the relevant aspects of ARV use among all stakeholders is essential to drive collaborative efforts to address irrational ARV use. The tackling of irrational ARV use should be prioritised to improve healthcare delivery towards ensuring patient safety and allowing for optimal utilisation of the ARVs. Irrational prescribing often derives from a wrong medical decision because of a lack of knowledge or inadequate training. Adverse clinical outcomes can be related to a lack of knowledge or skill. Even the simple act of transcribing previous medications and collecting information as part of the medication history requires knowledge of pharmacotherapy and adequate information about the patient's clinical condition. Equally, the choice of dose requires information about the patient's clinical status and immediate verification of the appropriateness of treatment. The provision of continuous in-service training and mentorship on the rational use of ARVs is pivotal for nurses in PHC settings. In addition, the hospital's Drug and Therapeutics Committee should regularly evaluate ARV usage patterns in these clinics [7].

14. Lessons learned from South African primary healthcare ART programmes

In South Africa, initiating ART in primary care is the responsibility of NIMART-trained professional nurses. It is no doubt that the availability of NIMART-trained nurses in PHC clinics has tremendously improved patients' access to HIV services [18, 72, 131]. Task-shifting has brought paediatric ART initiation and management into the practice of NIMART-trained nurses. Therefore, the nurses must be equipped with the knowledge and skills vital for this role. The country also introduced the clinical mentoring manual for integrated services through the Department of Health [132], targeted mentorship introduced for nurses in primary health care, and it was found to enhance clinical expertise. Doctors or nurses can become clinical mentors if they undergo mentoring training. In addition, supervisory and mentoring support is viewed necessary to help improve nurses' confidence in managing paediatric ART patients. Literature, however, reveals that the sustained success of this approach is dependent on factors such as adequate training and effective support systems [131]. Lessons learned from SA also revealed that training, mentorship, and clinical practice experience are associated with knowledge and confidence of NIMART-trained nurses regarding the provision of ART services to children. These studies therefore *recommended "the strengthening of the current training and mentoring and ensuring that NIMART-trained nurses are provided with regular updates and sufficient opportunities for clinical practice"* [71, 72, 131, 133–135].

15. Conclusions

The irrational use of medicines occurs at all levels of health care. This practice is also observed in hospital settings, and it contributes to a decrease in the patient's quality of treatment and often causes negative health consequences. For this reason, it is essential to consider the adoption of appropriate training, mentorship, and support methods as a strategy for promoting the rational use of ARVs. These can be introduced in rural PHC settings to increase the safety and effectiveness of antiretroviral use. This approach has been witnessed in practice to lead to increased quality of life, improved patient care and confidence, and professional development because appropriately trained nurses have been observed to experience work satisfaction due to the difference they make in patients' lives.

Quality improvement strategies such as mentorship, clinic medical record audits, and automated prescribing systems where possible can be used to address knowledge gaps in practice.

Acknowledgements

This project received funding from the University of Limpopo's Staff Capacity Development Programme (UCDP), as well as funding from the National Research Foundation Black Academics Advancement Programme (BAAP) (previously known as) National Research Foundation (NRF) - First Rand Foundation (FRF) Sabbatical Grant (Ref No: NFSG180605340566, Grant No: 116803).

Conflict of interest

The authors in this study declare that there is no conflict of interest, financial or otherwise.

Notes/thanks/other declarations

None.

Author details

Linneth Nkateko Mabila[1*], Patrick Hulisani Demana[2] and Tebogo Maria Mothiba[3]

1 Department of Pharmacy, University of Limpopo, Polokwane, South Africa

2 School of Pharmacy, Sefako Makgatho Health Sciences University, South Africa

3 Faculty of Health Sciences, University of Limpopo, Polokwane, South Africa

*Address all correspondence to: nkateko.mabila@ul.ac.za

References

[1] Shivhare SC, Kunjwani HK, Manikrao AM, et al. Drugs hazards and rational use of drugs: A review. Journal of Chemical and Pharmaceutical Research. 2010;**2**:106-112

[2] MSH. MDS-3: Managing Access to Medicines and Health Technologies. Arlington, VA: Management Sciences for Health; 2012

[3] Gopalakrishnan S, Udayshankar PM, Rama R. Standard treatment guidelines in primary healthcare practice. Journal of Family Medicine and Primary Care. 2014;**3**:424

[4] May F. Whither 'rational' use of drugs? Journal of Pharmacy Practice and Research. 2008;**38**:89-91

[5] Bissell P, Morgall Traulsen J. Sociology and Pharmacy Practice. London, UK: Pharmaceutical Press; 2005. ISBN 978-0853696131

[6] Brahma D, Marak M, Wahlang J. Rational use of drugs and irrational drug combinations. International Journal of Pharmacology. 2012;**10**:1-5

[7] Melku L, Wubetu M, Dessie B. Irrational drug use and its associated factors at Debre Markos referral Hospital's outpatient pharmacy in East Gojjam, Northwest Ethiopia. SAGE Open Medicine. 2021;**9**:20503121211025144

[8] Fatti G, Grimwood A, Bock P. Better antiretroviral therapy outcomes at primary healthcare facilities: An evaluation of three tiers of ART services in four South African provinces. PLoS One. 2010;**5**:e12888

[9] Fairall L, Bachmann MO, Lombard C, et al. Task shifting of antiretroviral treatment from doctors to primary-care nurses in South Africa (STRETCH): A pragmatic, parallel, cluster-randomised trial. The Lancet. 2012;**380**:889-898

[10] Long LC, Rosen SB, Brennan A, et al. Treatment outcomes and costs of providing antiretroviral therapy at a primary health clinic versus a hospital-based HIV clinic in South Africa. PLoS One. 2016;**11**:e0168118

[11] Rosen S, Long L, Sanne I. The outcomes and outpatient costs of different models of antiretroviral treatment delivery in South Africa. Tropical Medicine & International Health. 2008;**13**:1005-1015

[12] Martinson N, Mohapi L, Bakos D, et al. Costs of providing care for HIV-infected adults in an urban, HIV clinic in Soweto, South Africa. Journal of Acquired Immune Deficiency Syndromes. 2009;**50**:327

[13] Long L, Brennan A, Fox MP, et al. Treatment outcomes and cost-effectiveness of shifting management of stable ART patients to nurses in South Africa: An observational cohort. PLoS Medicine. 2011;**8**:e1001055

[14] Meyer-Rath G, Brennan A, Long L, et al. Cost and outcomes of paediatric antiretroviral treatment in South Africa. AIDS. 2013;**27**:243-250

[15] Dohrn J, Nzama B, Murrman M. The impact of HIV scale-up on the role of nurses in South Africa: Time for a new approach. JAIDS: Journal of Acquired Immune Deficiency Syndromes. 2009;**52**:S27-S29

[16] Cameron D, Gerber A, Mbatha M, et al. Nurse initiation and maintenance

of patients on antiretroviral therapy: Are nurses in primary care clinics initiating ART after attending NIMART training? South African Medical Journal;**102**(2):98-100

[17] Van Damme W, Kober K, Kegels G. Scaling-up antiretroviral treatment in southern African countries with human resource shortage: How will health systems adapt? Social Science & Medicine. 2008;**66**:2108-2121

[18] Nyasulu JCY, Muchiri E, Mazwi S, et al. NIMART rollout to primary healthcare facilities increases access to antiretrovirals in Johannesburg: An interrupted time series analysis. South African Medical Journal. 2013;**103**:232-236

[19] Morris MB, Chapula BT, Chi BH, et al. Use of task-shifting to rapidly scale-up HIV treatment services: Experiences from Lusaka, Zambia. BMC Health Services Research. 2009;**9**:1-9

[20] Stein J, Lewin S, Fairall L, et al. Building capacity for antiretroviral delivery in South Africa: A qualitative evaluation of the PALSA PLUS nurse training programme. BMC Health Services Research. 2008;**8**:1-11

[21] Crowley T, Stellenberg EL. Integrating HIV care and treatment into primary healthcare: Are clinics equipped? African Journal of Primary Health & Family Medicine. 2014;**6**:1-7

[22] Portillo CJ, Stringari-Murray S, Fox CB, et al. The HIV primary care workforce of tomorrow: The UCSF integrated HIV/AIDS primary care capacity nurse practitioner program. The Journal of the Association of Nurses in AIDS Care. 2016;**27**:214-222

[23] Meyers T, Moultrie H, Naidoo K, et al. Challenges to pediatric HIV care and treatment in South Africa. The Journal of Infectious Diseases. 2007;**196**:S474-S481

[24] Nyasulu JC, Maposa I, Sikhakhane BP, et al. Access to HIV services and viral load suppression among children during the 90-90-90 strategy implementation in South Africa: A time series analysis. Southern African Journal of HIV Medicine. 2021;**22**:1-8

[25] UNAIDS. 2015 Progress report on the global plan towards the elimination of new HIV infections among children and keeping their mothers alive

[26] Wessels J, Sherman G, Bamford L, et al. Southern African Journal of HIV Medicine. 2019;**21**. Epub ahead of print 8 July 2020. DOI: 10.4102/sajhivmed.v21i1.1079

[27] Stinson K, Jennings K, Myer L. Integration of antiretroviral therapy services into antenatal care increases treatment initiation during pregnancy: A cohort study. PLoS One. 2013;**8**:e63328

[28] Crowley T, Stellenberg EL. An evaluation of the adequacy of pharmaceutical services for the provision of antiretroviral treatment in primary health care clinics. Health SA Gesondheid. 2015;**20**:83-90

[29] Kekitiinwa A, Musiime V, Thomason MJ, et al. Acceptability of lopinavir/r pellets (minitabs), tablets and syrups in HIV-infected children. Antiviral Therapy. 2016;**21**:579-585

[30] Pasipanodya B, Kuwengwa R, Prust ML, et al. Assessing the adoption of lopinavir/ritonavir oral pellets for HIV-positive children in Zimbabwe. Journal of the International AIDS Society. 2018;**21**:e25214

[31] Levin LJ, Horak JL, Nuttall J. Looking back at paediatric HIV treatment in

South Africa. My, how we have grown! Southern African Journal of HIV Medicine. 2021;**22**:1-3

[32] Arts EJ, Hazuda DJ. HIV-1 antiretroviral drug therapy. Cold Spring Harbor Perspectives in Medicine. 2012;**2**:a007161

[33] Deeks SG, Overbaugh J, Phillips A, et al. HIV infection. Nature Reviews Disease Primers. 2015;**1**:1-22

[34] Eggleton JS, Nagalli S. Highly active antiretroviral therapy (HAART). In: StatPearls. Treasure Island (FL): StatPearls Publishing; 2022. PMID: 32119420

[35] Ward AR, Mota TM, Jones RB. Immunological approaches to HIV cure. In: Seminars in Immunology. Elsevier; 2021. p. 101412

[36] Ta TM, Malik S, Anderson EM, et al. Insights into persistent HIV-1 infection and functional cure: Novel capabilities and strategies. Frontiers in Microbiology. 2022;**13**:760:Article862270

[37] Oguntibeju OO. Quality of life of people living with HIV and AIDS and antiretroviral therapy. HIV/AIDS (Auckland, N.Z.). 2012;**4**:117

[38] Palma P, Foster C, Rojo P, et al. The EPIICAL project: An emerging global collaboration to investigate immunotherapeutic strategies in HIV-infected children. Journal of Virus Eradication. 2015;**1**:134-139

[39] Ásbjörnsdóttir KH, Hughes JP, Wamalwa D, et al. Differences in virologic and immunologic response to antiretroviral therapy among HIV-1 infected infants and children. AIDS (London, England). 2016;**30**:2835

[40] Barlow-Mosha L, Musiime V, Davies M-A, et al. Universal antiretroviral therapy for HIV-infected children: A review of the benefits and risks to consider during implementation. Journal of the International AIDS Society. 2017;**20**:21552

[41] Kannigan Y, Spicer KB, Naby F. The use of illustrated medication diaries to improve outcomes for children initiated on highly active antiretroviral therapy. Southern African Journal of HIV Medicine. 2018;**19**:1-7

[42] Violari A, Cotton MF, Kuhn L, et al. A child with perinatal HIV infection and long-term sustained virological control following antiretroviral treatment cessation. Nature Communications. 2019;**10**:1-11

[43] Gesesew HA, Ward P, Woldemichael K, et al. Early mortality among children and adults in antiretroviral therapy programs in Southwest Ethiopia, 2003-15. PLoS One. 2018;**13**:e0198815:1-17

[44] Zeng X, Chen H, Zhu Q, et al. Treatment outcomes of HIV infected children after initiation of antiretroviral therapy in Southwest China: An observational cohort study. Frontiers in Pediatrics. 2022;**10**:Article916740

[45] Bunupuradah T, Kosalaraksa P, Vibol U, et al. Impact of antiretroviral therapy on quality of life in HIV-infected southeast Asian children in the PREDICT study. AIDS Patient Care and STDs. 2013;**27**:596-603

[46] Embree J. The impact of HIV/AIDS on children in developing countries. Paediatrics & Child Health. 2005;**10**:261-263

[47] Dakshina S, Olaru I, Khan P, et al. Evaluation of weight-based prescription of antiretroviral therapy in children. HIV Medicine. 2019;**20**:248-253

[48] Memirie ST. Clinical outcome of children on HAART at police

referral hospital, Addis Ababa, Ethiopia. Ethiopian Medical Journal. 2009;**47**:159-164

[49] Vreeman RC, Nyandiko WM, Ayaya SO, et al. The perceived impact of disclosure of pediatric HIV status on pediatric antiretroviral therapy adherence, child well-being, and social relationships in a resource-limited setting. AIDS Patient Care and STDs. 2010;**24**:639-649

[50] Kabue MM, Buck WC, Wanless SR, et al. Mortality and clinical outcomes in HIV-infected children on antiretroviral therapy in Malawi, Lesotho, and Swaziland. Pediatrics. 2012;**130**:e591-e599

[51] DiMatteo MR. Variations in patients' adherence to medical recommendations: A quantitative review of 50 years of research. Medical Care. 2004;**42**:200-209

[52] Martin S, Elliott-DeSorbo DK, Wolters PL, et al. Patient, caregiver and regimen characteristics associated with adherence to highly active antiretroviral therapy among HIV-infected children and adolescents. The Pediatric Infectious Disease Journal. 2007;**26**:61-67

[53] Prendergast A, Tudor-Williams G, Jeena P, et al. International perspectives, progress, and future challenges of paediatric HIV infection. The Lancet. 2007;**370**:68-80

[54] Haberer J, Mellins C. Pediatric adherence to HIV antiretroviral therapy. Current HIV/AIDS Reports. 2009;**6**:194-200

[55] Buchanan AL, Montepiedra G, Sirois PA, et al. Barriers to medication adherence in HIV-infected children and youth based on self-and caregiver report. Pediatrics. 2012;**129**:e1244-e1251

[56] Gardiner P, Dvorkin L. Promoting medication adherence in children. American Family Physician. 2006;**74**:793-798

[57] Mehta D, Kohn B, Blumenfeld M, et al. To assess the success of computerized order sets and pharmacy education modules in improving antiretroviral prescribing. Journal of Pharmacy Practice. 2018;**31**:450-456

[58] Nachega JB, Marconi VC, van Zyl GU, et al. HIV treatment adherence, drug resistance, virologic failure: Evolving concepts. Infectious Disorders—Drug Targets (Formerly Current Drug Targets—Infectious Disorders). 2011;**11**:167-174

[59] Velo GP, Minuz P. Medication errors: Prescribing faults and prescription errors. British Journal of Clinical Pharmacology. 2009;**67**:624-628

[60] Chou YJ, Yip WC, Lee C-H, et al. Impact of separating drug prescribing and dispensing on provider behaviour: Taiwan's experience. Health Policy and Planning. 2003;**18**:316-329

[61] Lim D, Emery JD, Lewis J, et al. Australian dispensing doctors' prescribing: Quantitative and qualitative analysis. The Medical Journal of Australia. 2011;**195**:172-175

[62] Ofori-Asenso R, Agyeman AA. Irrational use of medicines—A summary of key concepts. Pharmacy. 2016;**4**:35

[63] Aronson JK. Balanced prescribing. British Journal of Clinical Pharmacology. 2006;**62**:629

[64] Aronson JK. Medication errors: Definitions and classification. British Journal of Clinical Pharmacology. 2009;**67**:599-604

[65] Nadeshkumar A, Sathiadas G, Pathmeswaran A, et al. Prescribing,

dispensing and administration indicators to describe rational use of oral dosage forms of medicines given to children. WHO South-East Asia. Journal of Public Health.2019;**8**:42-49

[66] Nadeshkumar A, Sathiadas G, Sri Ranganathan S. Rational dispensing of oral dosage forms of medicines to children at a teaching hospital in Sri Lanka. BMC Health Services Research. 2020;**20**:1-6

[67] Ahmed A, Saqlain M, Bashir N, et al. Health-related quality of life and its predictors among adults living with HIV/AIDS and receiving antiretroviral therapy in Pakistan. Quality of Life Research. 2021;**30**:1653-1664

[68] Kredo T, Ford N, Adeniyi FB, et al. Decentralising HIV treatment in lower- and middle-income countries. Cochrane Database of Systematic Reviews. Sao-Paulo Medical Journal. 2014;**132**:383

[69] Emdin CA, Chong NJ, Millson PE. Non-physician clinician provided HIV treatment results in equivalent outcomes as physician-provided care: A meta-analysis. Journal of the International AIDS Society. 2013;**16**:18445

[70] Kredo T, Adeniyi FB, Bateganya M, et al. Task shifting from doctors to non-doctors for initiation and maintenance of antiretroviral therapy. Cochrane Database of Systematic Reviews. 2014;**7**: Article No: CD007331

[71] Makhado L, Mboweni SH. Challenges influencing nurse-initiated management of antiretroviral therapy training and implementation in Ngaka Modiri Molema district, North West province. Health SA Gesondheid. 2020;**25**:1-11

[72] Makhado L, Davhana-Maselesele M, Lebese RT, et al. Factors facilitating trained NIMART nurses' adherence to treatment guidelines: A vital matter in the management of TB/HIV treatment in South Africa. BMC Nursing. 2020;**19**:1-8

[73] Potter P, Perry A, Stockert P, et al. Fundamentals of Nursing, St. Louis. Missouri: Mosby;

[74] Hogerzeil HV, Barnes KI, Henning RH, et al. Teacher's guide to good prescribing. World Health Organization, Department of Essential Drugs and Medicines Policy. Geneva, Switzerland; 2001:1-106. Available from: http://apps.who.int/iris/bitstream/handle/10665/67010/WHO_EDM_PAR_2001.2.pdf?sequence=1

[75] Hogerzeil HV. Promoting rational prescribing: An international perspective. British Journal of Clinical Pharmacology. 1995;**39**:1-6

[76] Kamarudin G, Penm J, Chaar B, et al. Educational interventions to improve prescribing competency: A systematic review. BMJ Open. 2013;**3**:e003291

[77] Religioni U, Pakulska T. Rational drug use in hospital settings–areas that can be changed. Journal of Medical Economics. 2020;**23**:1205-1208

[78] Wettermark B, Godman B, Jacobsson B, et al. Soft regulations in pharmaceutical policy making. Applied Health Economics and Health Policy. 2009;**7**:137-147

[79] Gustafsson LL, Wettermark B, Godman B, et al. The 'wise list'—a comprehensive concept to select, communicate and achieve adherence to recommendations of essential drugs in ambulatory care in Stockholm. Basic & Clinical Pharmacology & Toxicology. 2011;**108**:224-233

[80] Gurbani N. Problems and impact of irrational medicines: Use and tools &

interventions to improve medicines use. Pharma Times. 2011;**43**:23-24

[81] National Drug Policy South Africa. National Drug Policy for South Africa. 2001:1-31

[82] Sabuncu E, David J, Bernède-Bauduin C, et al. Significant reduction of antibiotic use in the community after a nationwide campaign in France, 2002-2007. PLoS Medicine. 2009;**6**:e1000084

[83] Fürst J, Čižman M, Mrak J, et al. The influence of a sustained multifaceted approach to improve antibiotic prescribing in Slovenia during the past decade: Findings and implications. Expert Review of Anti-Infective Therapy. 2015;**13**:279-289

[84] Keijsers CJ, Segers WS, De Wildt DJ, et al. Implementation of the WHO-6-step method in the medical curriculum to improve pharmacology knowledge and pharmacotherapy skills. British Journal of Clinical Pharmacology. 2015;**79**:896-906

[85] Osman FT, Yizengaw MA. Virological failure and associated risk factors among HIV/AIDS pediatric patients at the ART clinic of Jimma University Medical Center, Southwest Ethiopia. Open AIDS Journal. 2020;**14**:61-67

[86] Getawa S, Fentahun A, Adane T, et al. Antiretroviral treatment failure and associated factors among HIV-infected children on antiretroviral therapy: A retrospective study. HIV/AIDS—Research and Palliative Care. 2021;**13**:229-237

[87] Davies M-A, Moultrie H, Eley B, et al. Virologic failure and second-line antiretroviral therapy in children in South Africa-The IeDEA Southern Africa Collaboration. Journal of Acquired Immune Deficiency Syndromes. 2011;**56**:270

[88] Bunupuradah T, Puthanakit T, Kosalaraksa P, et al. Immunologic and virologic failure after first-line NNRTI-based antiretroviral therapy in Thai HIV-infected children. AIDS Research and Therapy. 2011;**8**:1-6

[89] Gupta P, Patel P, Horne R, et al. How to screen for non-adherence to antihypertensive therapy. Current Hypertension Reports. 2016;**18**:1-8

[90] Bernheimer JM, Patten G, Makeleni T, et al. Paediatric HIV treatment failure: A silent epidemic. Journal of the International AIDS Society. 2015;**18**:20090

[91] Williams M, Van Rooyen DR, Ricks EJ. Provision of antiretroviral therapy for children in Nelson Mandela Bay: Health care professionals' challenges. African Journal of Primary Health & Family Medicine. 2018;**10**:1-10

[92] Ford N, Wilson D, Chaves GC, et al. Sustaining access to antiretroviral therapy in the less-developed world: Lessons from Brazil and Thailand. AIDS. 2007;**21**:S21-S29

[93] Fetzer BC, Mupenda B, Lusiama J, et al. Barriers to and facilitators of adherence to pediatric antiretroviral therapy in a sub-Saharan setting: Insights from a qualitative study. AIDS Patient Care and STDs. 2011;**25**:611-621

[94] Frigati L, Cotton M, Rabie H. Antiretroviral therapy for the management of HIV in children. South African Medical Journal. 2014;**104**:898

[95] Munyayi FK, van Wyk B. Interventions for improving treatment outcomes in adolescents on antiretroviral therapy with unsuppressed viral loads: A systematic review protocol. BMJ Open. 2021;**11**:e049452

[96] Laurent C, Diakhaté N, Fatou Ngom Gueye N, et al. The Senegalese government's highly active antiretroviral therapy initiative: An 18-month follow-up study. AIDS. 2002;**16**:1363-1370

[97] Weidle PJ, Malamba S, Mwebaze R, et al. Assessment of a pilot antiretroviral drug therapy programme in Uganda: Patients' response, survival, and drug resistance. The Lancet. 2002;**360**:34-40

[98] Kumarasamy N, Solomon S, Chaguturu SK, et al. The safety, tolerability and effectiveness of generic antiretroviral drug regimens for HIV-infected patients in south India. AIDS. 2003;**17**:2267-2269

[99] Seyler C, Anglaret X, Dakoury-Dogbo N, et al. Medium-term survival, morbidity and Immunovirological evolution in HIV-infected adults receiving antiretroviral therapy, Abidjan, Côte D'Ivoire. Antiviral Therapy. 2003;**8**:385-393

[100] Tassie J-M, Szumilin E, Calmy A, et al. Highly active antiretroviral therapy in resource-poor settings: The experience of Me'decins Sans Frontiers. AIDS. 2003;**17**:1995-1997

[101] Coetzee D, Hildebrand K, Boulle A, et al. Outcomes after two years of providing antiretroviral treatment in Khayelitsha, South Africa. AIDS. 2004;**18**:887-895

[102] Ivers LC, Kendrick D, Doucette K. Efficacy of antiretroviral therapy programs in resource-poor settings: A meta-analysis of the published literature. Clinical Infectious Diseases. 2005;**41**:217-224

[103] Ferradini L, Jeannin A, Pinoges L, et al. Scaling up of highly active antiretroviral therapy in a rural district of Malawi: An effectiveness assessment. The Lancet. 2006;**367**:1335-1342

[104] Pujades M, Calmy A, O'Brien D, et al. Second-line antiretroviral therapy in resource-limited settings: the experience of Medecins Sans Frontieres. Aids. 2008;**22**:1305-1312

[105] Renaud-Théry F, Nguimfack BD, Vitoria M, et al. Use of antiretroviral therapy in resource-limited countries in 2006: Distribution and uptake of first- and second-line regimens. AIDS. 2007;**21**:S89-S95

[106] Orrell C, Harling G, Lawn SD, et al. Conservation of first-line antiretroviral treatment regimen where therapeutic options are limited. Antiviral Therapy. International Medical Press; 2007;**12**:83-88

[107] Galárraga O, O'Brien ME, Gutiérrez JP, et al. Forecast of demand for antiretroviral drugs in low and middle-income countries: 2007-2008. AIDS. 2007;**21**:S97-S103

[108] Freedberg KA, Kumarasamy N, Losina E, et al. Clinical impact and cost-effectiveness of antiretroviral therapy in India: Starting criteria and second-line therapy. AIDS. 2007;**21**:S117-S128

[109] Greco DB, Simão M. Brazilian policy of universal access to AIDS treatment: Sustainability challenges and perspectives. AIDS. 2007;**21**:S37-S45

[110] Over M, Revenga A, Masaki E, et al. The economics of effective AIDS treatment in Thailand. AIDS. 2007;**21**:S105-S116

[111] Elliott JH, Lynen L, Calmy A, et al. Rational use of antiretroviral therapy in low-income and middle-income countries: Optimizing regimen sequencing and switching. AIDS. 2008;**22**:2053-2067

[112] Rivera DM, Frye RE, Steele RW, Pediatric HIV. Infection: Practice essentials, background. Pathophysiology. Medscape Reference. 07 April 2016:1-13

[113] Calmy A, Ford N, Hirschel B, et al. HIV viral load monitoring in resource-limited regions: Optional or necessary? Clinical Infectious Diseases. 2007;**44**:128-134

[114] Rao N, Patel V, Grigoriu A, et al. Antiretroviral therapy prescribing in hospitalized HIV clinic patients. HIV Medicine. 2012;**13**:367-371

[115] File TM Jr, Solomkin JS, Cosgrove SE. Strategies for improving antimicrobial use and the role of antimicrobial stewardship programs. Clinical Infectious Diseases. 2011;**53**:S15-S22

[116] Hurford A, Morris AM, Fisman DN, et al. Linking antimicrobial prescribing to antimicrobial resistance in the ICU: Before and after an antimicrobial stewardship program. Epidemics. 2012;**4**:203-210

[117] McGowan JE. Antimicrobial stewardship—The state of the art in 2011 focus on outcome and methods. Infection Control and Hospital Epidemiology. 2012;**33**:331-337

[118] Spivak ES, Cosgrove SE, Srinivasan A. Measuring appropriate antimicrobial use: Attempts at opening the black box. Clinical Infectious Diseases. 2016;**63**:1-6

[119] Osowicki J, Gwee A, Noronha J, et al. Australia-wide point prevalence survey of antimicrobial prescribing in neonatal units: How much and how good? The Pediatric Infectious Disease Journal. 2015;**34**:e185-e190

[120] Kunin CM, Tupasi T, Craig WA. Use of antibiotics: A brief exposition of the problem and some tentative solutions. Annals of Internal Medicine. 1973;**79**:555-560

[121] Dailey YM, Martin MV. Are antibiotics being used appropriately for emergency dental treatment? British Dental Journal. 2001;**191**:391-393

[122] Bishara J, Hershkovitz D, Pitlik S. P2100 appropriateness of antibiotic therapy on weekends vs weekdays. International Journal of Antimicrobial Agents. 2007;**29**:S607

[123] van Bijnen EM, den Heijer CD, Paget WJ, et al. The appropriateness of prescribing antibiotics in the community in Europe: Study design. BMC Infectious Diseases. 2011;**11**:1-5

[124] Mutshatshi TE, Mothiba TM, Mamogobo PM, et al. Record-keeping: Challenges experienced by nurses in selected public hospitals. Curationis. 2018;**41**:1-6

[125] Muyakui E, Nuuyoma V, Amukugo HJ. Record-keeping: A qualitative exploration of challenges experienced by undergraduate nursing students in selected clinical settings. Global Journal of Health Science. 2019;**11**:53-59

[126] Britz RM. Medical record-keeping in South Africa: A medico-legal perspective [PhD thesis]. University of Pretoria; 2018

[127] Bali A, Bali D, Iyer N, et al. Management of medical records: Facts and figures for surgeons. Journal of Oral and Maxillofacial Surgery. 2011;**10**:199-202

[128] Mafune RV, Lebese RT, Nemathaga LH. Challenges faced by caregivers of children on antiretroviral therapy at Mutale Municipality selected

healthcare facilities, Vhembe District, Limpopo Province. Curationis. 2017;**40**:e1-e9. Epub ahead of print 28 August 2017. DOI: 10.4102/curationis.v40i1.1541

[129] Buthelezi SF, Modeste RRM, Phetlhu DR. Barriers to the management of children under five exposed to HIV in the rural areas of South Africa. Curationis. 2021;**44**:2073. Epub ahead of print 8 March 2021. DOI: 10.4102/curationis.v44i1.2073

[130] Moosa-Tayob S, Risenga PR. Challenges of caregivers providing care to children with disabilities at non-governmental organisations in Tshwane townships, South Africa. African Journal of Disability. 2022;**11**:930. Epub ahead of print 28 July 2022. DOI: 10.4102/ajod.v11i0.930

[131] Esterhuizen TM, Solomons DJ, Van der Merwe AS, et al. Factors influencing the confidence and knowledge of nurses prescribing antiretroviral treatment in a rural and urban district in the Western Cape province. Southern African Journal of HIV Medicine. 2019;**20**:1-7

[132] Georgeu D, Colvin CJ, Lewin S, et al. Implementing nurse-initiated and managed antiretroviral treatment (NIMART) in South Africa: A qualitative process evaluation of the STRETCH trial. Implementation Science. 2012;**7**:1-13

[133] Green A, de Azevedo V, Patten G, et al. Clinical mentorship of nurse initiated antiretroviral therapy in Khayelitsha, South Africa: A quality of care assessment. PLoS One. 2014;**9**:e98389

[134] Mashudu MM. An evaluation of the effectiveness of the nurse-initiated-and managed antiretroviral treatment (NIMART) programme, Waterberg District, Limpopo Province [PhD thesis], 2016

[135] Crowley T, Mokoka E, Geyer N. Ten years of nurse-initiated antiretroviral treatment in South Africa: A narrative review of enablers and barriers. Southern African Journal of HIV Medicine. 2021;**22**:1-13

Chapter 10

An Analysis of Institutional Maternal Death Audit Reports in the Western Region of Ghana

Marion Okoh-Owusu, George Kojo Owusu, Celia Brown and Frank Baiden

Abstract

Institutional maternal deaths in the Western Region of Ghana increased from 133 in 2011 to 150 deaths per 100,000 live births in 2014. We reviewed available audit reports on deaths that occurred in 2014 in order to identify priorities for improvement. We undertook a manual search for audit reports and used a structured questionnaire to extract information on the sociodemographic characteristics of patients and the circumstances of care and death. We entered and analyzed the data using EPI-INFO (v.7). Analysis was largely descriptive. Audit reports were available for 75% of the 93 deaths recorded in the region in 2014. The mean (SD) age of death was 28 (±8) yrs. The majority (80%) involved women who made at least three Antenatal Clinic (ANC) visits. Hypertensive diseases (35.8%), hemorrhage (31.3%) and sepsis (7.5%) were the leading causes of death. Most (82%) deaths occurred in hospitals, with almost 75% after 24 hours of arrival. Data completeness and consistency were the major limitations in the analysis. There is a need to improve institutional maternal health care in the region, with interventions designed to address the causes of maternal deaths and to improve the survival of mothers and babies ultimately.

Keywords: maternal deaths, audit, mortality, descriptive, evidence-informed

1. Introduction

Globally 830 women die daily from preventable causes related to pregnancy and childbirth. Nearly all of these deaths occur in developing countries. Despite considerable efforts, maternal mortality in sub-Saharan Africa remains unacceptably high and falls short of the target set in Millennium Development Goals (MDGs) [1–3].

According to the Ghana Demographic and Health Surveys, maternal mortality in the country declined from 634 per 1000 live births in 1990 to 319 in 2015 [4, 5]. This represented an average annual rate of decline of 2.7%. Ghana has achieved this level of reduction in maternal mortality through the deployment of interventions that have improved access to maternal health services, including emergency obstetric care and skilled attendants at delivery. The most notable of the interventions was introduction of the fee-free delivery policy (FEP) in the country in 2005. This is reported to have contributed to increased access to skilled attendants at delivery and reduced maternal deaths. Overall, however, Ghana failed to achieve the MDG target of attaining a maternal mortality ratio of 185 deaths per 100,000 live births by 2015 [6, 7].

A problem that has persisted throughout the implementation of the fee-free delivery policy has been high number of avoidable maternal deaths within health facilities, that is, institutional deaths. Progress in reducing institutional maternal deaths has been slow, with reports of sustained high numbers of avoidable deaths in health facilities in the country [8–11]. A case in point is the increase in institutional maternal deaths in the Western Region of Ghana from 133 to 150 deaths per 100,000 live births between 2011 and 2014. Reducing institutional maternal deaths will be important if Ghana is to achieve the target set in the Sustainable Development Goals (SDGs) of 70 maternal deaths per 100,000 live births or less by 2030.

2. Maternal death audits

An important intervention introduced in Ghana in the early 2000s is the conduct of audits on all maternal deaths in health facilities in the country [12]. Such audits must be conducted within four weeks of the death, and hard copies of reports must be shared with District and Regional Health Management Teams [10]. The audits aim to establish the circumstances of death and identify service delivery factors that must be improved to prevent future deaths. All deaths are simultaneous to be entered into the District Health Information Management System-2 (DHIMS-2), the backbone electronic data capture system of the Ghana Health Service (GHS).

While the information on all maternal health audits is expected to be shared at the regional and national levels, district and regional health management teams are also encouraged to periodically analyze the data that are made available to them to identify areas of generating generalizable knowledge and information to guide revisions to policies and guidelines. This paper is a descriptive analysis of data available in maternal death audit reports submitted to the Western Regional Health Directorate in Ghana in 2014.

3. Methods

3.1 Study site

The Western Region is one of the ten administrative regions of Ghana. The region covers a land area of 23,921 square kilometers and is the fourth-largest region in the country. It has a population of about two and half million people, 24% of whom are women of childbearing age. The entire western boundary of the region shares a border with La Cote D'Ivoire. The region experiences the highest level of rainfall in Ghana, and most parts of the region are forest that is traversed by very poor roads. The capital of the Western Region is Sekondi-Takoradi. The Effia Nkwanta Hospital in the Sekondi-Takoradi metropolis (STM) is the main referral health facility in the region. In addition, each of the 22 districts/municipalities in the region has a hospital or health center that offers comprehensive maternal health services. Consistent with the guidelines of the GHS, all maternal deaths in the region must be subjected to audit by facility management teams. Audits are required to cover the history of pregnancy, circumstances of death, and findings on the causes of death. The findings are to be reported on specially-designed maternal deaths audit forms. This information is expected to be entered into the District Health Information System Two (DHIMS-2) and transmitted to the regional and national levels. The DHIMS-2 is the electronic data capture system that serves as the backbone of institutional health service information management in Ghana. A copy of the report must also be sent to the regional level.

3.2 Data management, analysis, and limitations

The findings of the audit are recorded on specially-designed audit forms. The information is copied and transmitted to the district and regional health administration for collation and analysis. In addition, periodically teams from the regional health administration travel to the various districts and sub-district health facilities to verify submitted audit reports and follow-up on actions taken on the basis of the findings.

For the purpose of the work presented here, data were extracted from all audit forms submitted to the Regional Health Administration in 2014. Where feasible, information was corroborated with data in the DHIMS-2. The data from the forms were entered into computer using a platform created in EPI-INFO version 7. Analysis was largely descriptive and included computation of mean age of death, maternal mortality ratio, and extent of data adequacy.

An important limitation to the extent of analysis is the extent of data completeness for different variables. The effect of this is the use of different denominators for some variables (reported in the "Results" section). The absence of comparator data from overall (all pregnant women) maternal services against which the findings could be compared and inferences drawn was yet another limitation.

4. Results

A total of 93 maternal deaths occurred in 2014, and all the deaths were entered into the DHMIS-2 by December 2016. At least one maternal death was recorded in 15 out of the 22 districts in the region. However, at the Regional Health Directorate, audit reports were available for 67 (72%) of deaths, and all 67 were from 9 out of the 22 districts/municipalities (**Table 1**). The number of deaths recorded in the DHIMS and the number of deaths reported to have been audited as per the DHIMS were consistent with the number of actual reports available at the Regional Health Directorate in only 9 out of the 22 (41%) districts/municipalities. Among these nine district, seven had recorded no deaths (**Figure 1**).

The total number of audited maternal deaths for STM (60%) represents the highest number of deaths recorded in a district. It was followed by Ellembelle district, which also recorded 13 deaths in the DHIMS (DHIMS-2, 2017b) but reported 10 (15%) cases of audited maternal deaths. The highest maternal mortality ratios were recorded in the regional hospital in Sekondi-Takoradi (355/100,000 live births) and the districts hospitals Ellembelle (231) and Jomoro (146) (**Table 1**). Per population of women of childbearing age, however, the Ellembelle district recorded the highest of 45 deaths per 100,000 women, with the STM recording 25 deaths per 100,000 women.

The median and mean ages of women were 27 (range of 13–51 yrs) and 28 yrs., respectively. The age distribution was as follows: 10/67, 5% (less than 19 yrs); 45/67, 67% (20–35 yrs); and 12/67, 18% (above 36 years). In all the districts, deaths occurred among women who were regular Antenatal Clinic (ANC) attendants. Seven (18%)

District	WoCBA♣	No. of live births	No. of deaths	Maternal mortality ratio/100, 000 live births	Age/ Mean Age	No of cases attending ANC	No. of live births	Deaths within 24 hrs	Autopsy done	Time of death		Place of death		Parity			Period of death		
										pm	am	Facility	Home	Null	1–5	>5	Ante partum	Intra partum	Post partum
Bibiani Ahwiaso Bekwai	30,844	4201	2	48	18	2	2	2	0		1	1	1				0	2	0
Ellembelle	22,148	4329	10	231	28	10	7	2	0	5	5	9	1		6	1	0	2	8
Jomoro	38,145	2049	3	146	23	3	0	1	0	1	1				3		0	1	0
Nzema East	15,155	1362	1	73		1	0	1	0			1	0				0	1	0
Prestea Huni Valley	39,035	3701	5	135	27	5	3	1	1	4	1	3	2	1	1		0	1	2
Sekondi-Takoradi	158,170	11,279	40	355	29	33	22	7	2	19	15	29	6	2	28	1	4	7	24
Tarkwa Nsuaem	22,852	5466	3	55	35	3	1	1	0		2	2	1		2		0	1	0
Wiawso	34,406	4856	3	62	28	3	1	2	2		2	3	0		3		0	2	0
Total	360,755	35,764	67	187	28	60	36	17	5	29	27	48	11	3	43	2	4	17	34
Data completeness	N/A	N/A	72%		N/A	N/A	N/A	N/A	N/A	84%		88%			64%			82%	

♠*Based on the information provided in audit reports available at the Regional Health Directorate.*
♣*WoCBA – Women of childbearing age, that is, 15–49 yrs.*

Table 1.
Maternal deaths and related factors in the Western region of Ghana in 2014♠.

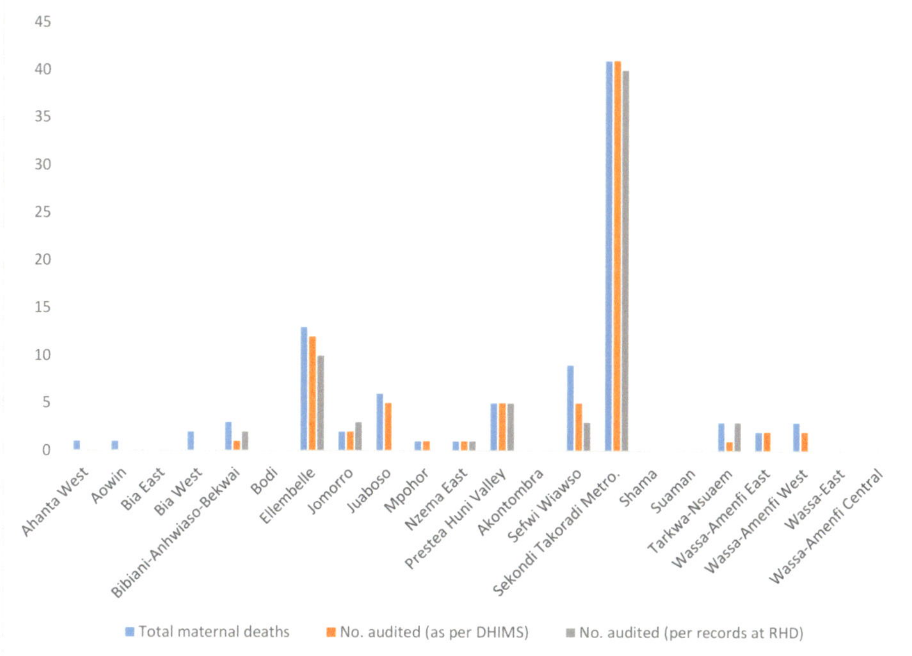

Figure 1.
Maternal deaths and number audited in 2014 as per different sources of record in the Western region of Ghana.

women in the cases in the Sekondi-Takoradi metropolis were non-ANC attendants. Overall, 80% of cases involved women who made at least three ANC visits.

The leading causes of death were hypertensive diseases (24 out of 67 cases, 36%), hemorrhage (31%), and sepsis (8%) (**Figure 2**). Nearly all (96%) of the cases of

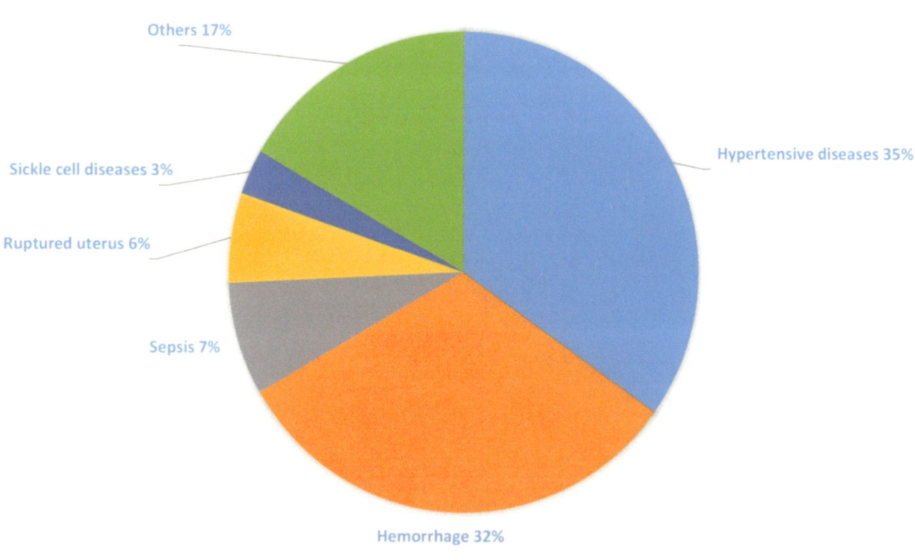

Figure 2.
Causes of maternal deaths in the Western region of Ghana in 2014.

District	No of cases with audit reports	Causes of maternal deaths								Audit report availability
		Hypertensive diseases	Hemorrhage	Sepsis	Ruptured uterus	Sickle cell diseases	Unsafe abortions	Ectopic gestation	Others	
Bibiani Ahwiaso Bekwai	2	0	2	0	0	0	0	0	0	100%
Ellembelle	10	4	5	0	0	1	0	0	0	100%
Jomoro	3	0	1	0	0	0	0	0	1	67%
Nzema East	1	0	1	0	0	0	0	0	0	100%
Prestea Huni Valley	5	1	1	0	0	1	0	0	2	100%
Sekondi-Takoradi	40	18	9	4	2	0	1	0	6	100%
Tarkwa Nsuaem	3	0	1	1	1	0	0	0	0	100%
Wiawso	3	0	1	0	1	0	0	1	0	100%
Total	67	23	21	5	4	2	1	1	9	99%

Table 2.
Causes of maternal deaths per district in 2014 in the Western region of Ghana.

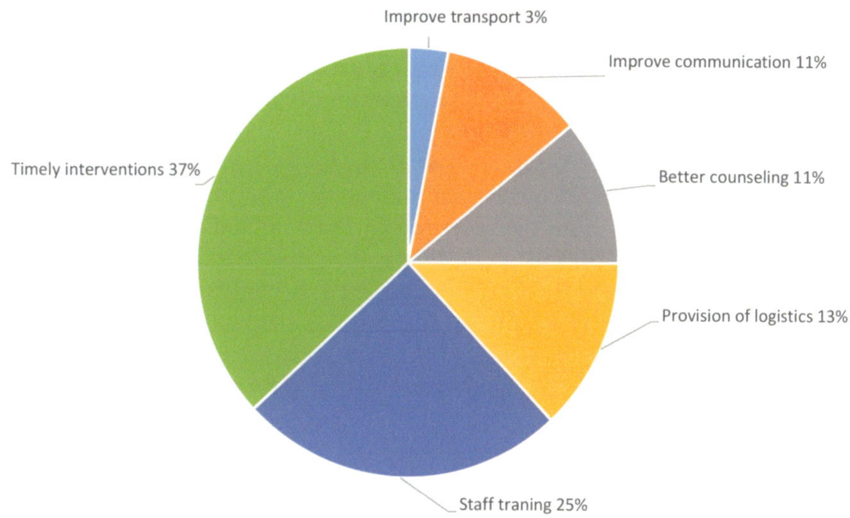

Figure 3.
Recommended actions following audit of maternal deaths in the Western region of Ghana – 2014.

hypertension-related deaths occurred in the Sekondi-Takoradi (18 cases, i.e., 78% of cases) and Ellembelle (4 cases, i.e., 17% of cases). In contrast, at least one hemorrhage-related death occurred in each district and municipality, with STM having the highest proportion of 43%, followed by 24% in Ellembelle (**Table 2**). All the cases of sepsis-related deaths occurred in the Sekondi-Takoradi municipality and Wiawso district. In 61% (34 out of 55) of cases, death occurred during the postpartum period. In 36 (54%) cases, deliveries resulted in live births.

The majority 82%, that is, 48 out of 59 cases of deaths, occurred in hospitals, with about a quarter (25%) occurring within 24 hours of arrival. Nearly an equal number of deaths during the day (29 out of 56 cases) occurred at night (27). The autopsy was conducted in only five (8%) cases in three districts or municipalities. The major interventions recommended by the audits were more timely intervention (38% of recommendations), improved staff competency through in-service training (25%), and improved logistics (11%) (**Figure 3**).

5. Discussion

The paper is a descriptive analysis of the causes and factors of maternal deaths in the Western Region of Ghana in 2014. A major limitation of this effort has been the quality of data available at the regional level. Although maternal death audits are mandatory and audits reports are required to be submitted to the region, it was in only 67 out of the 93 (73.1%) cases that such audit reports were submitted more than a year after the deaths occurred. Nationwide, out of 941 maternal deaths in 2014, only 81% had been audited by the end of the year (DHIMS-2, 2016).

It is apparent that the disparity between data on maternal deaths captured in the DHIMS-2 and physical records of audits at the Regional Health Directorate was quite considerable and is likely to be a national problem. This could be attributed to the fact that most health information officers have access to the online DHIMS-2 platform

(DHIMS-2, 2017c) and tend to make that data entry more prompt at the district level. The fact is the lack of completeness in the details required for the audit review process at the regional level. The lack of records on maternal health audits and hence lack of completeness in maternal health records was similarly reported in a recent review of maternal deaths at the regional hospital in the Eastern Region in 2012. In that review, it was found that audit reports were not available for 24% of cases [13].

Another level of data inadequacy that undermined the validity of the analysis is the lack of completeness in the data presented in various audit reports. Many fields on the audit forms were not filled, and the number of events did not add up. It was evident that audit teams or officers who completed the audit forms placed emphasis on filling out the section on the cause of death (99% completeness) and were less concerned when completing portions of the form that describe the circumstances of death. Data incompleteness ranged from 64 to 88% for parameters such as parity, time, place, and period of death. Given the basic nature of such information, the lack of completeness in these instances is unlikely due to a lack of familiarity or staff's lack of knowledge on how to complete these forms. It is more likely due to negligence buoyed by a lack of oversight and review of forms prior to submission to the regional level. In a study done in the era when mandatory audits had not been institutionalized, maternal health data at a district hospital in rural northern Ghana were similarly found to be grossly incomplete, inaccurate, and inconsistent. The era of audit and the introduction of an electronic data platform does not appear to have had much effect in these regards.

The current procedure where maternal health audits are conducted by the health teams at the facility where the death occurred needs to be reviewed. The approach appears overly self-serving and unlikely to engender the desired level of scrutiny and accountability. Consideration should be given to establishing a system of audits that routinely involves external and independent experts [8, 10]. It is critical that every maternal death is properly accounted for as a matter of public health records and as part of quality assurance in health institutions in the country. The lack of completeness of data on maternal death events is a serious issue that the authorities in the Ghana Health Service need to address urgently. A regime of responsibility and sanctions needs to be instituted.

This study found that the three main causes of death accounted for about 75% of all deaths. This pattern is consistent with findings in other studies and suggests that a precipitous drop in maternal deaths could be achieved if interventions could be targeted at these causes. Hypertensive diseases in pregnancy are overtaking hemorrhage as the leading cause of maternal mortality in Ghana [14–16]. Substantial reduction in these maternal deaths could be made in Ghana through widespread hypertension and proteinuria screening and early delivery of women with severe diseases [17]. Hemorrhage and sepsis are amenable to improved blood transfusion services and early and appropriate use of antibiotics. The positive impact of these has been demonstrated in a quality improvement program piloted at the Greater Accra Regional Hospital [18].

For many years, programs to reduce Ghana's maternal mortality ratio have predominantly focused on interventions at the community level. It has often been implied that when women attend ANC, the risk factors for maternal deaths will be identified, and the instituted interventions will lead to safe delivery. In this study, however, we find that 80% of deaths occurred among women who attended ANC at least thrice during pregnancy. We also found that most deaths occurred among women who had been at the facility beyond 24 hours. These findings support those made in a 2009 review of maternal deaths in the Upper West Region of Ghana [10] and in other countries with a high burden of maternal deaths [19, 20]. They put to question the long-held preposition (often advanced by health workers) that most maternal deaths result from women reporting late at the health facility [10, 13]. The quality of institutional maternal care should not be taken to be assured, and unless the issue of quality of institutional maternal care is rigorously addressed by the health service, substantial gains made in increasing antenatal attendance and skilled attendance will be undermined.

6. Conclusion

Hypertensive diseases in pregnancy, hemorrhage, and sepsis account for about 75% of institutional maternal deaths in the Western Region of Ghana. With most of the deaths occurring in women who were regular antenatal attendants and in women who were in health facilities for more than 24 hours, it is evident that most could have been prevented with appropriate and timely interventions at the various health facilities. Therefore, institutional maternal care strengthening should be a major priority in reducing maternal mortality in the Western Region of Ghana.

Acknowledgements

The authors dedicate this paper to the memory of all the women who died through childbirth in the Western Region in 2014 and to all the health workers who, under trying conditions, persevere to save maternal lives. The authors thank Mr. Lukeman Bamengzut, Ms. Georgina Ayepah, Mr. Pter Ntibeh, and Ms. Grace Afranie Toku for completing the data entries. We also thank the Public Health Unit and the Regional Health Directorate, who supported with access to the data.

Conflict of interest

The authors have no conflicts of interest.

Contribution of authors

Marion Okoh-Owusu MBChB MPH: Contribution: principal investigator, team leader, data collection, data entry and analyses, writing of manuscript.

George Kojo Owusu, MBCHB: Contribution: co-investigator, data collection, writing of manuscript, review of manuscript.

Celia Taylor BSoc Sc, PHD: Contribution: writing and critical review of manuscript.

Frank Baiden MBChB PhD: Contribution: project supervisor, data analyses, writing and critical review of manuscript.

Author details

Marion Okoh-Owusu[1*], George Kojo Owusu[2], Celia Brown[3] and Frank Baiden[4]

1 Ellembelle District Directorate of Health, Ghana Health Service, Western Region, Ghana

2 Effia Nkwanta Regional Hospital, Sekondi, Western Region, Ghana

3 The University of Warwick, Coventry, United Kingdom

4 Ensign College of Public Health, Eastern Region, Ghana

*Address all correspondence to: drokohowusu@gmail.com

References

[1] Chou D, Daelmans B, Jolivet RR, Kinney M, Say L. Every Newborn action P, ending preventable maternal mortality working g: Ending preventable maternal and newborn mortality and stillbirths. BMJ. 2015;**351**:h4255

[2] Alkema L, Chou D, Hogan D, Zhang S, Moller AB, Gemmill A, et al. Global, regional, and national levels and trends in maternal mortality between 1990 and 2015, with scenario-based projections to 2030: A systematic analysis by the UN maternal mortality estimation inter-agency group. Lancet. 2016;**387**(10017):462-474

[3] Lieberman A. Challenges for maternal health efforts. Lancet. 2016;**388**(10050):1146-1147

[4] Amoakoh HB, Klipstein-Grobusch K, Amoakoh-Coleman M, Agyepong IA, Kayode GA, Sarpong C, et al. The effect of a clinical decision-making mHealth support system on maternal and neonatal mortality and morbidity in Ghana: Study protocol for a cluster randomized controlled trial. Trials. 2017;**18**(1):157

[5] Amu H, Nyarko SH. Preparedness of health care professionals in preventing maternal mortality at a public health facility in Ghana: A qualitative study. BMC Health Services Research. 2016;**16**:252

[6] Kyei-Nimakoh M, Carolan-Olah M, McCann TV. Millennium development goal 5: Progress and challenges in reducing maternal deaths in Ghana. BMC Pregnancy and Childbirth. 2016;**16**:51

[7] Sofo S, Thompson E. Maternal mortality in Ghana: Impact of the fee-free delivery policy and the National Health Insurance Scheme. International Journal of Public Health Science. 2015;**4**(3):232-237

[8] Ansong-Tornui J, Armar-Klemesu M, Arhinful D, Penfold S, Hussein J. Hospital based maternity care in Ghana - findings of a confidential enquiry into maternal deaths. Ghana Medical Journal. 2007;**41**(3):125-132

[9] Bailey PE, Andualem W, Brun M, Freedman L, Gbangbade S, Kante M, et al. Institutional maternal and perinatal deaths: A review of 40 low and middle income countries. BMC Pregnancy and Childbirth. 2017;**17**(1):295

[10] Issah K, Nang-Beifubah A, Opoku CF. Maternal and neonatal survival and mortality in the upper west region of Ghana. International Journal of Gynaecology and Obstetrics. 2011;**113**(3):208-210

[11] Bosu W, Bell JS, Armar-Klemesu M, Tornui JA. Effect of delivery care user fee exemption policy on institutional maternal deaths in the central and Volta regions of Ghana. Ghana Medical Journal. 2007;**41**(3):118-124

[12] Wagaarachchi PT, Graham WJ, Penney GC, McCaw-Binns A, Yeboah Antwi K, Hall MH. Holding up a mirror: Changing obstetric practice through criterion-based clinical audit in developing countries. International Journal of Gynaecology and Obstetrics. 2001;**74**(2):119-130 discussion 131

[13] Akosua Owusu-Sarpong A, Boamah KA, Baiden F. Associated factors and quality of care received among maternal deaths at a regional hospital in Ghana: Maternal death audit review. African Journal of Reproductive Health. 2017;**21**(2):49-54

[14] Lee QY, Odoi AT, Opare-Addo H, Dassah ET. Maternal mortality in Ghana: A hospital-based review. Acta Obstetricia et Gynecologica Scandinavica. 2012;**91**(1):87-92

[15] Adu-Bonsaffoh K, Oppong SA, Binlinla G, Obed SA. Maternal deaths attributable to hypertensive disorders in a tertiary hospital in Ghana. International Journal of Gynaecology and Obstetrics. 2013;**123**(2):110-113

[16] Adu-Bonsaffoh K, Obed SA, Seffah JD. Maternal outcomes of hypertensive disorders in pregnancy at Korle Bu teaching hospital, Ghana. International Journal of Gynaecology and Obstetrics. 2014;**127**(3):238-242

[17] Goldenberg RL, McClure EM, Macguire ER, Kamath BD, Jobe AH. Lessons for low-income regions following the reduction in hypertension-related maternal mortality in high-income countries. International Journal of Gynaecology and Obstetrics. 2011;**113**(2):91-95

[18] Srofenyoh EK, Kassebaum NJ, Goodman DM, Olufolabi AJ, Owen MD. Measuring the impact of a quality improvement collaboration to decrease maternal mortality in a Ghanaian regional hospital. International Journal of Gynaecology and Obstetrics. 2016;**134**(2):181-185

[19] Oladapo OT, Adetoro OO, Ekele BA, Chama C, Etuk SJ, Aboyeji AP, et al. When getting there is not enough: A nationwide cross-sectional study of 998 maternal deaths and 1451 near-misses in public tertiary hospitals in a low-income country. BJOG. 2016;**123**(6):928-938

[20] Souza JP, Gulmezoglu AM, Vogel J, Carroli G, Lumbiganon P, Qureshi Z, et al. Moving beyond essential interventions for reduction of maternal mortality (the WHO multicountry survey on maternal and Newborn health): A cross-sectional study. Lancet. 2013;**381**(9879):1747-1755

Section 4

Essential Social Services as Health Enablers

Chapter 11

Access of Households to Arable Land and Nutritional Status of Children Aged 6–59 Months in Rural Areas of South Kivu, Case of the Health Zone of Minova, Eastern DRC

Emery Likaka, Espérant Kiangana and Gaylord Ngaboyeka

Abstract

Already knowing enough about the determinants of malnutrition, this study set itself the objective of verifying the influence of access to arable land on the nutritional status of children aged 6 to 59 months in a rural Health Zone of the DRC in South Kivu (Minova) with very high prevalence of malnutrition (62% CM and 7.1% AM). A cross-sectional quantitative study conducted on a representative sample of 424 children aged 6 to 59 months selected using the Lynch formula by probabilistic stratum sampling; using a structured questionnaire. Malnutrition (acute and chronic) assessed on the basis of WHO growth standards served as the dependent variable and access to arable land considered according to the FAO definition was the main independent variable. Chi-square or Ficher tests were used to compare proportions and logistic regressions were used to determine the factors associated with malnutrition; the significance threshold set at 5%. The frequency of less than 3 meals per day and the low socio-economic level of households were associated with chronic malnutrition (p-value 0.046 and 0.007). Exclusive breastfeeding and unimproved source of drinking water were associated with acute malnutrition. Finally, no statistically significant association was found between access to arable land and the nutritional status of children aged 6 to 59 months. How land production and household incomes are allocated for other needs would also be part of the problem.

Keywords: arable land, chronic malnutrition, acute malnutrition, Minova, Sud-Kivu, DR Congo

1. Introduction

Globally, nearly two billion people, or about 30% of the population, suffer from invisible hunger, that is, deficiencies in micronutrients and other macronutrients [1].

Efforts to achieve food security for all in order to combat malnutrition are hampered by emerging issues that threaten the food system [2]. Undernutrition is the single most important risk factor for mortality and morbidity in developing countries [3].

One in three children (200 million worldwide) does not realize their full physical, cognitive, psychological, and/or socio-emotional potential due to poverty, poor nutrition, poor health, insufficient care, and stimulation associated with other risk factors for early childhood development [4–6]. Scientific studies carried out on maternal and child health have revealed that 45% of cases of death of children under five are directly or indirectly due to malnutrition [4]; The cost of prematurely developed diseases and deaths directly caused by hunger in the world is estimated at 30 billion per year according to the FAO.

In Africa, there was a time when land seemed almost inexhaustible, but population growth and market development are creating increased competition for land resources, especially near villages and towns and in rural areas. High-value productive areas. According to the FAO, about 65 percent of agricultural land in Africa is degraded, costing the continent nearly $68 million each year and affecting 180 million people, mainly poor rural populations already struggling to meet their needs. With demographic pressure on natural resources such as access to land and water, to which are added the indirect effects of the Covid-19 pandemic and climate change, deforestation, recurrent armed conflicts and the rate of high unemployment favoring the rural exodus; the number of people suffering from malnutrition in Africa and the DRC is likely to double or even triple over the next few years. A profound change in the global food and agriculture system is, therefore, necessary to hope to feed millions of people who suffer from malnutrition hunger today and the 2 billion additional people that the world will have by 2050 [7], Asia and Africa are the most affected.

In the Democratic Republic of Congo, evidence from nutritional surveys of major DHS and MICS studies report alarming prevalence of deficiency malnutrition in chronic and acute forms, while paradoxically the country has about 80 million hectares of arable land, including Barely 10% developed and occupies the second place in the world in terms of cultivable arable land after Brazil and an unprecedented hydrographic network [8].

Despite some progress recorded in the prevention and fight against malnutrition, the DRC is to date deviating in order of severity, the first country in the world with such a high number of people affected by food insecurity.

The incidence of poverty for the whole country is very high (71.34%) if we compare it to that of the other countries of Central Africa [9]. Deficiency malnutrition in all its forms remains a worrying public health problem [10] with 43% chronic malnutrition and the prevalence of GAM ranging from 6.5 to 15% in the provinces and an average of 2% acute malnutrition strict; ranking the DRC as 1 of 10 countries that account for 60% of the global burden of wasting in children under 5.

In South Kivu, about 9% of children aged 6–59 months only have access to a minimum acceptable diet and 14.9% for the Minova Health Zone [11] and the 2018 MICS survey revealed 48% chronic malnutrition (about one in two children), a proportion far above the national average (43%).

Still in South Kivu, in the territory of Kalehe, the prevalence of stunting in children under five in the ZS of Minova was estimated at 62.1% in 2018 against 51% in 2020 according to the results of the surveys conducted by the NGO Graines and the National Nutrition Program as well as global acute malnutrition at 7%.

Recurrent armed conflicts force people to move outside their natural living environment (rural exodus) in search of peace and employment to urban centers that are poorly prepared for rapid urbanization and demographic explosion.

It should also be noted that the large land concessions in South Kivu and Minova in the territory of Kalehe are strongly solicited by personalities and businessmen who want to invest in land. This seems to constitute a kind of heaviness for the rural population who rely only on agricultural life for their survival, yet without financial means to compete with purchases or limit sales.

A study carried out in 2008 by the INGO ACF in the territory of Kalehe revealed that access to land for women and other inhabitants of Minova is very limited and constitutes one of the major sources of conflict between herders and farmers. According to this study, the total cultivated areas vary between 0.02 and 12.7 Ha, with an average of 1.5 Ha for the ZS of Kalehe and 1.7 Ha for the ZS of Minova per agricultural practitioner [12].

The survey conducted by the National Nutrition Program in South Kivu with the support of UNICEF, WFP and FAO found that the average cultivated area per inhabitant in the Minova Health Zone varies between 13.1 and 30 ares.

Having found no studies focused on in-depth research into the causes of the persistence of malnutrition in this area despite the joint interventions carried out by Humanitarian Organizations; we estimated that there would be a problem of household access to arable land, which would influence these high prevalence of malnutrition alongside other underlying factors. Thus, this justified our study to explore the association between access to land and the nutritional status of young children in rural areas, given that for the low-income peasant population; it has been affirmed by certain literature that agriculture represents an important part of the food ration of families [13, 14] while other authors think that the simple fact of having access to arable land does not guarantee advances a good nutritional status.

In view of the above, our study mainly addressed the following research question: "Is there an association between having or not having access to arable land and the nutritional status of children aged 6–59 months in rural areas, the case of the Minova Health Zone given the high prevalence of stunting and acute malnutrition?" If not, what are the other factors associated with this malnutrition in the Zone?

Generally, this study aims to verify the influence of rural households' access to arable land on the nutritional status of children aged 6–59 months in order to better guide control strategies and actions to improve their health.

Specifically, this involves identifying the proportion of households without access to arable land in this health zone; assess/determine the level of exposure of households without arable land to acute and chronic malnutrition in children under 6–59 months; determine the prevalence of chronic and acute malnutrition among the target population of Minova Health Zone and other associated factors.

Three hypotheses have thus been formulated to verify these objectives: the proportion of households in the Minova Zone that do not have access to arable land will be close to 50%; the prevalence of chronic and acute malnutrition will be significantly higher in households without access to land compared to those with access; then the large size of households and closely spaced births will be one of the main factors associated with acute and chronic malnutrition in children aged 6–59 months in this area considering the low purchasing power of the population.

2. Methodological framework

2.1 Materials and method

This cross-sectional quantitative study was conducted in 11 Health Areas randomly selected out of the 21 in the Minova Health Zone (Bobandana, Bulenga, Cheya Chebumba, Kalungu, Karango, Kishinji, Minova, Muchibwe, Numbi and Ruhunde) in the province of Sud Kivu (Eastern DRC) during the period from June to November 2021.

The study population is made up of children aged 6–59 months residing in the households of the chosen Health Areas; the size of our sample was 375 children but we added 15% or 426 children in total surveyed to prevent the risk of non-response and possible incomplete data when cleaning the database.

Inclusion criteria: to be a resident child aged 6–59 months in the survey household whose father or mother has given consent for anthropometric measurements and is willing to answer the questionnaire. The mother of each selected child was also concerned by the measurement of the Brachial Circumference.

Was excluded from the study, the child from 6 to 59 months concerned whose parent did not give the consent for his participation or residing less than 6 months in the household.

2.2 Sample and sampling technique

Systematic and proportional stratified sampling was used at several stages in strict compliance with statistical standards (Health area at 1st stage, Village at 2nd stage).

In the village, households with children aged 6–59 months were identified with the help of parcel surveys from Community Relays then the choice of children was made by the technique of systematic random drawing with reference to the table of proportion of Health Areas.

The sampling interval was equal to the number of children aged 6–59 months in the village divided by the number of children to be surveyed in this village.

The sample size was calculated with the following Lynch formula:

$$
\begin{aligned}
n &= \frac{NZ\alpha^2 \bullet P \bullet (1-P)}{N \bullet a^2 + Z\alpha^2(1-P)} \\
&= \frac{211163 \bullet 1.96^2 \bullet 0.43(1-0.62)}{211163 \bullet 0.05^2 + 1.96^2(1-0.62)} \\
&= \frac{211163 \bullet 3.8416 \bullet 0.43 \bullet 0.38}{211163 \bullet 0.0025 + 3.8416 \bullet 0.38} \\
n &= 375 \\
n &= 375 \text{ Respondents}
\end{aligned} \tag{1}
$$

where N = total population of the 11 health care; n = sample; Z alpha = constant = 1.96 (for 95% CI); a = the margin of error; P = the prevalence of malnutrition in the health zone; P = 62% of Chronic Malnutrition [15].

2.3 Malnutrition in its chronic and acute forms was the dependent variable of our study

After exclusion of outliers, the two forms of malnutrition were defined according to WHO growth standards.

Regarding the Independent Variables, we considered:

Access to arable land:

Defined according to the FAO as the set of processes by which citizens, individually or collectively, acquire the rights and opportunities allowing them to occupy and use land (for production and for economic and social purposes), whether on a temporary or permanent basis [16, 17].

These processes include participation in formal and informal markets, access to land through family or social networks, including transmission of land rights by in heritance and within families, and allocation of land by the state and other authorities, with control over them.

According to the Provincial Inspection of Agriculture of South Kivu (direction of production and protection of plants), an agricultural household must have on average an area of 50 ares (1/2 hectare) for the cultivation of cassava and at least 30 ares for other speculations such as (legumes, cereals, vegetables, potatoes) in order to consider that he has access to arable land to meet his most basic needs.

Conveniently, to express the area of arable land owned by a household during this study; the head of the household of the child surveyed presented the land purchase document, or he expressed it according to locally recognized conventional measures (kamba moya = one hectare of land, nusu ya kamba =1/2 hectare; kipandé = between 30 and less than 50 ares).

The other independent variables were evaluated taking into account their standard values (birth weight in Kg, child's age in months, male or female sex, arm circumference in millimeters, exclusive Breastfeeding in 6 months, the daily frequency of meals greater than or equal to 3, their composition of at least four essential food groups, the level of education attained by the head of the household, and his profession, the size of the household, the marital status of the parent of the child, religion, birth interval, child vaccination status, source of drinking water, socio-economic status or constituted wealth index.

2.4 Data collection

The subjects of study were randomly identified by a systematic technique of drawing from households after having constituted a sampling base as indicated above. The biological mothers (or father of the child) served directly as respondents to the questions asked.

To identify the survey households, the interviewers used the home visit notebooks and local count notebooks from the Village Community Relays. Data was collected electronically on Android tablets using Open Data Kit (ODK) and stored remotely on the server. This collection in the field was facilitated by qualified staff, with medical and non-medical profiles (two nutritionists, a public health graduate, a primary school teacher and two agricultural engineers) making up three paired teams; all supervised by the Principal Investigator. A refresher course preceded the collection to strengthen the investigators' understanding of the mastery of the tools and the technique, followed by a pre-survey.

High-precision anthropometric equipment provided by UNICEF, including SECA electronic scales, Shakir measuring rods and strips, was used to take various measurements (weight, height, MUAC) in addition to the search for nutritional edema.

In terms of ethical consideration, the request for consent was read and requested from each respondent before completing the questionnaire and taking measurements. No act contrary to the ethics and methodology of the research was practiced. Parents of children suspected of malnutrition were advised to take them to the Health Centers of their choice for confirmation and appropriate action.

2.5 Data analysis

The data collected from a structured and digitized questionnaire with the Kobo toolbox platform were analyzed with Stata version 14.

Descriptive statistics (medians and interquartile ranges (IQR) for continuous variables, and frequencies with percentages for variables categorical) were used to describe the study sample according to the shape of the distribution and then the chi-square test was used for comparison.

To determine the associated factors, we constructed logistic regression models (univaried and multi-varied) and to introduce the variables into the multi-varied analysis, the step-by-step selection method with a forced entry of plausible factors was used.

The measures of association were reported by the unadjusted odds ratios (ORna) and the adjusted odds ratios (ORa) with their 95% confidence intervals, ie the significance level set at 5%.

3. Results of the study

The majority of people in the Minova Health Zone (86.60%) is self-employed and live in self-employed activities (agriculture, livestock, petty trade, etc.). 39.10% of households include more than 7 people and the majority of houses are built of boards (44.12%). Mostly monogamous (74.19%), almost a third of the population has no level of education (34.82%) and the Protestant religion is dominant, followed by Catholics.

The median age of our respondents was 26 years and for children under five, this was 24 months, dominated by the 24–59 month age group (**Table 1**).

The results of the analyses show in the histogram in **Figure 1** that 52.6% of households in Minova do not have access to arable land. There was also a high prevalence of acute malnutrition in households without access to land (9.1%) compared to those with access (5.1%) but this difference was not statistically significant.

Regarding the mode of acquisition of arable land by households, sharecropping and inheritance are the most dominant means of acquisition found in Minova with 39.49 and 26.15%, respectively. With regard to the crops cultivated, 44.30% of farmers practice mono-cropping. With regard to provisions, only 8% of households have food stocks in their homes. 29% practice livestock farming, dominated by backyard animals and 84.63% of households spend an average of between two and twenty thousand Congolese francs, or $1 to $10 per week, to supplement market needs, which indicates a kind of precariousness in living conditions (**Table 2**).

Table 3 shows that the prevalence of global acute malnutrition in the Minova Health Zone is 7.92% based on the weight/height ratio associated with other measures taken among children aged 6-59 months, and that chronic malnutrition (stunting) affects at least one out of every two children in the area, i.e. 50.38%. In addition,

Variables	*n* (%) or Med (min–max) or Avg (SD)
Profession of Head of Household (*n* = 418)	
Non-employees	362 (86.60)
State employees/Private sector	56 (13.40)
Age of respondent in years (*n* = 424)	26 (14–70)
Gender of Respondent (*n* = 424)	
Female	401 (94.58)
Male	23 (5.42)
Respondent's marital status (*n* = 424)	
Singles	98 (23.11)
Separared	22 (5.18)
The bride and groom	304 (71.70)
Level of education of the respondent (*n* = 424)	
No studies	148 (34.82)
Primary studies	135 (31.85)
Studies high school and more	141 (33.33)
Household size (*n* = 422)	
Median size (Min–Max)	7 (2–19)
1–7 peoples	257 (60.90)
More than 7 people	165 (39.10)
Age of children in months (*n* = 422)	24 (6–59)*
Children from 6 to 11	10.43
Children from 12 to 23	27.01
Children from 24 to 59	62.56
Gender child (*n* = 424)	
Girls	52.36
Boys	47.64
Intergenerational interval in months (*n* = 422)	19.92 (13.60)**
Less than 2 years old	54.26
2 years or more	45.70
Number of children under 5 in the household (*n* = 424)	2 (1–6)*
1 child	33.65
2 and more	66.35
Religion practiced by respondent (*n* = 424)	
Catholic	24.06
Protestant	53.77
Kimbanguist	1.42
Muslim	2.59
Other religions	18.16

Variables	n (%) or Med (min–max) or Avg (SD)
Tribe/nature of study population (n = 423)	
Non-aboriginal	39
Aboriginal	61
Last 3 months household income (n = 313) Median (Min–Max)	
	45 (1–600)*
≤ 100$	78.91
>100$	21.08
Socio economic status, n = 313	
Poor	52.08
Medium	41.85
Rich	6.07

*Med = Median; n = number; % = percentage in column.
**Average = mean; SD = standard deviation.

Table 1.
Sociodemographic characteristics of households surveyed in the Minova health zone.

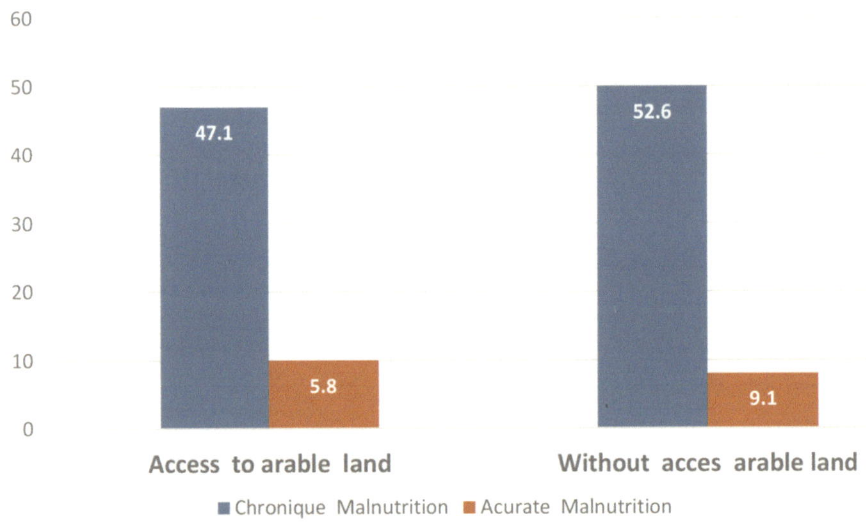

Figure 1.
Distribution of malnourished children according to access to land in the Zone (p *value GAM = 0.269 and* p *value CM = 0.337).*

Variables	% or Med (min–max)
Area of land owned by households in hectares (n = 195)	1 (0.01–15)
Less than one hectare of arable land	45.13
One to two hectares of arable land	28.72
More than two hectares of arable land	26.15
Means/mode of household arable land acquisition (n = 195)	

Variables	% or Med (min–max)
Purchase	9.74
Legacy	26.15
Rental	21.54
Metayage	39.49
Others means	3.08
Types of crops planted in the fields (n = 307)	
Various crops (manioc/potatoes, market gardening)	55.70
Non-varied crops (only one type in the field)	44.30
Weekly market spending by household (n = 397)	5.25 (1–50)
From 1 to 10 dollars	84.63
From $ 11 to 20 dollars	12.59
From $ 21 to 50 dollars	2.77
Households with food stocks (provisions), n = 423	
No provisions	91.96
Available provisions	8.04
Types of food stocks (household provisions), n = 33	
At least 3 types of food (legumes, staples, oil/animal food)	30.30
Two types of food in stock (basic food + other)	15.15
Only one type of feed in stock	54.55
Household livestock practice (n = 423)	
No	70.69
Yes	29.31
Type of farming practiced by the household (n = 124)	
Backyard breeding (poultry, guinea pigs, rabbits)	54.84
Small livestock (goats, sheep, pigs)	33.87
Mixed breeding (all species)	10.48
Breeding of large livestock (cattle)	0.81

Table 2.
Agricultural practices of surveyed households in the Minova Health Zone.

7.91% of children were born with a low birth weight according to the WHO reference and more than half of children (65.48%) were exclusively breastfed for six months. Only 5.45% of households have access to a diversified diet (4-star foods) that can meet their essential nutrient intake needs. A significant proportion of households (40.63%) consume their livestock products occasionally.

The results of the univariate analysis presented in the following **Table 4** show that the factors associated with acute malnutrition in children aged 6-59 months are low birth weight, household socioeconomic status, daily meal frequency, exclusive breastfeeding, and immunization status.

Variables	% or Med (min–max)
Diagnosis of GAM with Weight-Height, Nut Edema, PB (n = 404)	7.7
Weight-height index (n = 404)	0.03 (−4.96; 3.91)
Acute global malnutrition (<−2 Z-score)	7.20
Normal child ≥−2Z-score)	92.8
Nutritional edema (n = 309)	
Yes	7.12
No	92.88
Branchial perimeter (n = 401)	143 (110–180)
Acute global malnutrition (<125)	6.56
Normal child (≥125)	93.44
Weight-for-age index (n = 401)	1.06 (5.7; 2.43)
Underweight	24.01
Normal child	75.99
According to the Size-Age Index (n = 401)	−2.03 (−5.92; 2.87)
Growth delay	50.38
Normal growth	49.62
Children who were exclusively breastfed (n = 424)	
No	36.32
Yes	63.68
Continuous breastfeeding at 24 months or older (n = 423)	
No	34.52
Yes	65.48
Birth weight (kg) (n = 417)	3 (1–5.8) Moy 3.201
Child born with low weight (<2.500 kg)	7.91
Child born with normal weight (2.500–3.500 kg)	66.43
Child born overweight (>3.500 kg)	25.66
4 star food consumption in the household (n = 422)	
Consume the 4 star meal	5.45
Does not consume 4 stars	94.55
Frequency of consumption of livestock products (n = 124)	
Regularly (1 week to 1 month)	23.96
Occasionally (3–6 months)	40.63
Rarely	35.42
Meal frequency (24-hour recall) (n = 423)	
<3 meals	85.31
≥3 meals	14.69
Nutritional status of mother and child by PB (mm), n = 410	260 (150–442)
Thinness (≤ 230 mm)	11.79

Variables	% or Med (min–max)
Good nutritional status (≥230 mm)	88.21
Source of drinking water for the household (*n* = 423)	
Developed water point	86.05
Undeveloped water point	13.95
Complete child immunization by age (*n* = 420)	
Child not fully vaccinated by age	20.24
Child fully vaccinated according to age	79.76

GAM = global acute malnutrition, Min = minimum value, Max = maximum value, Med = median.

Table 3.
Nutritional status of children under 5 years of age in households surveyed in the Minova Health Zone.

After adjustment by multivariate analysis (**Table 5**), only the variables exclusive breastfeeding, low birth weight and source of drinking water remained associated with acute malnutrition.

With respect to chronic malnutrition, the results of the bivariate analysis (**Table 6(a)** and **(b)**) reveal that meal frequency and household socioeconomic status are significantly associated with chronic malnutrition in children aged 6–59 months in the study area ($p < 0.05$ with 95% CI).

Variables	% de GAM	ORna (95% CI)	*p*
Access to land			
Yes (*n* = 138)	5.8	1	
No (*n* = 175)	9.1	1.63 (0.64–4.55)	0.269
Exclusive breastfeeding			
Yes (*n* = 205)	3.4	1	
No (*n* = 108)	15.7	5.28 (1.98–5.53)	<0,001
Food consumption at 4 stars			
Yes (*n* = 37)	2.7	1	
No (*n* = 276)	8.3	3.27 (0.50–138.48)	0.227
Child sex			
Girls (*n* = 168)	8.9	1	
Boys (*n* = 145)	6.2	0.67 (0.25–1.71)	0.367
Frequency of meals per day			
<3 (*n* = 267)	10.7	1.51 (1.13–5.98)	<0,002
≥3 (*n* = 46)	6.5	1	
Reproductive interval in months			
Less than 2 years (*n* = 164)	8.5	1.19 (0.47–3.12)	0.68
2 years or more (*n* = 138)	7.2	1	
Birth weight (kg)			
<2.500 kg (*n* = 23)	26.1	3.97 (1.12–12.34)	0.007

Variables	% de GAM	ORna (95% CI)	*p*
2.500 kg and more (*n* = 208)	8.2	1	
Branchial perimeter of the mother (mm)			
<230 mm (*n* = 33)	9.1	1.23 (0.22–4.51)	0.745
≥230 mm (*n* = 280)	7.5	1	
Household size			
≤7 people (*n* = 187)	6.4	1	
>7 people (*n* = 126)	9.5	1.54 (0.61–3.87)	0.311
Socio economic status			
Low (*n* = 162)	6.8	13.31 (1.89–576.09)	0.001
Average (*n* = 131)	9.2	18.55 (2.66–797.22)	0.001
High (*n* = 19)	5.3	1	
Childhood immunization by age			
Up to date (*n* = 256)	6.3	1	
Not current (*n* = 57)	14	2.45 (1.85–6.45)	0.046
Drinking water source			
Fitted (*n* = 219)	5	1	
Undeveloped (*n* = 94)	13.8	3.03 (1.19–7.79)	0.007
Number of children under 5 years old			
1 child (*n* = 87)	8	1	
More than one child (*n* = 226)	7.5	0.93 (0.35–2.75)	0.876
Level of education of the respondent			
Without (*n* = 104)	10.6	3.05 (0.86–13.50)	0.053
Primary (*n* = 102)	8.8	2.49 (0.66–11.40)	0.128
High school and above (*n* = 107)	3.7	1	
Tribe			
Non-aboriginal (*n* = 118)	10.2	1.73 (0.68–4.36)	0.196
Aboriginal (*n* = 195)	6.2	1	

GAM = global acute malnutrition; ORna = unadjusted odds ratio; CI = 95% confidence interval.

Table 4.
Factors associated with acute malnutrition (AM) in children 6–59 months of age in the Minova health zone (simple logistic regression).

Variables	ORa (95% CI)	*p*
EBM less than 6 months	3.03 (1.19–7.79)	<0.001
Low birth weight	3.50 (1.09–12.15)	0.049
Undeveloped water source	3.21 (1.10–9.32)	0.032

GAM = global acute malnutrition; ORa = adjusted odds ratio; CI = confidence interval; EBM = exclusive breastfeeding.

Table 5.
Multivariate analysis: factors associated with acute malnutrition (am) in children 6–59 months of age in the Minova health zone.

In **Table 7**, it is found that even after adjustment for all factors by multiple regressions, daily meal frequency and low household socioeconomic status remained statistically associated with chronic malnutrition as found in the bivariate analyses.

Children from households that consumed less than three meals per day were twice as likely to be chronically malnourished compared to other children and those from households with low socioeconomic status were 3.97 times more likely to be

(a)			
Variables	**% de CM**	**ORna (95% CI)**	***p***
Access to land			
Yes (*n* = 138)	47.1	1	
No (*n* = 175)	52.6	1.24 (0.78–2.00)	0.337
Exclusive breastfeeding			
Yes (*n* = 215)	48.4	1	
No (*n* = 98)	54.1	1.26 (0.76–2.09)	0.349
Consumption of food at 4 stars			
Yes (*n* = 37)	48.6	1	
No (*n* = 276)	50.4	1.07 (0.51–2.27)	0.845
Frequency of meals per day			
<3 (*n* = 267)	48.7	3.03 (1.19–7.79)	0.007
≥ 3 (*n* = 46)	58.7	1	
Child sex			
Girls (*n* = 162)	53.7	1	
Boys (*n* = 151)	53.6	0.87 (0.54–1.39)	0.535
Marital status of Respondent			
Single (*n* = 74)	43.2	0.70 (0.40–1.22)	0.181
Separated (*n* = 13)	53.8	1.07 (0.30–3.97)	0.909
Married (*n* = 226)	52.2	1	
Reproductive interval in months			
Less than 2 years (*n* = 164)	48.8	0.92 (0.57–1.49)	0.736
2 years or more (*n* = 138)	50.7	1	
Birth weight (kg)			
< 2.500Kg (*n* = 23)	65.2	1.99 (0.75–5.63)	0.129
2.500–3.500Kg (*n* = 208)	48.6	1	
> 3.500Kg (*n* = 82)	50	1.06 (0.61–1.82)	0.825
Brachial perimeter of the Mother (mm)			
< 230 mm (*n* = 33)	45.5	0.81 (0.36–1.78)	0.568
> = 230 mm (280)	50.7	1	
Household size			
<=7 people (*n* = 187)	47.1	1	
> 7 people (*n* = 126)	54.8	1.36 (0.84–2.20)	0.181

Socio economic status				
Law (n = 163)		46.6	5.28 (1.98–5.53)	<0,001
Average (n = 131)		53.4	3.97 (1.12–12.34)	0.006
High (n = 19)		57.9	1	
(b)				
Variables	**% de CM**	**None**	**ORna (95% IC)**	***p***
Childhood immunization by age				
Up to date (n = 256)	49.6	129 (82.69)	1	
Not current (n = 57)	52.6	27 (17.31)	1.12 (0.61–2.09)	0.680
Source of drinking water				
Fitted (n = 219)	93.6	114 (73.08)	1	
Undeveloped (n = 94)	55.3	42 (26.92)	1.34 (0.80–2.25)	0.232
Number of children under 5 years old				
1 Child (n = 284)	14.8	45 (28.85)	1	
More than one child (n = 226)	50.9	111 (71.15)	1.11 (0.66–1.88)	0.679
Food stock (Provisions)				
No provisions (n = 284)	50.3	141 (90.38)	1.08 (0.47–2.53)	0.831
Available provisions (n = 29)	48.3	15 (9.62)	1	
Level of education				
Without (n = 104)	54.8	47 (30.13)	1.33 (0.75–2.37)	0.299
Primary (n = 102)	48	53 (33.97)	1.01 (0.57–1.81)	0.957
High school and above (n = 107)	47.7	56 (35.90)	1	
Tribe				
Non-aboriginal (n = 118)	54.2	54 (34.62)	1.30 (0.80–2.11)	0.262
aboriginal (n = 195)	47.7	102 (65.38)	1	
Household land area				
Less than one hectare (n = 104)	48.1	54 (73.97)	1.17 (0.50–2.77)	0.688
1 hectare or more (n = 34)	44.1	19 (26.03)	1	

CM = chronic malnutrition, ORna = unadjusted odds ratio, CI = confidence interval.

Table 6.
Factors associated with chronic malnutrition in children aged 6–59 months in the Minova HZ: simple logistic regression.

Variables	**ORa (95% CI)**	***p***
Frequency of less than three meals/day	2.46 (1.85–6.45)	0.046
Low socio economic status	3.97 (1.12–12.34)	0.007

ORa = unadjusted odds ratio, CI = confidence interval.

Table 7.
Multivariate analysis: Factors associated with chronic malnutrition in children 6–59 months of age in the Minova health zone.

chronically malnourished compared to children from households with high socioeconomic status.

4. Discussions from results

4.1 Access to arable land

This study shows that more than half of households, or 54%, live without access to arable land, while agriculture in rural areas is an important source of income for the population, as stated by Coulibaly B. and Berkhout ED. in their studies carried out in Mali and in certain countries of Sub-Saharan Africa [18, 19].

The international NGO ACF in its study conducted in the Minova Health Zone in 2008 confirms that of all the main constraints linked to agriculture in this zone; limited access to arable land alone occupies 22% and the practice of sharecropping comes first as a mode of accession, followed by inheritance. According to studies by the National Nutrition Program of South Kivu and the UNICEF-WFP-FAO agencies, at least 45% of the households surveyed have no means of accessing land and that the purchase of food constitutes up to 75% of object of family expenses. This reality, which is not, however, unique to Minova alone, remains a major concern for the population, especially when it is necessary to take into account the speed of population growth experienced by the country.

4.2 Malnutrition and access to land

With a prevalence of chronic malnutrition of 50.38% in Minova, that is, one in two children, against GAM at 7.7%; malnutrition remains one of the worrying factors in the health of children in terms of the risk of morbidity and mortality. These results are not far from those found in the MISC 2018 surveys (48% chronic malnutrition for South Kivu against 43% for the whole of the DRC), EDS 2014 (MC 53% and MAG 6.5%) and the survey the most recent (2021) from Pronanut the three UN Agencies which found that the prevalence of GAM in Minova in children under five increased from 7.5% in 2018 to 5.8% in 2021, 95% CI (4.1–8.1) and that of MC decreased from 67.6 in 2018 to 51.0 (30.1–34.4) as a result of ongoing joint response interventions in the Area.

Several factors discussed below justify this high prevalence and further require a holistic response to continue to reverse the trends.. Even though some of the articles read claim that food security and hunger presented strong evidence of qualitative and quantitative links between land tenure, household food security and nutritional status [11, 13, 20] and that the reduction or a loss of access to land in an agrarian society leads directly to a reduction in income; access to food and impact on the nutritional status of populations [11, 13, 18, 20–22]; we found that there is no statistically significant association between having access to arable land and improved nutritional status.

Our results also diverge from the findings of the study carried out by Eide WB and Nahalomo on the situation of adequate food and the nutritional status of people evicted from the land in 2018 in Uganda, which found that out of 187 children followed 1 child in 2 of mothers evicted from arable land had developed wasting. The results of the similar study conducted by Tefft and Kelly had however also found the results close to those of Eide and Nahalomo.

By comparing the nutritional status of children in the rice-growing areas with that of children in the cotton-growing areas Tefft and Kelly 2002 [23] in Mali, Tefft and Kelly found a lower prevalence of wasting and stunting (*p*-value less than 0.05) among children from households in the irrigated rice-growing areas of Macina and Niono (19–25%) compared to children in the cotton-growing area (35–48%), which signified a positive influence of the access to arable land.

Andrew D Jones in the study on agricultural biodiversity, dietary diversity and nutritional status in low and middle income countries concurred with the findings that, agricultural biodiversity (as a result of access to arable land) was consistently positively associated with improved height-for-age (HAZ) Z-score of preschool children. He says, "A one-unit increase in the number of cultured species was associated with a 0.03 and 0.05 increase in HAZ, respectively, in children aged 24–59 months. He also found that land evictions become a public health problem because limited or non-existent land ownership is linked to about 80% of cases of hunger and under nutrition among people living in rural areas." The same is true for Azka Rehman et al. in Pakistan who in turn stated that women's land ownership has a significant positive effect on children's height/age z-score (HAZ score): if a woman owns land, the height-age score of her child may be 0.94 points higher than that of landless women [24].

Despite this continuation of previous results, our study found rather high proportions of malnutrition among children from households without access to arable land (52.6% of MC and 9.1% of MAG) compared to those with access but this without any association statistically significant.

For us, this difference due to an effect of chance in the two categories of households can be explained on the one hand by the way in which the production of the land and the incomes of the households are affected there for other needs and other apart from the heterogeneity of predictors of malnutrition such as socioeconomic status, breastfeeding and infant feeding practices, which have shown statistically significant as sociations in other studies.

Gamuchirai Chakona and Charlie M. Shackleton also confirm this thinking when they state that intra-household food allocation is one of the important factors affecting the nutritional status of children in South Africa.

4.3 Factors associated with malnutrition

Low birth weight (LBW), non-practice of exclusive breastfeeding and water consumption from undeveloped sources were significantly associated with the occurrence of acute malnutrition in children aged 6–59 months in the ZS of Minova even after adjusting for any confounding factors by multiple logistic regression.

This observation has already been made by several other researchers such as Mbalenhle Mkhize and M. Sibanda in South Africa in their study examining the factors associated with the nutritional status of children under five who found that low Birth weight contributed 25.92% to the occurrence of both acute and chronic malnutrition in children and similar observations were found in numerous articles used [3, 5, 6, 25, 26]. On the other hand, F. Diawara in Mali found in his study conducted in 2006 that only the age of the child, the parity of the mother and the family meal were associated with wasting in children aged 6–59 months with a value $p < 0.05$.

For our part, we are of the opinion that the low birth weight being a reflection of intrauterine growth retardation due to the prolonged under nutrition of the pregnant woman, the child born of this household is not spared to develop sooner or later, other forms of deficiency malnutrition such as emaciation, especially if other factors coexist such as diarrhea often caused in children by the ingestion of unclean water and early feeding.

Regarding the benefit of exclusive breastfeeding, several studies conducted by Experts have argued that early breastfeeding of the child at the hour following birth, exclusive breastfeeding before the first 6 months after birth and the continuity of breast-feeding until more or less 24 months constitutes a powerful line of defense against any form of infant malnutrition, including cachexia and obesity in adulthood.

In our study, we found in the bivariate analyzes that the further a child moved away from the age of breastfeeding, the more he had the chance of being affected by chronic malnutrition (less than 12 months: 20.59%, between 12 and 24 months: 44.30% and over 24 months: 57.50% with p-value <0.001) which further supports the thesis that breast milk effectively protects young children against different forms of malnutrition [27–31].

In relation to chronic malnutrition, the results analyzed after adjustment show that in households where children consume less than 3 meals a day, they were 2.46 times more likely to be affected by chronic malnutrition compared to those who have a frequency superior.

This result meets the opinion of several Experts in Nutrition (chrono nutrition) who affirm that the more a diet is adequate (quality, quantity, frequency); the more the child is protected from the risk of under nutrition although this is divergent from the results found by Stephen Kofi et al. in Ghana [19, 32].

This we, this is true by the fact that the more the child consumes meals during the day, the more it increases the chance to vary the foods that can bring together the different nutrients that the body needs for its growth. Our study also revealed that in households with low socio-economic status, children were 3.97 times more likely to have chronic malnutrition before age five ORa 3.97, 95% CI (1.12–12.34), p value = 0.007.

Our results thus join those found by D.Karageorgou who cites among the main factors of change in chronic malnutrition, the wealth index with 4% [33].

Célestin Bucekuderhwa and S. Mapatano also demonstrate in their study on understanding the dynamics of food vulnerability in South Kivu that the capacity to take charge is the ability to mobilize human, economic and institutional resources for the benefit of the household; and this ability therefore depends on education, knowledge, culture, time and control over resources, including socio-economic status or income [22].

5. Conclusions

Considering the very high prevalence of multiple forms of deficiency malnutrition in the Provinces of the DRC despite its potential, this study examined the influence of access to arable land on the nutritional status of a sample of children. From 6 to 59 months in the HZ of Minova (South Kivu) with specific reference to cases of chronic malnutrition and acute malnutrition. Malnutrition (chronic and acute) which constituted our outcome was discussed in relation to access to arable land as the main explanatory variable associated with other factors sensitive to nutrition including breastfeeding and feeding practices. Infant and young child feeding, mother's age, household socio-economic status, level of education of mothers and household heads, water-hygiene-sanitation, vaccination, agricultural practices.

After analyzing the data, it was found that:

- The prevalence of chronic malnutrition and global acute malnutrition were observed to be relatively higher in households without access to arable land compared to those with access, but there was no proven statistically significant association. The simple fact of having access to arable land for a household in Minova therefore does not guarantee the improvement of the nutritional status of children aged 6–59 months residing there.

- 54% of households in Minova do not have access to arable land that can meet their production needs and of consumption;

- The frequency of less than 3 daily meals in the household and the low socio-economic level were significantly associated with the occurrence of chronic malnutrition in children aged 6–59 months. In addition, low birth weight, exclusive breastfeeding and undeveloped source of drinking water are variables that have been significantly associated with global acute malnutrition.

Compared to research perspectives and recommendations, we did not carry out the study on soil fertility in our study to assess the influence that this could have on production per sown area and the content of nutrients in food; this could be an important confounding factor.

We thus suggest to future researchers or organizations to be able to carry out studies on the physicochemical and biological analysis of the soil of the ZS of Minova in order to determine its level of fertility and better orientate on the consequent actions (types of appropriate speculations, bio fortification possibly, etc.).

Thus, we recommend:

- to the Government of the Republic:

    - To structure and ensure the strict application of the structure of food prices throughout the national territory in order to guarantee the minimum of food security to households and contribute to the fight against undernutrition considering that the latter do not have sufficient access to arable land and obtain their supplies from markets.

    - To put in place adequate strategies to improve farmers' access to arable land and their protection against land misuse (Ministries of Agriculture and that of Land Affairs).

    - Initiate a general grassroots development program alongside the determinants of health already known (improvement of drinking water supply, access to quality health care for all, job creation for young people and facilitation of access). More investment should be made in improving the food system to achieve better nutrition.

    - "No panis nec pax", no peace, no bread too: having to ensure the safety of people and their property throughout the national territory is one of the prerequisites for the nutrition and health of the population.

- To the community of the Health Zone of Minova:

To understand that despite the efforts made to redress chronic and acute malnutrition, much remains to be done. With or without access to land, we can fight malnutrition in our households.

The fight is essentially based on prevention. Our life practices and the way our household incomes are distributed (their use) greatly depend on it. Let us learn to consume in quantity and quality what we produce locally.

Author details

Emery Likaka[1*], Espérant Kiangana[2] and Gaylord Ngaboyeka[2]

1 UNIKIS-ERSP-UCB, Bukavu, Democratic Republic of the Congo

2 ERSP-UCB, Bukavu, Democratic Republic of the Congo

*Address all correspondence to: lokitaemery@gmail.com

References

[1] Feyder J, Hunger LA, Tue LAF. Hunger. 2012;**782**:343

[2] Brondeau F. How to secure access to land to ensure food security for African populations: Elements for reflection. How to secure access to land to ensure food security for African populations: Elements for reflection. 2021;1-14

[3] Kibr G. A narrative review of poor nutritional practices, motivators and consequences in pregnant women: Evidence from recent literature and program implications. 2021;**82**

[4] General Secretariat of the United Nations. The Global Strategy for Women's, Children's and Adolescent's Health (2016–2030)2015. p. 108

[5] Anin SK, Saaka M, Fischer F, Kraemer A. Association between infant and young child feeding (IYCF) indicators and nutritional status of children (6–23 months) in northern Ghana. 2020;**12**(9):29

[6] Akombi BJ, Agho KE, Hall JJ, Merom D. Stunting and severe stunting among children under 5 in Nigeria: A multilevel analysis. 2017;**57**

[7] Andre Croppenstedt F, Medhat El-Helepi C, Laila Lokosang C. African Commission on Agricultural Statistics 2019; 1-14

[8] DRC Agricultural Code2008. p. 52

[9] Guengant Pierre, José Mangalu Mobhe, Agbada NMB. Benefiting from the dividend D Putting people back at the center of development trajectories Democratic Republic OF THE DEMOGRAPHIC DIVIDEND? Put the population back at the center of the development trajectories of the Democratic Republic of the Congo. 2014

[10] PAM. Second Regular Session Interim Country Strategic Plan – Yemen (2019–2020)2020. p. 45 Available from: https://executiveboard.wfp.org/fr%0D

[11] Eide WB, Marais M, Wamala E, Kabahenda M. Realizing the right to adequate food and nutritional status of land evictees: A case for mothers/caregivers and their children in rural central Uganda. 2018;**33**

[12] ACF-D. Suivi-évaluation D. Rapport de la mission d' évaluation dans les zones de santé de Minovaet Kalehe, Territoired e Kalehe, Province du Sud Kivu, République Démocratique du C2008. pp. 1-41

[13] Jones AD. Critical review of emerging research evidence on agricultural biodiversity, diet diversity and nutritional status in low- and middle-income countries. 2017;**75**(10):31

[14] Paz L. Urban agriculture - food autonomy. 1993;**21**(3)

[15] Ministry of MS & PRONANUT SK. End-line nutritional survey report of the ZS of Bunyakiri Minova in South Kivu-DRC. 2021;1-7

[16] Boto I, Peccerella C La, Researcher J, Brasesco F, Access to Land and Rural Development. 2012

[17] Diagourou E, Jacques C. Youth Access to Land: Women's Visions. 2009

[18] Coulibaly B, Sagoe G, Piwowar A. Towards poverty reduction in developing countries: An empirical study of the impact of land reforms in Kati, Mali. 2021;**16**(3)

[19] Berkhout ED. Better soils for a healthier life? An econometric

assessment of the link between soil nutrients and malnutrition in sub-Saharan Africa. 2019;**14**(1)

[20] Chakona G, Shackleton CM. Household food insecurity along an agro-ecological gradient influences the nutritional status of children in South Africa. 2018;**34**

[21] Thareau B. Regulating Access to Land, the Local Reinvention of Agricultural Corporatism. 2014

[22] Bucekuderhwa C, Mapatano S. Understanding the dynamics of vulnerability to food insecurity in South Kivu

[23] Tefft J, Kelly V. Understanding and reducing malnutrition in Mali. 2003;1-8

[24] Rehman A, Ping Q, Razzaq A. Pathways and associations between women's land ownership and children's food and nutrition security in AU

[25] Africa E. A review of some studies on factors associated with the nutritional status of children under five in South Africa. 2020;**17**(21)

[26] Ayoubi M El. Intrauterine growth retardation and extreme prematurity: Impact on mortality and morbidity in the short and medium term. 2017;

[27] Mshida HA, Kassim N, Mpolya E, Kimanya M. Water, sanitation and hygiene practices associated with the nutritional status of children under five in semi-pastoral communities Tanzania. 2018;**98**(5):21

[28] Morrison C, Linskens C. Explanatory factors of malnutrition in sub-Saharan Africa;**167**(167):39

[29] Fournier T, Jarty J, Lapeyre N. Food, weapon of its kind. 2019;19-49

[30] Nu F. New Report on the State of Food Security and Nutrition in the World 20212021. p. 264

[31] Wigle JM, Akseer N, Mogilevskii R, Brar S, Conway K. Stunting reduction factors in the Kyrgyz Republic: A country case study. 2020;**112**(Suppl 2)

[32] Singh S, De A. Regional differences in agricultural and socio-economic factors associated with dietary diversity of farming households in India. 2020; **15**:4

[33] Karageorgou D. Assessing food intake from household budget surveys: A national analysis in Bangladesh. 2018; **13**(8)

Chapter 12

Older Adults in Co-Residential Family Care: Circumstances Precipitating Rural Older Adults for Co-Residential Family Care Arrangements

Kidus Yenealem Mefteh

Abstract

Using a phenomenological study design, this study attempts to investigate the factors that lead rural older adults to seek out co-residential family care arrangements. Twelve older adults from rural areas were interviewed in-depth; the data were then inductively categorized and organized into themes. The circumstances that lead older adults to give up their independent life and move in with their offspring in the research area include physical limits and health issues, separation and divorce, the loss of a spouse, economic troubles, neglect, inheritance disputes, and inaccessible places. The result recommends decision-makers and other interested parties that measures must be focused on preserving a favorable living environment for elderly people living in rural areas and addressing issues that are crucial in co-residential family care settings developing senior/adult care facilities and expanding access to health care.

Keywords: co-residential care, rural ethiopia, older adults, qualitative study, family caregivers

1. Introduction

An increasing number of older adults are living and receiving support and care from diverse sources. Older adults can organize their living arrangements in official institutions, with other people, or by themselves, according to Li [1]. However, compared to those living alone or in institutions, the majority of older adults live with their family members [1–4]. In Ethiopia, there are 3,568,810 million persons over the age of 60 or 4.8% of the country's total population [5]. In 2022, the number is anticipated to reach 5,325,652 million. Among them, 78% of them would reside in rural areas, while 22% will do so in cities (CSA as given in Ministry of Labor and Social Affairs, [6]). In Ethiopia, the majority of senior citizens reside in their own or family houses and are supported by their families [7–10]. In rural Ethiopia, older people primarily get care and support from their extended family network, which cannot be properly replaced by any other body [9].

The traditional system of care through familial ties is essential for the well-being of older adults in underdeveloped nations like Ethiopia where the system of public transfer for supporting older adults is inadequately established. However, studies frequently concentrate on older adults in residential care institutions with little attention to older adults living with their relatives [11], particularly to those who are dependent and in a co-residential living arrangement with their kin. This is despite the fact that the majority of older adults in Ethiopia receive care and support through their kinship ties [7, 8, 12]. When an elderly person can no longer handle necessary daily tasks on their own, care is required. Health, environmental, and economic changes spur support within families [13]. Many elderly people see an increase in family support as their sickness progresses [14]. Additionally, older adults may need care due to physical issues and psychological difficulties [15]. According to the vast majority of studies, physical limitations, especially those that affect ADL, increase the need for family care and the chance that older adults will live with family members [1, 16, 17]. Likewise, emotional closeness or bonding, as well as reciprocity of care [18–20], play important roles in co-residential family care [21, 22].

Widowed, divorced, and never married older people are more likely to live with and rely on their offspring than married older people [2, 16, 23, 24]. When elderly people lack the funds to cover their basic necessities and medical care, they must rely on their families [25]. On the other hand, older adults with great physical and mental health and the ability to give back appear to be prerequisites for care and support. According to a study conducted in Ethiopia, older adults who are financially independent, physically fit, and in good health are more likely to receive assistance [10].

Studies have also highlighted the socioeconomic, psychological, and spiritual requirements of older people in rural areas. Older adults deal with a variety of physical and psychological issues [26], such as joint discomfort and dependency-inducing sight impairment [27]. The context of caregiving in a co-residential care setting is determined by a variety of characteristics, including the caregiver's relationship to the care receiver, gender, age, and socioeconomic status [28]. Older adults with little financial resources are more likely to be marginalized and have low social status [29], which can lead to isolation (neglect) and eventual loneliness. In addition, rural older adults have socioeconomic difficulty, low income, and a lack of land ownership [30–32].

Care choices for older adults are influenced by factors such as the number of children, educational level, residential area, availability of health infrastructure and care facilities, and filial piety-related values [33]. In Ethiopia, facilities offer older people essential services, health care, and recreational activities [34, 35]. Studies on the effects of institutional care and the requirements of senior citizens living in residential care facilities have also been done by Alemnesh and Adamek [36], Eskedar [37], Tigist [38], and Bruck [39]. Older adults benefit from the fundamental healthcare services offered in institutions, although they are insufficient [36, 37].

In Ethiopia, older adults receiving institutional care are more likely to experience depression, isolation from friends and relatives, a lack of daily activities, and a lack of social engagement [36–39]. Getachew [40] and Aynshet [41] each conducted a study on the conditions of elderly persons who are homeless and older adults who are beggars. The research concluded that factors contributing to bad living conditions included poverty, death, separation from immediate family, and a lack of social support.

In her investigation of the care provided to Italo-Ethiopian war veterans (1935–1941), Hosseana [42] discovered that both formal and informal care providers offer financial, material, transportation, health, and informational support. The research on older adults in rural locations in Ethiopia received little attention from Abraham [43], Noguchi [44], Fantahun et al. [45], and Kifle [8]. However, elderly people in rural areas and those who live in communities remain a population group in Ethiopia that has received little attention [8, 11, 43].

In sub-Saharan Africa, where the majority of older adults live and receive support from their informal networks, families are strong and familial ties are still present despite the strain [46]. In Ethiopia, it is a widespread family system custom to look after older parents, especially in rural areas [7–9, 12]. In addition to this, the majority of the scholarly literature focuses on urban older adults who reside in institutions. Society has the propensity to view elderly people as helpless and dependent, which opens the door to abuse such as exploitation and neglect.

Older people make up 9.1% (11,103) of Bassona Warana Woreda's total population, according to CSA [5]. According to the Woreda Finance and Economic Development Office report from 2021, the proportion of older people aged 60 and over in the total population is predicted to be 9.5%, which is significantly higher than the national share of older people (4.8%) in the total population of the nation as measured by the 2007 Census. This project will significantly advance knowledge, practice, and policy in the field of geriatrics in general and geriatric social work in particular given the paucity of literature on family care and support for older adults in Ethiopia. It will address the knowledge gap regarding aging rural Ethiopians receiving family care, which currently exists in the literature. The study's baseline data on geriatrics and family care was what the researcher hoped would spark more research on informal care. This study aims to explore study participants' experiences with the conditions that lead them to co-residential family care and is motivated by the paucity of studies on elder adults living in family care arrangements in rural areas.

2. Objective of the study

The main goal of this study is to examine and explain older adults' lived experiences in rural areas in relation to the circumstances that led them to seek family care in a co-residential family care setting. This study specifically attempts to describe the socioeconomic and health-related factors that lead rural older adults to co-residential family care arrangements.

2.1 Research questions

1. What are the physical and health-related circumstances that precipitate rural older adults for co-residential family care in the study area?

2. What are the socio-economic circumstances that precipitate rural older adults for co-residential family care in the study area?

2.2 Scope of the study

Only older adults who were receiving co-residential family care at the time the study was done are included in the study. The study also specifically focused on the conditions that lead older people in rural areas to require co-residential family care in order to represent the lived experience of older adults.

3. Methods

3.1 Study area

Although the meticulous number of older adults in Gudoberet Kebele (the smallest administrative unit in Ethiopia) is unknown, it is estimated that 438 (46,089.5%) older adults live there based on estimates from the Bassona Werrana Wereda (the third-level administrative division of Ethiopia—after zones and regional states). The choice of Gudoberet Kebele to conduct the study is influenced by the practicality of the Kebele in terms of time and expense as well as the researcher's familiarity with the area. The population is agrarians who depend on agriculture for their living, according to the manager of the kebele. Residents who belong to the Amhara ethnic group and are Ethiopian Orthodox Christians make up more than 99% of the population.

3.2 Study design

In-depth interviews with rural older study participants were conducted by the researcher to get the data. The lived experience of older adults in rural areas was investigated and described using a descriptive phenomenology approach, with an emphasis on the factors that lead to co-residential family care. According to Sloan and Bowe [47], the researcher selected this approach to examine and explain older adults' experiences as they actually were. In a phenomenological study, it is typical to put away thinking and prior interpretation and place more attention on the lived experiences of older adults because these experiences make more sense to those who are living them. The study's intrinsic structural experience belongs to older adults because of their lived experiences with it (Husserl, n.d. as cited in [48]). In addition, descriptive phenomenology employs bracketing or separating the researcher's perspective, values, and comprehension of older adults' experiences in co-residential family care [49]. So, the researcher used language to convey their personal experience that mimics how rural older adults' facial emotions become psychological expressions [50]. Additionally, bracketing was used for the study's analysis and interview. The study has received approval from the Mizan-Tepi institutional review board, and informed consent and confidentiality were properly acknowledged when interview data was being gathered.

3.3 The sample

The researcher has taken into consideration several phenomenologically recommended concerns when determining sample size. As Dukes [48] pointed out, the researcher placed a lot of emphasis on avoiding making assumptions about what they wanted to observe and paying attention to what was actually visible. Furthermore, samplings were also taken into account based on the research topics [51]. These factors guided the interviewing of 12 rural older adults receiving co-residence care who were available during the data collection.

Older adults who live with their families in a rural Kebele of Gudoberet and receive care from them are the study's participants. The inclusion criteria for choosing participants older adults are developed in accordance with the study's goal. The criteria utilized to identify participants are (1) older adults aged 60 and above based on the UN definition, (2) older adults who are co-residing with their family carers receiving care, and (3) older adults who are willing and capable of supplying information with consent.

3.4 Data collection procedure

This study employed in-depth interviews to get data from rural older adults by creating an interview guide. After the interviewer establishes a casual, engaging relationship with rural older adults, the phenomenology design calls for a lengthy interview in which data are gathered through open-ended questions [52]. The Mizan-Tepi University Institutional Review Board granted the study's ethical approval (IRB). Additionally, the researcher adhered to [53] Ethical and Safety Recommendations when investigating delicate subjects. In addition, this study followed the Declaration of Helsinki's guidelines. The older adults in rural areas were scheduled for interviews at a time that worked best for them. They were made aware of their ability to decline to take part in or not reply to particular interview questions.

Likewise, older adults were made aware of their right to privacy and secrecy, and they were advised that neither their names nor the information they provided would be utilized in any other way. About 40–75 minutes were allotted for the interviews. The participants' native language of Amharic was used for all of the interviews. With the elder people's permission, the interviews were audio recorded.

3.5 Data analysis

The first step in the data analysis method was arranging the older adult interview data and phenomenologically transcribing the audio recordings. The researcher has horizonalized the interview data by assuming that each statement is pertinent to the study. Listing the meaning or meaning units was done after the horizonalized sentences. After that, meanings were grouped into common themes (a group of related data arranged in the same location) and categories, resulting in a meaningful "essence" that permeates the data. This was accomplished by eliminating overlapping and repeating statements [54]. The textural descriptions of rural older adults in a co-residential family care setting were then developed using these grouped themes and categories. Construction of the circumstances for co-residential family care is based on the textural descriptions, structural descriptions, and integration of textures and structures into the meanings and essences of rural older adults' lived experiences [52]. This study's goal is not to theorize using previous interpretation, as was discussed in the study design. So, information gathered from older people in rural areas is inductively coded.

The researcher has carefully listened to the audio recordings of all of the participants older adults in order to improve the quality of the data. Peer debriefing involved disclosing part of the data and analysis to coworkers in order to solicit their helpful feedback. In order to confirm that the analysis accurately reflects the lived experiences of the study's rural older adult participants, the researcher also presented the analysis to them.

4. Findings

The study participants who are older adults move out of their own homes or locations and into co-residential family care. For a variety of reasons, they moved away from their initial residence, and they spent between about 2 months to 23 years living in the houses of their offspring. The older adult participants' socio-demographic characteristics (**Table 1**) are listed below for a better understanding of their background. Additionally, the studies use pseudonyms to characterize the experiences of older adults.

Participants (pseudonym)	Sex	Age (years)	Education	Religion	Marital status	Source of livelihood	Number of children alive	Relationship with current caregiver	Number of years lived in their current living arrangement
Almaz	F	89	No education	Orthodox	Divorced	Agriculture	1	Mother	23
Emebet	F	65	Read and write	Orthodox	Widow	Agriculture	3	Mother	14
Asegedech	F	67	No education	Orthodox	Divorced	Agriculture	1	Mother	Since married
Abebe	M	69	No education	Orthodox	Remarried	Collecting fire woods	2	Father	5
Mulu	F	61	No education	Orthodox	Remarried	Local liquor sale	2	Mother	20
Bogale	M	88	No education	Orthodox	Widow	Agriculture	4	Father	5
Mekonen	M	89	Fourth grade and church education	Orthodox	Widow	Agriculture and pension	5 (adoptees)	Father (not biological)	Since married
Haile	M	92	Church education	Orthodox	Widow	Agriculture and pension	8	Father	Since married
Desta	M	82	No education	Orthodox	Married	Agriculture	5	Father	Since married
Gizachew	M	75	Read and write	Orthodox	Separated	Agriculture	1	Father	3
Yeshemebet	F	73	No education	Orthodox	Widow	Agriculture	7	Mother	2 months
Gete	F	70	No education	Orthodox	Widow	Agriculture	8	Mother	5

Table 1.
Socio-demographic characteristics of older adult participants.

4.1 Physical limitations and health problems

The functional limitations of older adults to carry out tasks is one of the justifications for shared living. Among the participants, *Bogale*, *Haile*, *Mekonen*, *Desta*, and *Yeshemebet* claimed that their choice to live with their adult children was motivated by a physical inability to manage daily tasks on their own. Their primary means of subsistence is agriculture, which involves hard physical labor. However, when they grew older, they found it difficult to handle the demands of agricultural labor. They, therefore, made the decision to leave all of their assets, including their land, to their children who lived close by in the hope that they would manage them and take good care of them.

> *I started to lose my strength as I grew older. I was unable to tend to the animals while also cultivating the stony farmlands. I then made the decision to sell the cattle and give one of my daughters the farmland in exchange. I also let my two girls use the empty space in my compound. They built their own home and share residence with us. (Desta, 13 April 2021)*

Nevertheless, due to temporary and bedridden health issues, some older adults are unable to maintain their independent living. Even though they were physically fit when it started, their condition forces them to depend on their children. Before they begin to cohabit with their children, *Emebet*, *Abebe*, *Bogale*, and *Yeshemebet* each give a brief description of their health.

> *I plunged into a little gorge twelve years ago. Then my hand and one part of my leg went numb. My kids drove me to the hospital and got me some holy water. I am unable to regain my health, though, because nothing is possible apart from God's approval. I therefore stay here and sleep in the midst of my kids as I wait for God to either heal me or take my life. (Emebet, 24 March 2021).*

> *Due to an eye condition that made it difficult for me to cook, fetch water, and perform other household tasks, I was unable to work. Consequently, two months before to the date of this interview, I made the decision to move in with my married daughter. I do not have a female child living with me who helps with household duties. (Yeshemebet, 18 April, 2021)*

According to interview data from older adults in the study area, their physical health and strength are decreasing, forcing them to look for co-residential family care.

4.2 Inaccessible location

The decision of older adults to relocate their living arrangements to their offspring, who are located in a relatively accessible location, is influenced by the location of their home or neighborhood being inaccessible. Their inability to access the institutions they deemed essential for the old age period is a result of the remoteness of their former location as well as their physical deterioration. Some older adults find it difficult to complete their old age activity because of the distance to a church and the rough terrain.

> *The environment made it difficult for me to move into the location I wanted when I was at home. I find it challenging to consistently travel to church due to the slick roads. When I get older, that's when I need to connect with God. I therefore require a convenient place*

where I may locate a church close by. Because it's convenient for me to attend church and is closer to town, this is where I've chosen to live. (Bogale, 29 March 2021)

Gete also notes the terrain and how to get to the church, but she also stresses out how the weather and lack of medical facilities have an impact on her health and force her to change her living situation.

I formerly resided in a warm, sunny lowland area. I struggle with hypertension. Additionally, there isn't a clinic where people can get examinations and medical care. My children warned me that the warm, sunny weather might make my condition worse. I made the decision to come here because it is a highland location and is close to health centers. (Gete, 15 April 2021)

As a result, the necessity for co-residential family care in rural older adults is influenced by external circumstances. Regardless of the quality of family caregiving, older adults are encouraged to live with their families in co-residence by the neighborhood's generally favorable physical environment, which allows them access to religious and medical institutions.

4.3 Separation and divorce

One of the circumstances that lead to co-residential family care is conflict with a spouse that results in legal separation or divorce. Some of their reasons for divorcing their spouse and choosing a new living situation for their children include behavioral issues with their spouse, complications with their husband and adoptee, and disputes over children born outside of marriage.

We shared a home for 35 years. We are currently residing in different locations due to our inconsistent behavior. I moved to Addis Abeba and stayed there for eighteen years as a result of her behavior. I built a house once I got home. I imagined that we would cohabitate. But she walked away from me. I became sick because I was upset. Then, when I arrived here, my sister assisted me in obtaining medication and recovering from my sickness. She warned me not to go back to my house again, so I made this my home. (Gizachewu, 12 April 2021)

Due to tension between her husband and the adoptee, *Almaz*, 89, and her husband split 23 years ago. Her husband planned to give the adopted child ownership of their farmland.

We had one adopted child and my spouse had been sterile. My husband wished to give the adoptee the farmland. He intended to take the farmland, according to my adoptee. I informed him that since he is not a member of my blood family, he cannot take my land. Our argument became very heated. He gave me some little barley. I instructed him to consume the barley. I divorced at that point. I eventually got to my biological child. (Almaz, 23 March 2021)

Asegedech also says that she made the decision to live with her child because her spouse had an extramarital child. She was angry and made the decision to move in with her married daughter.

4.4 Death of spouse

Emebet, *Yeshemebet*, *Gete*, *Bogale*, *Mekonen*, and *Haile* are among the older participants who are widowed. All of them, with the exception of *Emebet*, lost their spouses when they turned 60. If their spouses were still alive, some of the participants who switched to co-residential family care said they would prefer to live alone. They must relocate their living situation with their children due to the loss of their partner, their ensuing isolation, and the difficulties they face at work.

> *Upon the death of my wife, I encountered difficulties in living because there is no one with me to cook and do other domestic work. Then, I decided to live with my child after the 7th year of my wife's death. (Bogale, 25 April, 2021)*

After turning 80, *Mekonen* and *Haile* lost their wife. They could not support themselves on their own. They made the decision to welcome their married son and daughter into their own house as a result. When their spouse passed away, they moved in with their children.

4.5 Economic problem

Because they lack the resources to live alone, some older adults must rely on and live with their children in order to be healthy. They have no other option for living but sharing a home with their children, especially if they lack farmland. *Abebe*, *Mulu*, and *Asegedech* spoke about a financial issue that led to co-residence with their children.

> *During the Derg regime, the local administration took my farm. After that, I got a job renting land from nearby farms. However, when my physical fitness declined, I was unable to continue, and the cost of renting land increased such that I could no longer compete with other farmers. These made me dependent on my son, then I had to switch to my daughter. (Abebe, 20 May, 2021)*

> *The main cause of my daughter's dependence on me is the financial situation. I have no source of income and have instead spent the majority of my life working for others. I moved in with my daughter because I was having financial trouble. (Mulu, 26 April, 2021)*

Asegedech further notes that her reliance on her daughter is a result of the financial difficulties she encountered following her divorce from her husband.

> *I didn't receive a portion of the land or any other property when my spouse and I got divorced. After that, I ran into financial problems. My daughter was my final hope. I arrived here because I lack any sources of support. If I had a source of income, like farmland, I believe I am capable of surviving on my own. (Asegedech, 27 April, 2021)*

Men are the primary breadwinners in the study area, and if a husband dies, the wife will find it difficult to maintain her usual lifestyle on her alone, forcing her to move for co-residential family care.

4.6 Neglect and inheritance dispute

Among the various factors that lead older adults to leave their house and move in with another child is neglect by nearby children and possible abuse threats. Participants who are older adults who have moved away from their former homes note that they may be threatened and neglected by their children if they share a house or live in the same area. When there is a conflict of interest, children who are supposed to be a source of protection can end up being a threat to older people. Children and the surviving parent clash when one of the parents pass away about who will inherit what. Sometimes the argument is intensified to make older people fear their children and leave or move in with another child who can take care of them and protect them.

> *One of my children begged me to give her a half of her father's property after my spouse passed away. I complied with her request and collected my village's elders and youngsters. I instructed my kids to split up their father's assets evenly. Then, one of my daughters steadfastly refused to split the acreage because she wanted to take all of her father's land by herself. We argue over this as a result, and I filed a lawsuit. I was permitted to use the land by the court. I gave her permission to take her share even after the court's ruling, but she persisted in pestering me. She intended to murder me. Due to the fact that I was living alone, I began to fear for my life. I left my house as a result and moved here to be with my children. (Gete, 15 April 2021)*

Some of the older adults were compelled to move out of their home and live with another child or relative due to abuse by a son who shared a residence with them. *Bogale* and *Yeshemebet* emphasize how frustrating it is that their sons have been neglecting them at home. They complained about how their married son, who lived in the same compound, was treated.

> *My child displays challenging conduct and lives with me in one compound. I gave her a blessing because his wife is a lovely person. But my kid treated me badly. He ignored me for the first three and a half years after the loss of my wife. He never encourages me to approach close to the fire, even when I start to get cold, while he relaxes there. I become upset as a result, and I ask my other son to take me to him. (Bogale, 29 March 2021)*

Although older adults in this study want their children to provide them with care and safety, there are occasions when difficult relationships arise as a result of financial considerations and caregivers' abusive behavior toward older people. By escaping this toxic and violent relationship, the older adult's decision to move to a new co-residential family care setting is mediated by the presence of an adult child with a stronger emotional attachment.

5. Discussion

The likelihood of co-residence is determined by the parents' financial dependence on their children, their marital status, and their capacity to perform activities of daily living (ADL) independently [17]. The move to co-residence is linked to older adults who are widowed having declining health [55]. As older adults with health issues are more likely to depend on others for a living, their physical and mental state affects whether they choose co-residential family care. Changes in functional health status result in a requirement for additional family support and an increase in the possibility that older adults will live with children [1, 16, 17].

This study also shows that independent living is impossible for older adults due to their physical limitations in doing daily tasks. As a result, they are compelled to live together with their adult children since they require help with daily tasks.

The co-residence of older adults with their children was also found to be influenced by their marital status. Ruggles and Heggeness [24] observed that changes in older adults' marital status owing to separation, divorce, and widowhood enhance older people's need to co-reside with their offspring. This conclusion is consistent with the study's findings. The likelihood of co-residential living with children grows as a result of the change in marital status experienced during a period of widowhood [16]. The results also showed that the requirement for co-residence is not solely caused by a change in marital status, as older adults' decisions to do so may also be influenced by financial pressures and physical limitations that prevent them from living alone. Accordingly, a study by Audinaryana et al. [2] found that socioeconomically disadvantaged women, widows without jobs, and those who have had physical disabilities are more likely to live with their adult children.

Challenges arise for older adults who want to keep their independence due to economic issues. Due to their financial struggles, they are forced to change their living situation to co-residential care. According to earlier research [17], economic factors influence informal family care, and indicators of older adults living situations include their degree of education, occupation, and pension [1, 2, 17]. Owning material goods and working in the economy helps older adults keep their independence, but economic hardship makes it more necessary for them to live with children. While older people with high occupational levels and pension coverage live alone, shared living is more likely to occur when one's financial capacity is lower [1, 2]. In this study, agriculture is the main source of income for older adults, who also have lower literacy rates. Age-related financial pressures force them to rely on co-residential family care.

Older adults in the study area are vulnerable to challenges with their ability to support themselves due to the lack of social security programs. For people without access to farms, the economic burden is too great. The choice of older adults will be influenced by a variety of factors, therefore having financial resources does not ensure independent living. This study demonstrated that, despite having adequate financial resources, older adults often need to live with their adult children due to physical restrictions and inaccessibility of their residence. Some senior citizens who are unable to manage their property and live independently move their married adult children into their own homes.

This study also identifies other factors that lead rural older adults to change their living arrangements, including inheritance conflicts, abuse, and neglect by their shared child. However, earlier research has shown that older adults who experience violence or family conflict tend to live alone or stop sharing housing, contradicting this conclusion [56]. It is advantageous for older adults who have been mistreated or neglected to move to other co-residential care when other children are available who have stronger emotional bonds with them. Older adults move in with their adult children for emotional connection and a healthier parent–child bond [17]. The results showed that older adults who experience abuse usually arrange their living situation with a caring, close-knit adult child.

5.1 Conclusion and implication for practice

Older adults decide to co-reside for family care for a variety of reasons, including physical limitations and health issues, an inaccessible location, separation and divorce, the loss of a spouse, economic difficulties, neglect, and disputes over inheritance. Future policy initiatives for the care of older people in rural areas should think about making local infrastructure development accessible, bolstering the family system, and extending support services. Physical, psychological, and social difficulties are forcing older adults in the research region to relocate for co-residential family care.

In Ethiopia, social work is still a relatively new profession. Higher education institutions should seek to open and expand gerontology social work education by developing faculty, curriculum, attracting a large number of students, and disseminating research findings in order to satisfy the requirements of older adults [57]. To offer care for this population group that is becoming more and more demanding, social work education generally and geriatrics social work training in particular should be increased.

Addressing older adults' social and psychological needs is just as important as meeting their bodily requirements. Interdisciplinary education must be prioritized if gerontological social workers are to be qualified. Geriatric social work interventions should include a biopsychosocial approach and interdisciplinary teamwork, especially with health experts, to address the complex needs of older adults and their family caregivers [58].

Senior centers should be built because they provide a number of advantages, including opportunities for older people to make new friends and find joy in life [59]. Additionally, the establishment of senior centers in rural areas would encourage self-care and health management among older people living there [60]. Senior centers also encourage older people's involvement in the community through social interaction and friendships with other older people, both of which have been found to be important in other studies [61].

The creation of daycare facilities helped older adults live better lives by addressing their loneliness and sense of isolation [62– 64]. Additionally, because older adults in nuclear families are more likely to suffer from depression than those in joint families, the importance of family caregivers for older adults should not be minimized [65]. Besides that, it is important to recognize the role that family support plays in reducing loneliness in old age, especially for people who do not get enough family time [63]. It is also important to offer assistance to rural older adults' family caregivers in order to lessen their burden of caregiving. Training in caregiving [66], financial assistance and reimbursement for the care given to senior citizens [67], and provision of farmlands for family caregivers are significant.

The creation and implementation of home care for senior citizens, which is currently a favored style of care, should involve social workers significantly [28]. It is essential to increase older adults' access to healthcare. Additionally, daycare and family care arrangements could be combined with services like health education and entertainment programs.

It is important to provide material assistance and expand community health insurance programs. The quality of life for older people in rural areas will improve thanks to gerotechnology or the provision of assistive gadgets for incapacitating medical issues. To support older people in rural areas and lessen the strain on family caregivers, it is crucial that all stakeholders—including governmental and non-governmental organizations, religious institutions, and human service professionals—play their part.

5.2 Limitations of the study

"Why do older adults in rural areas in the research region seek co-residential family care?" is the topic that this study seeks to address. A co-residential family care arrangement's sorts of services, older adults' needs, interactions, and problems are not examined in this study. Furthermore, conclusions from the study should not be extrapolated to apply to other older adults receiving co-residential family care outside the study area.

Acknowledgements

I would want to show my gratitude to all the respectable senior citizens who took part and shared their expertise, opinions, and experience by sparing their time and energy. Without their gracious attitude and active participation, the study may not have been able to be completed. They were incredibly cooperative and supportive. Because of them, my time in the field was really intriguing and enlightening. Fourthly, I would like to express my gratitude for the assistance and collaboration of the Gudoberet Kebele Administration, the Bassona Werrana Woreda Administration Office, and the North Shoa Zone Labor and Social Affairs Office during the data collection process.

Funding

The author received no financial support for the research, authorship, and/or publication of this article.

Declaration of conflicting interests

The author declared no potential conflicts of interest with respect to the research, authorship, and/or publication of this article.

Ethical approval and consent to participate

Ethical clearance was obtained from Mizan-Tepi University research directorate. The aim and potential benefits of the study were discussed with all older adult participants. Written informed consent was taken before involved with participants.

Author details

Kidus Yenealem Mefteh
Department of Social Work, Mizan-Tepi University, Mizan-Aman, Ethiopia

*Address all correspondence to: yenealemkidus@gmail.com

References

[1] Li Z. Determinants of living arrangements among the Chinese elderly: New evidence from the CLHLS 2011 wave. Chinese Studies. 2015;**4**:32-43. DOI: 10.4236/chnstd.2015.41006

[2] Audinaryana N, Sheela J, Kavitha N. Living arrangements of the elderly women in a rural setting of South India: Patterns, differentials and determinants. International Journal. 1999;**29**(2):37-48. Available from: http://www.jstor.org/stable/41421174 [Accessed: February 24, 2021]

[3] Govil P, Gupta S. Domestic violence against elderly people: A case study of India. Advances in Aging Research. 2016;**5**:110-121. DOI: 10.4236/aar.2016.55011

[4] Sereny MD. Living arrangement of older adult in China: The interplay among preferences, realities and health. Research on Aging. 2011;**33**(2):172-204. DOI: 10.1177/0164027510392387

[5] Central Statistical Agency. Population and Housing Census Report. Addis Ababa: Author; 2007

[6] Ministry of Labor and Social Affairs. Government of the Federal Democratic Republic of Ethiopia Draft National Plan of Action on Older Persons (2008-2017) E.C. Addis Ababa: Author; 2017

[7] Abdi A. Who Takes Care of the Elderly in Ethiopia When Reciprocal Relationships Breakdown? [master thesis]. Lund, Sweden: Lund University; 2012. Retrieved from: https://lup.lub.lu.se/student-papers/record/3054302/file/3054304.pdf

[8] Kifle M. Old Age and Social Change: An Anthropological Study of the Lives of the Elderly Among the Amhara of Ensaro [master's thesis]. Addis Ababa University; 2002

[9] Ministry of Labor and Social Affairs. Government of the Federal Democratic Republic of Ethiopia National Plan of Action on Older Persons (1998-2007) E.C. Addis Ababa: Author; 2006

[10] Samson C. Domestic Elder Abuse: A Phenomenological Study of the Lived Experiences of Abused Elders in Dangila Town Administration, Ethiopia [doctoral dissertation]. Addis Ababa University; 2014

[11] Messay GK. Examining Quality of Life of Community-Dwelling Older People in Addis Ababa, Ethiopia [doctoral dissertation]. Addis Ababa University; 2015

[12] Help Age International. Vulnerability of Older People in Ethiopia: The Case of Oromia, Amhara and SNNP Regional States. Author; 2013

[13] Knodel J, Chayovan N. Intergenerational family care for and by older people in Thailand (Report 11-732). Population Studies Center, University of Michigan, Institute of Social Research. 2012;**32**:682-694. DOI: 10.1108/01443331211280719

[14] Center for Policy on Aging-Rapid Review. The Care and Support of Older People: An International Perspective. 2014. Available from: http://www.cpa.org.uk [Accessed: November 23, 2021]

[15] Sigurðardottir SH. Patterns of Care and Support in Old Age [dissertation series NO. 40, 2013]. School of Health Sciences, Jönköping University; 2013. Available from: http://www.diva-portal.org [Accessed: December 25, 2021]

[16] Korinek K, Zimmer Z, Gu D. Transitions in marital status and functional health and patterns of intergenerational co-residence among China's elderly population. Journal of Gerontology: Social Sciences. 2011;**66B**(2):260-270. DOI: 10.1093/geronb/gbq107

[17] Zhang Z, Gu D, Luo Y. Co-residence with elderly parents in contemporary China: The role of filial piety, reciprocity, socioeconomic resources, and parental needs. Journal of Cross-Cultural Gerontology. 2014;**29**(3):259-276. DOI: 10.1007/s10823-014-9239-4

[18] Hsu H-C, Shyu Y-IL. Implicit exchanges in family caregiving for frail elders in Taiwan. Qualitative Health Research. 2003;**13**(8):1078-1093. DOI: 10.1177/1049732303256370

[19] Mitchell BA. Would I share a home with an elderly parent? Exploring ethnocultural diversity and intergenerational support relations during young adulthood. Canadian Journal on Aging. 2003;**22**:69-82. DOI: 10.1017/S0714980800003743

[20] Ugargol AP, Bailey A. Reciprocity between older adults and their care-givers in emigrant households of Kerala, India. Ageing and Society. 2020;**41**:1699-1725. DOI: 10.1017/s0144686x19001685

[21] Firbank OE, Johnson-Lafleur J. Older persons relocating with a family caregiver: Processes, stages, and motives. Journal of Applied Gerontology. 2007;**26**(2):182-207. DOI: 10.1177/0733464807300224

[22] Romero-Moreno R, Márquez-González M, Losada A, López J. Motives for caring: Relationship to stress and coping dimensions. International Psychogeriatrics. 2010;**23**(4):573-582. DOI: 10.1017/s1041610210001821

[23] Meng D, Xu G, He L, Zhang M, Lin D. What determines the preference for future living arrangements of middle-aged and older people in urban China? PLoS One. 2017;**12**(7):1-14. DOI: 10.1371/journal.pone.0180764

[24] Ruggles S, Heggeness M. Intergenerationalco-residenceindeveloping countries. The case of rural Thailand. Population and Development Review. 2008;**34**(2):253-281. DOI: 10.1111/j.1728-4457.2008.00219.x

[25] Chirwa M, Kalinda R. Challenges of the elderly in Zambia. A systematic review study. European Scientific Journal. 2016;**12**(2):351. DOI: 10.19044/esj.2016.v12n2p351

[26] Hiremath SS. The health status of rural elderly women in India: A case study. International Journal of Criminology and Sociological Theory. 2012;**5**(3):960-963. Available from: https://ijcst.journals.yorku.ca/index.php/ijcst/article/download/36067/32745 [Accessed: January 15, 2021]

[27] Tiwari S, Sinha A, Patwardhan K, Gehlot S, Gambhir IS, Mohapatra S. Prevalence of health problems among elderly: A study in a rural population of Varanasi. Indian Journal of Preventive and Social Medicine. 2010;**41**(3):226-230. Available from: https://www.academia.edu/download/84850344/iblt10i3p226.pdf [Accessed: March 15, 2021]

[28] Greenberg J, Seltzer M, Brewer E. Caregivers to older adults. In: Berkman B, editor. Family and Intergenerational Social Work Practice in Special Caregiving Situations. New York: Oxford University Press; 2006. pp. 339-354

[29] Cao F. Elderly Care, Intergenerational Relationships and Social Change in Rural China. Singapore: Springer Nature; 2019. DOI: 10.1007/978-981-13-2962-3_6

[30] Li H, Tracy MB. Family support, financial needs, and health care needs of rural elderly in China: A field study. Journal of Cross-Cultural Gerontology. 1999;**14**(4):357-371. DOI: 10.1023/A:1006607707655

[31] Lowry D. Aging, Social Change and Elderly Wellbeing in China: Insight from Mixed Method Village Research (Report 09-691). Population Study Center, University of Michigan, Institute of Social Research; 2009. Available from: https://www.psc.isr.umich.edu/pubs/pdf/rr09-691.pdf [Accessed: December 10, 2021]

[32] Panda KP. The elderly in rural Orissa: Alone in distress. Economic and Political Weekly. 1998;**33**(25):1545-1550. Available from: http://www.jstor.org/stable/4406908 [Accessed February 24, 2021]

[33] Lu J, Zhang L, Zhang K. Care preferences among Chinese older adults with daily care needs: Individual and community factors. Research on Aging. 2020;**43**:166-179. DOI: 10.1177/0164027520939321

[34] Segniwork L. Experiences and Practices of Old Age Home Care and Support to the Elderly Living in the Institutions: Assessment at Three Selected Institutions in Addis Ababa [master's thesis]. Addis Ababa University; 2014

[35] Tewodros H. Institutional Care Provided for the Elderly and Residents Perception of the Quality of Care Provided by Mekedonia Home for the Elderly and Mentally Disabled [master's thesis]. Addis Ababa University; 2016

[36] Alemnesh T, Adamek ME. "We prefer greeting rather than eating": Life in an elder care center in Ethiopia. Journal of Cross-Cultural Gerontology. 2014;**29**(4):389-404. DOI: 10.1007/s10823-0149244-7

[37] Eskedar S. Exploring Effects of Institutional Care on the Life of Elderly: The Case of Mekedonia Humanitarian Association [master's thesis]. Addis Ababa University; 2015

[38] Tigist D. Assessment of Psychosocial Wellbeing and Meaning of Life Among the Elderly in the Elders' Home Setting at Addis Ababa, Ethiopia [master's thesis]. Addis Ababa University; 2015

[39] Bruck A. Psychological Effects of Institutional Care for the Older Persons: A Study at Kibre Aregawyan Megbare Senay Derejet (KAMSD) [master's thesis]. Addis Ababa University; 2016

[40] Getachew G. Homeless Older People Living Conditions and Their Coping Strategies: The Case of Kobo Town, North Wollo Zone, Amhara Regional State [master's thesis]. Addis Ababa University; 2017

[41] Aynshet W. Elders Engaged in Begging as a Means of Livelihood in Debre Birhan Town: An Exploration of Major Push Factors and Their Challenges [master's thesis]. Addis Ababa University; 2017

[42] Hosseana S. The Perspective of Older War Veterans of Italo-Abyssinian War of 1935-41, on the Nature of Care They Receive in Addis Ababa, Ethiopia [master's thesis]. Addis Ababa University; 2017

[43] Abraham Z. Aging in Rural Ethiopia: The Lived Experiences of Older People in Agrarian Community with Particular Reference to Sedika Kersa Community, Arsi, and Oromia [master's thesis]. Addis Ababa University; 2017

[44] Noguchi M. Aging among the Aari in rural southwestern Ethiopia: Livelihood

and daily interactions of the "GAltA". African Study Monographs. 2013;**46**:135-154. DOI: 10.14989/173537 [Accessed: November 23, 2021]

[45] Fantahun M, Berhane Y, Högberg U, Wall S, Byass P. Ageing of a rural Ethiopian population: Who are the survivors? Journal of Public Health. 2009;**123**(4):330

[46] Cohen B, Menken J, editors. Aging in Sub-Saharan Africa: Recommendations for Furthering Research. National Academy of Sciences; 2006. Available from: http://www.nap.edu/catalog/11708.html [Accessed: June 24, 2021]

[47] Sloan A, Bowe B. Phenomenology and hermeneutic phenomenology: the philosophy, the methodologies, and using hermeneutic phenomenology to investigate lecturers' experiences of curriculum design. Qual Quant. 2014;**48**(3):1291-1303. DOI: 10.1007/s11135-013-9835-3

[48] Dukes S. Phenomenological methodology in the human sciences. Journal of Religion and Health. 1984;**23**(3):197-203

[49] Nawaz M, Jariko MA, Mushtaque T. Phenomenological research, A reflex account. International Journal of Quantitative and Qualitative Research Methods. 2017;**5**(2):1-9. Available from: www.eajournals.org

[50] Giorgi A. The Descriptive Phenomenological Method in Psychology: A Modified Husserlian Approach. Duquesne University Press; 2009

[51] Bartholomew TT, Joy EE, Kang E, Brown J. A choir or cacophony? Sample sizes and quality of conveying participants' voices in phenomenological research. Methodological Innovations. 2021;**14**(2):1-14. DOI: 10.1177/20597991211040063

[52] Moustakas C. Phenomenological Research Methods. Thousand Oaks: SAGE; 1994

[53] WHO. Ethical and Safety Recommendations for Researching, Documenting and Monitoring Sexual Violence in Emergencies. World Health Organization; 2007. Available from: https://apps.who.int/iris/bitstream/handle/10665/43709/9789241595681_eng.pdf

[54] Morse JM. Confusing categories and themes. Qualitative Health Research. 2008;**18**(6):727-728. DOI: 10.1177/1049732308314930

[55] Silverstein M. Stability and change in temporal distance between the elderly and their children. Demography. 1995;**32**(1):29-45. DOI: 10.2307/2061895

[56] Jadhav A, Sathyanarayana KM, Kumar S, James KS. Living Arrangements of the Elderly in India: Who Lives Alone and What are the Patterns of Familial Support. Population Studies Center, University of Pennsylvania, UNFPA India and Institute for Social and Economic Change; 2013. Available from: https://iussp.org/sites/default/files/event_call_for_papers/301_Jadhav%20et%20al_0.pdf [Accessed: March 15, 2021]

[57] Scharlach A, Damron-Rodriguez J, Robinson B, Feldman R. Educating social workers for an aging society. Journal of Social Work Education. 2000;**36**(3):521-538. DOI: 10.1080/10437797.2000.10779026

[58] Damron-rodriguez J, Corley CS. Social work education for interdisciplinary practice with older

adults and their families. Journal of Gerontological Social Work. 2003;**39**(1-2):37-55. DOI: 10.1300/j083v39n01_05

[59] Beisgen B, Kraitchman M. Senior Centers: Opportunities for Successful Aging. New York: Springer Publishing Company; 2003. Available from: https://books.google.com/books?hl=en&lr=&id=yzb2IWhPunYC&oi=fnd&pg=PR9&dq=related:2WOljdSkMNgJ:scholar.google.com/&ots=m4TfR_QSSU&sig=CYvsrcqM6UNWvugDYSKsKc-uiwM

[60] Casteel C, Nocera M, Runyan CW. Health promotion and physical activity programs in senior centers. Activities, Adaptation, & Aging. 2013;**37**(3):213-223. DOI: 10.1080/01924788.2013.784853

[61] Bacsu J-DR, Jeffery B, Abonyi S, Johnson S, Novik N, Martz D, et al. Healthy aging in place: Perceptions of rural older adults. Educational Gerentology. 2014;**40**(5):327-337. DOI: 10.1080/03601277.2013.802191

[62] Giles R. The Experience of Attending a Day Care Centre: A Study into Older Adults' Quality of Life. MA in Social Work. University of London; 2015. Available from: https://www.ageuk.org.uk/bp-assets/globalassets/lewisham-and-southwark/documents/2015-goldsmith-university-research-dissertation-on-stones-end-day-centre.pdf

[63] Khalaila R, Vitman-Schorr A. Social support and loneliness among frail older adults attending daycare centers: A multicultural study in Israel. Archives of Gerontology and Geriatrics. 2021;**97**:104486. DOI: 10.1016/j.archger.2021.104486

[64] Valaitis R, Cleghorn L, Ploeg J, Risdon C, Mangin D, Dolovich L, et al. Disconnected relationships between primary care and community-based health and social services and system navigation for older adults: A qualitative descriptive study. BMC Family Practice. 2020;**21**:69. DOI: 10.1186/s12875-020-01143-8

[65] Taqui AM, Itrat A, Qidwai W, Qadri Z. Depression in the elderly: Does family system play a role? A cross-sectional study. BMC Psychiatry. 2007;**7**(1):57. DOI: 10.1186/1471-244x-7-57

[66] Tirrito T, Spencer-Amado J. Older adults willingness to use social services in places of worship. Journal of Religious Gerontology. 2000;**11**(2):29-42. DOI: 10.1300/J078v11n02_03

[67] Gerald LB. Paid family caregiving. Journal of Aging & Social Policy. 1993;**5**(1-2):73-89. DOI: 10.1300/j031v05n01_06

Chapter 13

Remodeling the Web: Supporting the Needs of Older Women Experiencing Intimate Partner Violence in Rural Contexts

Heather Helpard and Lori E. Weeks

Abstract

Researchers and health care providers know little about older, diverse women who experience intimate partner violence (IPV) within rural contexts and their service and support needs. In addition, rural older women experience significant geographic disparities in health status and outcomes, socioeconomic inequities, and access to appropriate services, creating unique challenges. In this study, we sought to contribute knowledge and innovative approaches to conceptualize and respond to identified specific needs and challenges older women experiencing IPV in rural contexts face. This study draws on the thematic analysis of 14 interviews with diverse rural New Brunswick and Nova Scotian women who experienced IPV or service providers supporting older rural women who experienced IPV. Findings from this study culminated in the following themes: *retaining the traditional web, breaking threads, spinning new connections, and remodeling the web*. All these patterns played out within rural contexts where identified supports and challenges encouraged or hindered older rural women's agency and supportive workers' abilities to spin supportive connections and create innovative solutions to meet the needs of older, diverse rural women experiencing IPV. These findings will serve to inform future person-centered, supportive, and collaborative approaches and strategies for future and relevant service provision, education, and research for this population.

Keywords: intimate partner violence, older women, diverse women, rural, Canada

1. Introduction

Within Canada, women are victims in approximately 80% of reported intimate partner violence (IPV) cases [1]. IPV "refers to any type of abusive behavior that occurs between intimate partners, such as spouses or common-law partners" [2]. While researchers and service providers have paid more attention to IPV in younger women, a global aging population warrants a closer look at IPV rates in older women [3]. While accurate prevalence data is challenging to obtain, global data suggests that 16.5–54.5% of women over 45 years of age may experience IPV [3]. Researchers suggest that older women may experience IPV differently than younger women due to an increased likelihood of comorbidities and dependency on a perpetrator for physical care and financial support [3]. Our knowledge of IPV rates and experience in a diverse cohort of women remains inadequate [2].

What complicates the matter even further is that in many rural and remote areas in Canada, including those in Atlantic Canada, women comprise a higher proportion of the rapidly aging residents [4]. New Brunswick (NB) and Nova Scotia (NS) are credited as two of the oldest Canadian provinces. Researchers estimate that almost half of the population of New Brunswick (NB) and over two-thirds of the people in Nova Scotia (NS) live in rural areas, and many who live in these places are older women with different languages, ethnicities, and comorbidities [5–8]. Across Atlantic Canada, many of these diverse older rural women live alone, are widowed, married, or live with a common-law partner, experiencing significant differences from those living in urban areas in terms of illness burden, mortality, and socioeconomic status [5–8].

IPV incidence between rural and urban Canadian women exists in Atlantic Canada, with rural women experiencing the highest overall rates of IPV compared to their urban counterparts in recent years [9]. Many older rural women live in low-income situations with poor health outcomes [10] with experiences of geographic isolation, inaccessibility to healthcare services, and unique sociocultural characteristics that may shape decisions, self-esteem, and health behaviors [10, 11]. However, such statistics often do not capture diverse groups of women at different phases of their lifespans or in various contexts in which these women live [12, 13]. Often, researchers describe women who have experienced IPV as a homogeneous group in reports and studies, leading to the development and implementation of supports and resources that may not meet the unique needs and circumstances of older and diverse groups of women living in rural settings [2, 11, 14].

Many define rural areas in terms of population or distance from the closest urban center, implying, to some degree, social isolation and inaccessibility to healthcare services and resources [15, 16]. These significant geographic disparities in health status and health outcomes, socioeconomic inequities, and limited technological and transportation access to appropriate services create unique challenges to providing supportive services [17]. The literature suggests that factors such as a lack of human and material resources and large geographical distances between communities [17] can create unique challenges for supporters working with this population. To address rural healthcare resource availability and accessibility issues, researchers have called for the formation of comprehensive rural health frameworks, recommendations, and innovations among critical stakeholders in the community, rural communities, and healthcare providers [17]. However, what remains are struggles with funding, housing, and culturally appropriate care [18].

From a geographical standpoint, "rural" was defined in this study as an area with fewer than 10,000 people [19]. However, rurality embodies more than population density and geographical distance to the nearest urban center. Within these geographically defined and designated areas exist eclectic ways of life created and maintained by patriarchal family structures, resilient attitudes, cultural and religious values, and stereotypes [20, 21]. Such attitudes, values, and ways of life may shape self-worth, purpose, and behaviors [11] in older, diverse rural women in Atlantic Canada and their attitudes, behaviors, and supportive needs in response to IPV experiences. Within this rural context, one can experience being embraced or "othered," depending on the degree to which one identifies with valued and revered ways of rural life and membership [14].

Researchers and healthcare providers know little about how older women experience IPV in rural contexts and their service and support needs. In addition, rural older women experience significant geographic disparities in health status and health outcomes, socioeconomic inequities, and limited technological and transportation access to appropriate services, creating unique challenges to providing supportive services [10]. While it is clear that intimate partner violence can occur with women in any context and at any stage of their lifespan, older women's experiences of intimate partner violence are both a significant and understudied phenomenon [3, 22–25]. In addition, little is known about the needs of diverse older rural women aged 50 years or older who are living in rural contexts [26]. Without such knowledge, it is very difficult to understand how rurality and living within a rural geographical area facilitate or create barriers for older, diverse women seeking support for intimate partner violence and to determine what supports are needed to address gaps within rural contexts for women living with IPV that are different than what may be required in urban settings.

Our research team identified the need to understand how rural contexts facilitate or create barriers for these women and their service providers, who supported them in a paid or unpaid capacity. Thus, this study aims to gain insights into the needs of rural, diverse older women who had experienced IPV.

2. Methodology and methods

As part of a study funded by the Justice Partnership and Innovation Program-Family Violence Initiative by Justice Canada, "Identifying and Responding to the Needs of Diverse Older Women Who Experience Intimate Partner Violence: The RESPOND Study," [27, 28], team members conducted interviews with diverse and older NB and NS women who experienced IPV and service providers supporting these women who had experienced intimate partner violence (IPV). The research team accessed interviewed participants by extending invitations to surveyed service providers in the project's second phase and distributing created study recruitment posters through organizations that provide services to women with IPV [28]. Also, women who experienced IPV could find these recruitment posters on public bulletin boards (e.g., health centers) and social media (e.g., Facebook and Twitter) [28]. Within these interviews and for this study, the research team identified the need to understand how rural contexts facilitate or create barriers for these women and their service providers, who supported them in a paid or unpaid capacity.

The inclusion criteria for participants included: (a) individuals who identified as a woman, including transwomen and femmes, (b) individuals who self-identified as a member of a visible minority or identify as an official Francophone language minority, (c) women who experienced IPV in midlife or older who are not currently in an abusive relationship or residing with an abusive individual, (d) women who were currently residing within a New Brunswick or Nova Scotia rural community and not a care facility, and (e) those who could be interviewed in French or English. Data collection resulted in a thematic analysis of 14 interviews (2 women and 12 supporters of older women who have experienced IPV in rural NB or NS) (**Table 1**). The study sample included six bilingual service providers from New Brunswick and six supporters of older women in Nova Scotia who supported older women who had experienced IPV in a rural setting. In addition, 1 NS Arabic woman and 1 NB Francophone woman, who both experienced IPV, participated in interviews.

Participant pseudonym	Description of participant
Denise	An outreach worker from NS
Nathan	A counselor at a shelter in NS
Pat	A worker at a shelter in NS
Britney	A worker with police and victim services in NS
Katelyn	A staff nurse who works with IPV victims in NS
Irene	A support worker with black women in NS
Cathy	An IPV outreach worked from NB
Penelope	A victim service worker from NB
Lenore	An NB victim services coordinator from NB
Harriett	An executive director for a rural women's resource center in NB
Linda	A community social worker from NB
Janice	A manager at an adult program in NB
Mary	A 48-year-old NB Francophone woman who experienced IPV
Raj	A 53-year-old NS Muslim woman who experienced IPV

Table 1.
Description of interview participants.

A feminist theoretical perspective informed this qualitative research analysis, supporting participants' involvement in the knowledge co-creation process and providing a lens to observe and consider how factors and structures within the rural context facilitate or create barriers for study participants. It was also rooted in constructivist approaches, which support relativist ontological views (e.g., different observers may have different viewpoints about what counts as truth) and underpinnings of pragmatism (e.g., human knowledge and values are situated in events and services to address practical issues in the everyday world), symbolic interactionism (e.g., subjective meanings of and realities through constant social interaction, language, and communications) and constructivism (e.g., truth and knowledge are constructed by humans as they engage with the world they interpret [29–31].

Inductive thematic analysis is a highly flexible method amenable to a range of epistemologies and research questions. Themes, often defined as abstract entities, capture or unify individuals' experiences into meanings and patterns [32], offering a rich and detailed account of participant voices by highlighting similarities, differences, and surprising insights within the data. Using Braun and Clarke's six-phased iterative [32] and reflexive process, the research team initially read through interview data stored in well-organized and labeled archives. In biweekly research meetings, phone conversations, and a couple of workshops, the research team annotated data items in the interviews to document ideas of potential codes and then refined these codes further in team meetings and discussions. The research team used the initial codes to organize meaningful concepts found within the data. Then, the research team interpreted the codes to develop data themes and subthemes, with the aid of theoretical and reflexive memos and field notes about potential codes and themes within the data. Finally, the research team organized the themes, subthemes, and codes into a thematic map to visualize relationships and patterns among the data. Themes were continually reviewed and refined by the research team (collapsing or breaking apart

DOI: http://dx.doi.org/10.5772/intechopen.109767

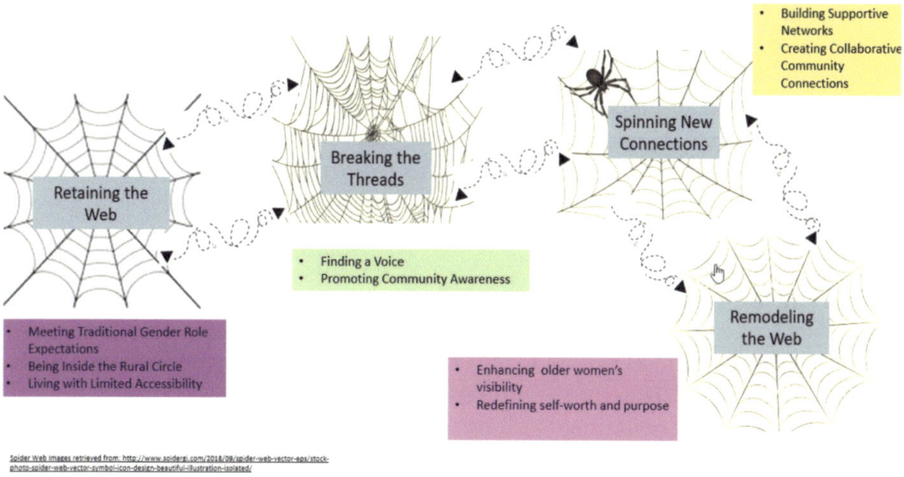

Figure 1.
Remodeling the web: the experiences and needs of older diverse women who had experienced IPV and unpaid and paid support workers.

some themes) for referential adequacy to the raw interview data and written observations and field notes during the interviews, leading to the final definition and naming of themes. The completed thematic diagram (**Figure 1**) tells the story of the data. One-third of the interview transcripts were in French, so the expertise of two bilingual research team members took the lead in documenting English translations of the French transcripts, using detailed memos to capture inherent meanings and patterns relevant to the francophone culture. In the interview with the Arabic woman, an Arabic interviewer included notes and explanations in the transcript to clarify aspects of Muslim culture. A research member on the team offered insight and expertise during discussions about interview content shared by black Canadian support workers.

Due to time limitations, the research team did not complete member checking during the data analysis. However, member checking was sought during the presentation of findings at national and international conferences. In summary, according to Lincoln and Guba's [33] trustworthiness criteria, many members of the diverse research team were involved with prolonged engagement with the data and data analysis process, interview translation, as well as peer debriefing at regular research team members and retreats, leading to logical, detailed, traceable and clearly documented analysis processes supporting interpretations and findings derived from the interview, data analysis decisions, personal reflections and insights from the interview data.

The Research Ethics Boards granted ethical approval for this study at Dalhousie University, the University of New Brunswick, the Université de Moncton, and the University of Prince Edward Island. All participants provided informed consent before the interviews began and received a $25 honorarium.

3. Results

Four overarching themes emerged during the data analysis process. Themes of "Retaining the Web," "Breaking the Threads," "Spinning New Connections," and

"Remodeling the Web,", and related subthemes (**Figure 1**) provide an interpretation of diverse older women's as well as paid and unpaid supporters' experiences, challenges, needs, and opportunities regarding IPV support and service needs within complex and ever-changing rural settings within Atlantic Canada. These findings and a diagram (**Figure 1**) evolved from secured interviews between members of the research team and study participants, as well as researcher memos during an analysis process guided by Braun and Clarke's [32] six phases of thematic analysis. **Figure 1** depicts the relationship between these themes and subthemes.

3.1 Retaining the Web

"Retaining the Web" (**Figure 1**) is a theme that represents the chronic barriers faced by study participants. The perceived present reality for participants in Atlantic Canada is living or working in a contained and restraining web. Societal structures, stigma, trauma and invisibility, discriminatory and oppressive gender roles and hierarchies, age, racial, and language stereotypes, and inaccessible human and material resources to assist with IPV shape this web. This theme also captures the perceived barriers that older, diverse women experience when attempting to access IPV services in rural settings. This theme subdivides into the subthemes, 'meeting traditional gender role expectations,' 'being inside the rural circle,' and 'living with limited accessibility.'

3.1.1 Meeting traditional gender role expectations

Many study participants described older, rural women as entrenched within a present-day web of power inequity shaped by patriarchal ideals and the need to meet traditional gender role expectations. Denise, an outreach worker from NS, reveals, "For older women, the kind of deal was the husband is the breadwinner, and the wife took care of the home." This division of roles and responsibilities within the home places older, rural women in a vulnerable and dependent physical, emotional, social, and financial position within their relationships, a reality that may promote and escalate feelings of helplessness, isolation, and oppression. Mary, a 48-year-old francophone woman who experienced IPV, echoes these sediments, saying, "If you can't beat him, keep quiet, so you don't upset the boat."

Meeting traditional gender roles means accepting and upholding a climate of self-sacrifice for older, rural women in preference to others' needs. Within such an atmosphere, older, rural women's potential physical and emotional isolation may escalate when IPV occurs within the home. Reflecting on her IPV experience, Mary remembers such feelings, saying, "I realized how my life was going to go. You can insult me and beat me to the point of killing me if you want. I accept it, I love you, but you must never get your hands on one of our children." Compatible cultural and religious beliefs can further reinforce patriarchal ideologies and gender role expectations. Denise comments, "Certain religions encourage couples to work out things no matter what ... such a damaging power differential. And I think there is a lot of shame and stigma". Raj, a 53-year-old Muslim woman who experienced IPV, shares, "in my religion, when a wife is patient and tolerates whatever happens with her in the marriage life, she will go to heaven" (Raj). Raj further describes what toleration entails, sharing,

> *We [the wives] allowed our husbands to trampling and stepping on our dignity. Trampling on our emotions. Trampling on our comfort and trampling on you [the wife] ... If not, you will lose your life and your children and family*

Also, older women's feelings of self-worth align with meeting traditional gender role expectations within rural contexts. Cathy, an IPV outreach worker from NB, explains, "They [older women] are often told [by their husbands or partners] that they can't make it on their own." Denise agrees, considering the older, rural woman who has been a caretaker and homemaker "might not have any savings at all." This limited ability to make it on their own may also come from little formal education and work opportunities.

3.1.2 Being inside the rural circle

Penelope, a victim service worker from NB, describes the rural context as comprised of "little cliques which define a degree of acceptance of how you will be treated." Lenore, an NB victim services coordinator, reveals, "The level of secrecy here is huge ... senior women have the burden of the well-being of the family on their backs; the honor of the family ... We mustn't break up the family." The health and supportive benefits of living in a rural context apply if one is part of the inner circle that ascribes to and embraces these gender role expectations, beliefs, and secrecy related to IPV. Nathan, a counselor at a shelter in NS, reflects, "Diverse women face additional challenges in a rural community. They feel shamed when discussing their case with anyone, and many do not understand their culture ... they suffer a lot" (Nathan).

Discussion and acknowledgment of IPV happening in rural households are subject to stigma and discrimination. Older, diverse women can erode the rural culture of secrecy by speaking out about IPV experiences. In that case, they risk stigma, racism, potential rejection and isolation from family, friends, and the community, and social exclusion from membership and support offered to those within the rural circle. Lenore shares, "There were horrible rumors out in the community about who was accessing the shelter." Such stories spread throughout a rural community not only threaten older women's self-esteem and how they will be viewed and accepted by others but also create a barrier to their comfort level in accessing services. Therefore, for an older, diverse woman to be outside the circle in a rural community because exposing the secret of IPV means risking rejection from supportive networks, cultural groups, relationships, financial security, dignity, and personal safety. Harriett, an executive director for a rural women's resource center in NB, believes that such aspects of a rural way of life hinder older, diverse women's sense of security. She indicates that these vulnerable women must have the "ability to feel safe in reaching out both within the community and outside the community as they [older, diverse rural women who experienced IPV] have a real lack of anonymity and a lack of privacy."

3.1.3 Living with limited availability

Within the rural context, Linda, a community social worker from NB, reveals that paid and unpaid support workers continually strive to find culturally relevant human and healthcare resources for older, diverse women experiencing IPV from "a pool that is getting shallower and shallower." Many study participants shared that IPV services in rural communities were directed "mostly towards younger women ... those are the women that suffer domestic violence the most" (Harriett). It was not common among study participants to consider older women with IPV as a distinct population requiring unique resources and services because "they [older women] do not want to go to where they are known" (Linda). Janice, a manager at an adult program in NB, spoke about the lack of specific IPV services for older women.

She explains, "There are no services specifically for older women ... we don't see them. Young women are open to different services ... older women are the opposite ... they want to keep everything a secret." The lack of visibility and attention to older women with IPV in rural contexts resulted in the development of generic programs and the construction of shelters that did not consider modifications such women with illnesses or disabilities may need. Pat, a worker at a shelter in NS, discloses, "We do not have a lot of staff or facilities or the money to put equipment in for or care for older women with illnesses and disabilities... They can try to get a room on the main floor to avoid stairs."

Moreover, Harriett comments, "It is difficult to find someone who wants to work but also speaks French at the same time. It's a constant, constant battle." While NB is a bilingual province, Francophone providers and resources are often in short supply. Mary claims, "services are not as available to Francophone women everywhere, and that affects who I go talk to and if I decide if it is worth the time to go through that to try and find someone who understands." Linda expands further on language issues for immigrant women in rural contexts who speak neither French nor English:

> *Speaking neither English or French makes it a big challenge and unfortunately, in this case, it was not the priority to deal with the violence she [a client] was experiencing. We could not do therapy with this person, you understand, because the language barrier was just too big ... We couldn't understand each other enough.*

In rural contexts, there exists limited accessibility to providers, services, and resources to meet the specific needs of older, diverse rural women and for those who are trying to help them from a counseling, treatment, supportive, or legal perspective. Linda shares, "We have to contact many people to help with translation ... it's a big challenge, and most times we can't get the help, and we can't offer the help and support we usually offer to other clients." In addition, study participants raised concerns about older, rural women's limited accessibility to centrally located and distant IPV services in rural contexts and support workers' ability to access them in their homes. Linda divulges, "Isolation is a big obstacle. Transport and isolation in the region [rural settings]. There is nothing close, and there are no other services here [rural town] that offer domestic violence services." Therefore, Linda discloses that older, diverse women must rely on others within the rural circle for support, even if they are the perpetrators of abuse. She shares, "There are no buses in Kent County. A client of mine had to depend on a taxi where, at one point, it was the abuser driving her. The fact that we had a client, and it was her ex-spouse."

Janice spoke about the "lack of protection and privacy for the elderly in rural areas from the eyes of rural residents if they are made to access local programs and shelters." Linda expands on this point, saying, "Adult protection can do nothing to help them [older women] as long as they understand what is happening ... there is nothing they can do. Police services are also the same thing." Mary, an older Francophone woman, claims, "Without any care of the hard time to find help and get there, no one comes to me." This need for service within the home environment may be an important consideration for older, diverse women in rural settings who have, as Janice asserts, "lived in their homes for decades, and it is all they have ever known." It may not always be easy for older women to relocate to another place, such as a nursing home, when, as Linda notes, "You've been through 60 years of abuse, and there is no counseling offered there." What also makes it hard for rural, older women to leave their homes, families, and communities to access outside services and alternative housing arrangements is to leave their animals. Linda acknowledges, "We can't have animals at our shelter, you know … there are other services for animals, but it is not good for their [older women] dog or cat or horses to go to the other side of the province or for women to leave them behind."

3.1.4 Summary

"Retaining the Web" represents how older, diverse rural women and unpaid and paid supporters continue to live, work, and exist within a societal structure shaped by patriarchal ideals and traditional gender role expectations that are accepted and supported inside the rural circle. These ideologies, as well as cultural practices and religious beliefs that align with them, permeate and influence healthcare provision and planning, family and community relationships, and political and legal systems. With the rural inside circle being a primary means of support, older, diverse women with IPV risk isolation, alienation from their home, family, and community, further poverty, stigma, and shame in a rural context that provides limited access to outside services and resources supportive of language and cultural needs, as well as financial and legal protection.

3.2 Breaking the Threads

"Breaking the Threads" (**Figure 1**) is a theme that captures actions identified by study participants that are needed to fracture the retained web in rural settings, such as the patriarchal societal structures, traditional gender role expectations, stereotypes, and age, racial, and language discrimination. The theme subdivides into two subthemes, 'finding a voice' and 'promoting community awareness.'

3.2.1 Finding a voice

Within present-day rural contexts, study participants have found that older, diverse women who have experienced or are experiencing IPV have been silenced and oppressed within their homes and communities. Britney, a worker with victim and police services in NS, observes, "Older women do not often realize that they have been abused … they think that is just the way life is … so they accept it as the norm." Linda concurs that "the elderly more than the young do not realize it is violence."

To 'break the threads' that perpetuate this silence and oppression requires re-awakening and reflection before an onslaught of education. There is a need for these women to 'find a voice' through storytelling with a trusted healthcare provider, family member, friend, or cultural representative in a safe and secure place. Raj recommends, "Don't be silent … Women should share their pain with someone and get someone they trust involved." However, Cathy cautions, "It's just taboo… they [older women] want to hide more … they want to keep everything secret to avoid backlash, embarrassment, loss of home, and hurting others" (Cathy). Denise agrees, "Women might feel too embarrassed to tell their story to someone that's so close in the community, or they might not trust that privacy will be kept." In addition, Lenore, an NB victim services coordinator, agrees, "It's an obstacle to go and show them they have the right to be someone, to be understood, to be loved and to have support." To address these concerns, Katelyn, a staff nurse from NS, shares, "I listen to their story. I hear what they have to say … reading between the lines, looking at their gestures. I always leave the door open for them to share and express." Linda believes trust can be gained by:

> *Sending them messages and assuring them [older women] they are beautiful, intelligent, and strong ... asking them to write in a journal or share pictures to discuss ... encouraging them to tell a bit of their story and taking the time to listen ...*

Furthermore, in a rural context, Linda proposes, "attention to a location, like beside a hospital or connected to a business, would not let others see them come into my office, and it ensures client confidentiality." However, other study participants felt that a primary consideration of gaining trust in older, diverse women with different cultural backgrounds and languages was to advocate for more support workers and care providers who could identify with their background and lived experiences. Irene, a support worker with black women in NS, recommends "Having people that look like those individuals who are providing service ... making sure they are culturally relevant, making sure they're grounded in that person's culture." Nathan expands on this point, noting, "It is also important to have providers of the same generation as the victim ... the same age range ... which may help with trust for victims to tell the story to someone relatable."

3.2.2 Promoting community awareness

When questioned about specific IPV services and supports for older, diverse women in rural contexts, many study participants indicated that there were few or none. Penelope shares, "We offer the same services as we can, regardless of age group." Denise agrees, saying, "First of all, we just do all the same things that we do with all women." Nathan discloses, "I find that we never treat anyone of any age difference, but I find there are more resources allocated for younger women experiencing violence or intimate partner violence than older women." Older, diverse women experiencing IPV were generally not thought of by participating support workers as a group with unique needs and were invisible. Mary divulges, "I feel many have turned their backs on me ... You fall on your own" (Mary). To 'break the threads,' there need to be ways to channel older, diverse women's voices so that community members can be informed about intimate partner violence and change some previous mindsets. Denise suggests:

> *There needs to be changes to support this population in general, I think that other service providers like doctors, nurses, lawyers, judges, social workers, community leaders, like everyone in the public needs to be trained and aware of intimate partner violence needs in all groups within the older generation ... like generational and cultural competence.*

Harriett, an executive for a rural women's resource center in NB, believes community awareness starts with "a lot of social media, going out and talking about it and getting information out ... We have to widen our scope and try to get the word out in these ways." While older, diverse women are less visible on social media, Penelope reflects:

> *Awareness, our young people have it. Older women are less on social media ... but this mustn't stop us all from getting their words and messages out. We must keep going because putting out the message can narrow the gap between the generations in our rural communities.*

While such actions to educate and inform others in the rural community are essential, Irene implies the message is more complex. She cautions that in rural contexts, "it is important to acknowledge that systemic racism has impacted how other people outside the community interpreted the community of black older women where intimate partner violence is an issue." The training and messages to healthcare providers and rural community members must also be authentic. "Whenever there is a type of forum that's organized within the community, talks about community experience or community needs with intimate partner violence, they [older, diverse women] need to be there to participate and give those first voice stories" (Irene). Katelyn stresses the need also to "get the information down or getting research, having research guide the messages for the community and even having focus groups ... getting it down accurately on paper. Getting it written and shared." Nathan outlines a role for himself in this process, saying, "As a man, I feel there need to be support groups with men to raise awareness with men about violence... stand up against violence, ... support the cause ... to balance the process."

3.2.3 Summary

"Breaking the Threads" represents an initial starting point to unravel the constraints of the present-day web to help older, diverse women in rural contexts reawaken and 'find a voice' to help them recognize and understand they are victims of IPV and to feel comfortable and safe to share their stories with trusted health care providers and, preferably, with those who look like and can identify with their cultural backgrounds and generation. The rural community, and public, including health care providers, men groups, and community leaders, may need to participate in training as well as research and knowledge dissemination of first-hand stories from older, diverse women to raise community awareness that they experience intimate partner violence and systemic racism in rural communities.

3.3 Spinning New Connections

"Spinning New Connections" (**Figure 1**) is a theme that represents the study participants' perceptions of the need for the creation of new threads and connections within their immediate surroundings, as well as with local and distant communities and intersectoral and healthcare partners. Participants suggest that such innovation, re-imagination, and creativity are required to build a new foundation for future initiatives and models of care that better meet their needs to cope, live with, and address IPV in rural settings. The theme subdivides into two subthemes, 'building supportive networks,' and 'creating collaborative community connections.'

3.3.1 Building supportive networks

In present-day rural settings in Atlantic Canada, study participants spoke of the social and geographic isolation experienced by older, diverse women who had experienced or are experiencing IPV. Linda observes, "the elderly often have nobody. You know we see that often." Mary shares, "It is so important for me to be well surrounded with whom I share strong bonds like family and friends and others who can understand you... it is amazing how good it makes you. It reassures you."

What complicates social and geographical isolation with the need for informal, supportive networks is that many IPV services and resources for women are outside the home and local, rural community. Denise shares, "Many services providers are stretched too thin in rural areas and prefer women meet them where they are for service regardless of if they [older women] live far out of town and have no vehicle." For these reasons, Harriett imparts, "they [older women] need someone they trust, like family or friends or a support person, to kind of lead them to services and resources or come with them ... or learn do this on the Internet." On the other hand, older women uncomfortable with technology or with no support persons may require healthcare providers also travel to meet these women where they live or steer them in a direction where they can meet others with similar interests and backgrounds. Denise discloses, "Specifically with the older population, I find I do more home visits than meeting in the office" (Denise). Nathan suggests that "it would be great if a group from an institute goes to where those older women are in their home and supports them to stay there." Social support networks make older and diverse women feel more connected and closer to home in rural settings. Groups within the local community can be found in places such as "within churches to pray, sing, or hum" (Katelyn) or homes. Irene, a supporter of black women in NS, elaborates further, sharing:

> *We have done women's circles, where it gives them the Opportunity to share resources that have helped them. We have also had long kitchen table talks, specifically about being a survivor, what that looks like, and providing some peer support.*

Older and diverse women who do not speak French or English could create informal support networks using "apps and writing and non-verbal communication to get to the place with others who do not speak their language" (Irene). Irene further elaborates, "social networking can involve something as simple as a senior's group or women's circles in the community where they [older diverse women] can crochet and knit and talk and eat ... incorporate mental health." Also, Raj feels that building supportive networks with older and diverse women in rural settings needed to incorporate culturally based rituals and practices of expression to bring people together. She states:

> *I want to say rituals. A lot of women use their rituals ... Like one of the ladies did henna on her hands and feet. And it was around her coming through her journey. There are things like Bollywood dancing and activities from the Muslim community. They get together and talk about their experiences, but it's through dance, and expression of creativity like plays and different things like that (Raj).*

3.3.2 Creating collaborative community connections

To 'spin new connections' requires forming and nurturing collaborative partnerships between older, diverse rural women who have experienced or are experiencing IPV, their advocates, community organizations, and the justice system. The strength of community connections in rural settings is imperative to offset the issues surrounding limited accessibility to others and resources. Within rural contexts, Raj believes, "Partnership is power!!! I think civil society and the government need to work together hand in hand with us without any hierarchy or power struggle for change."

A key priority identified by study participants is to be "part of reworking the puzzle of resources within the community" (Katelyn). The involvement of older, diverse women and their advocates to streamline and connect multiple IPV referral processes, healthcare providers, resources, and related services in private yet accessible, "central multiservice locations, satellite clinics, mini prevention offices and virtual programs across and between rural contexts" (Denise). Also, it is imperative to educate older, diverse women and advocates about their availability and how to access healthcare resources and services, as well as to "understand legal statutes and navigate judicial processes" (Britney). Irene sees "huge barriers to older women when there is a lack of knowledge about where services are, who providers are, and what can be offered in rural communities." Lenore suggests:

> *We need to reach them [older diverse women] more ... for discussion and education. Perhaps, ... going to their homes to offer them little presentations on supports and services, laws, policies, and healthy relationships.*

In rural contexts, there are diminished RCMP services, communication, and safety concerns. Denise mentions, "There's often only one RCMP officer patrolling like a rural area ... it takes police what seems like forever to them [older women] to get there." Lenore reveals, "Older women are very sensitive to police comments... bad attitudes of police regress women in their efforts to make statements or press charges." Linda expands on such experiences, sharing, "Women can be vulnerable as laws and judicial processes often punish the victim and put all the responsibility on the victim." More work is needed to "improve laws, policies, and justice for vulnerable victims and populations of IPV crime and helping judges understand the issues of complexity and violence." Lenore contends, "We all work for the people" (Lenore). Katelyn reveals, "There's not a lot of trust with agencies and organizations.... most of the time they are not staffed with black people." Irene asserts:

> *I think some of the recommendations would be we need more people in support roles that look like us, that are trained to... Because I mean the thing about it is that we know the African-Nova Scotian experience. But having the supports through that experience are lacking.*

Therefore, older, diverse women and their advocates must work toward forming collaborative partnerships with Multicultural Associations, diverse elected counselors, healthcare providers, and the judicial system in developing more culturally appropriate IPV healthcare, police, and judicial services, as well as language translation and educational resources.

Other forms of health care delivery from health care providers and support workers could involve case-based management approaches and partnerships with local church organizations. Denise reveals," A lot of times older women are more connected with church organizations... like in a counseling capacity, a friendship capacity, and for food, shelter, transportation, and financial aid." However, Harriett maintains, "What we are noticing with older women ... is that there is no affordable housing for them to meet their needs, including mobility issues .... they are on Income Assistance." Older women, often in more dire financial situations, do not have the means to work. Without provided secondary housing, there are only the "shelters with the bare minimum with no special beds, and not very accessible at times with ... at our place having to walk up at least 6 stairs to get into the building itself" (Nathan). For older women who choose to stay in their homes, Lenore indicates, "They [older, diverse women] should continue to receive services ... as well as resources to equip them to be safe and to defend themselves."

On a positive note, to address financial aid needs, Denise insists, "Older women so a really good job with fundraising initiatives and getting their name out in rural communities ... using social media platforms more." Harriett shares, "Some of us [support workers] have really good fundraising campaigns ... like toonie draws and ... a Chase the Ace champaign raising $300,000.00 ... and a safer pets program ... Not one penny of government funding." Linda advocates for "more subsidized funding for programs for older women from the government." In particular, Linda indicates, "If we had subsidies, we could have more specific IPV programs for older, diverse women ... to touch more on the problems they are experiencing."

3.3.3 Summary

"Spinning New Connections" represents and addresses mechanisms and strategies to facilitate building eclectic informal, supportive networks and creating multiple collaborative community connections. Both will thread together as a solid foundation for creating a new web that better serves the unique needs of older, diverse women who have experienced or are experiencing IPV and paid and unpaid support workers in rural Atlantic Canada. There is a need to facilitate and strengthen meaningful informal networks with family, friends, and groups of older women that share experiences and support generational and cultural roots within the home, local rural settings, and between rural settings. The involvement of community churches, judicial, multicultural, and fundraising organizations, government subsidy funding, police, and health care providers and support workers in partnership with community leaders and advocates, and older, diverse rural women who experienced or are experiencing IPV is paramount to facilitating a collaborative, inclusive, and connected approach that serves to dismantle previous power and oppressive hierarchies that serve to silence and isolate these women within their rural communities.

3.4 Remodeling the Web

"Remodeling the Web" is a theme that represents the study participants' vision for a new, supportive web. This remodeled web, created in partnership with older and diverse women and support workers, has a supportive infrastructure more attuned to the needs of the study participants. This unique and evolving web supports transparency, equitable voices, preventative and meaningful services, appropriate human and material resources, and connections that meet the needs of diverse older women and support workers in rural Atlantic Canadian settings. The theme subdivides into two subthemes, 'enhancing older women's visibility,' and "redefining self-worth and purpose."

3.4.1 Enhancing older women's visibility

In the present-day web, older and diverse women are invisible and devalued within the family and rural context. Denise observes, "While all services welcome access by older women ... Like you see people taking in cutsie voices to older women, or like infantilizing them." Irene feels:

> *It is not appropriate for me to assume I know the answers for them ... I ask permission, and I encourage them to self-advocate or play an engaged role in our talk, so the real person in front of me appears in a space of conversations that are the bigger picture.*

Older and diverse women who have experienced or are experiencing IPV should be visible at the center of the remodeling web. Traditionally, there has been a "top-down" approach to developing resources and services for women experiencing IPV, with little attention to older and diverse women in rural contexts. Irene reasons that "women end up accessing and receiving services and even kind of controlling what those services are by influencing what those services are is by having someone endorse that service." The people that favor these services are, as Harriett describes, "Government officials and a community board ... who imply what they do is what this the community wants. But it doesn't mean that they are representing the women themselves." Instead, opportunities for "dialogue and different understanding with older and diverse women is needed, asking a lot of questions ... and exploring all the possibilities of choices and resources and services to follow" (Irene).

It is also essential to have, as Irene states, "Diversity on our board of directors .... and advocates available for women of color ... diversity of service.. with opportunities to expand and grow and learn and to reach out in new ways." Raj says, "I advise the bigger society to seek the truth. To see women and return and maintain women's right." Katelyn believes, "People who understand this population [older and diverse women] have an understanding then, some insight into their IPV experiences, community concerns, and needs." Irene also contends, "They [older and diverse women] need to be seen and at the center making sure the resources are relevant to their experiences, generation, making sure they're culturally relevant ... grounded in their culture."

What is also really important is to show respect to the older and diverse women who have taken the steps, with the support of their advocates, informal, supportive networks, and community partners, to become visible in rural settings. In a remodeling web, let resources and services "center around the women who are IPV victims, not the abusers" (Katelyn). Katelyn thinks, "These women should be honoured ... there needs to be respect and admiration ... not stigma, shame, or discrimination." Linda advocates:

> *We need to from their [older and diverse women] resourcefulness and sense of caring for people who have been through a similar situation ... making visible themselves and sharing the information and experience they received.*

3.4.2 Re-defining self-worth and purpose

Within a remodeled web of resources and support with the older and diverse rural women at the visible center, there is a renewed opportunity for them to redefine a sense of self-worth and purpose for the future. Raj recalls, "He made me weak and not trusting myself. He was always humiliating me. He let me feel that I am a weak woman, and I am nothing." Mary pleads for others like her to "Run! Run! Get out of it! Because it never gets better" (Mary). Denise feels that a supportive, collaborative approach with this population in a remodeled web can help these women realize "it's me first, it's my health first. And I need to be here to be present for the rest of my family." Harriett agrees, saying:

> *We could see their strength, but they [the older, diverse women] don't see it. I think they could see it; it would make much more of a difference. If there was a way we could help them see that, it could give them a sense of worth and purpose. Because they really have gotten to this point, they are by being strong (Harriett).*

A remodeled web allows these women to recognize their resilience and resourcefulness and use those strengths to move forward after "so much shock and heartbreak." Denise contends, "Finding themselves [older and diverse women] after IPV means kind of coming out on the other side of that and developing self-esteem and self-love." Within the remodeled web that is forever changing, these women have the opportunity to "recreate themselves after thinking like it's too late for that ... inspiring others like them of what resiliency truly is" (Denise). Katelyn shares that this process is "peeling away the layers and seeing a purpose ... and saying, 'I'm going to do for myself'" (Katelyn). Linda shares, "We [support workers] can bring out their [older and diverse women] by bringing out their qualities that don't see themselves, you know ... with tools to boost their self-esteem." Katelyn agrees, saying:

> *Giving women the empowerment or letting them know that, yes, you do have power, yes, you can do something, you're not a victim, you've overcome much, you know ... I honour you ... You have a part in this too ... there's some things you can do ... receive the help you need to build up the self-esteem and to build up the self-worth.*

3.4.3 Summary

"Remodeling the Web," represents the supportive and openly changing environment that centrally locates, shapes, and gives visibility to older and diverse women's presence within rural communities, their role as partners with advocates, health care providers, support workers, community organizations, stakeholders, and leaders. From a grassroots versus "top-down" approach, older and diverse women are at the center of their IPV program and service development, research, and mentorship of others with similar experiences and their continual personal self-growth journey.

4. Conclusions

This study aimed to understand how rural contexts facilitate or create barriers for older and diverse women and their service providers, who supported them in a paid or unpaid capacity. The results of a thematic analysis of 14 interviews (2 women and 12 supporters of older women who have experienced IPV in rural settings of Nova Scotia or New Brunswick, provinces located in Atlantic Canada. Four overarching themes, "Retaining the Web," Breaking the Threads," Spinning New Connections," and "Remodeling the Web," and related subthemes (**Figure 1**) emerged. These findings interpret study participants' experiences, challenges, needs, and opportunities regarding IPV support and service needs within complex and ever-changing rural settings within Atlantic Canada. The study findings suggest future practice, education, and research considerations for further discussion and attention.

4.1 Practice implications

The study's findings support the need to change or augment present-day ways that healthcare providers, resources, and community supports can be aligned and accessed for older, diverse rural women who have or are experiencing IPV. Previous study findings suggest that, for older women, geographic isolation, patriarchal and religious values, mistrust of health care and service providers, and traditional gender role expectations may complicate leaving an abusive relationship [34]. Study findings suggest that health care, support providers, and trusted community leaders may be vital in facilitating social networking, mentoring, multidisciplinary, intersectoral, and rural community partnerships with populations of older and diverse women who have experienced IPV in rural contexts.

First, there needs to be more recruitment of culturally diverse healthcare providers and a partnership with community leaders and organizations who represent older, diverse women, whether in language or cultural differences. Past research findings on older and diverse women experiencing IPV suggest mixed reactions to trusting the genuineness of health care and service providers and police, particularly if they did not look like or come from the same cultural background [34, 35]. Second, social networking strategies need to encompass cultural traditions and creative and innovative expressions which resonate with this diverse population. Health care and service providers may need to meet older and diverse women's needs where they are located instead of expecting them to travel to them. Often travel to centrally located facilities, such as known shelters within rural settings, may compromise older and diverse women's anonymity, confidentiality, and privacy. Research findings support that older women in rural locations face significant challenges in leaving IPV relationships, such as social and geographic isolation and fear of consequences of retribution by the abuser if they access services in their hometown [2, 27, 34].

Third, service providers need to engage more with these women to determine how to ensure their safety in their homes with their animals and decide which type of housing, financial, cultural, educational, and support are required if they must relocate. Study participants also preferred to have IPV services and resources, as well as other accessible services, under one roof in a confidential location. Researchers have uncovered similar suggestions in previous studies where older women in rural settings fear leaving IPV relationships and the only way of life they have known [2, 27, 34]. Fourth, there needs to be the development of more local rural collaborative forums and workshops for healthcare providers to understand rural life's unique challenges and benefits, including the additional challenges older, diverse women face in these areas. Past researchers confirm this to be an understudied area in literature [27]. Fifth, there needs to be further discussion of how older, diverse women access translation services in health care and the justice system and knowledge about what services or not qualify them if they are not Canadian citizens. Again, past researchers have identified that research and intervention in this subject area have yet to be widely studied [27].

Sixth, there also needs to be programmed to promote self-worth in women, not only at their stage of life now but for future generations of women, which includes men's supportive voices. Past research on the engagement of rural Nova Scotian women in physical activity behavior post-myocardial infarction suggest that the level of self-worth may significantly impact health behavior decisions of putting oneself first [11]. Seventh, study participants suggested there need to be better accommodations for older women with disabilities in shelters, which did not have wheelchair ramps and safety measures or assistance with disabilities and medications, and secondary affordable and accessible housing options. This lack of attention to providing adequate support for women in the design of affordable and accessible housing may be due to previous study findings that support little attention has been paid to older women in creating IPV interventions [27].

Eighth, service providers need to advocate for changes in safety, transportation, legal services, laws, and policies to support the victim versus the abuser. Past researchers have shared similar findings related to rural women's hesitancy to approach police officers to report IPV for fear that the judicial system will have further victimized them and that they will have severe consequences from their abuser [34]. Finally, healthcare and service providers, community leaders, government officials, and researchers need to direct future efforts toward discovering flexible employment options and re-examining needed financial aid, safety and protection, affordable housing, and resources to help diverse and older women remain in the home, including considering animal and pet support.

4.2 Education implications

Study findings suggest that health care and service providers should work with community partners, government officials, and stakeholders to develop, fund, and include more rural content in professional education curriculums and increase rural preceptorship opportunities for students. In particular, study findings suggest a need to educate health service providers and promote community awareness of the incidence and unique service and resource needs of older, diverse rural women who have experienced or are experiencing IPV. To date, government, and community IPV services and resources have primarily focused on younger women and children inside and outside rural areas [27, 34]. Consistent with previous research findings, study participants expressed little awareness that older and diverse women who had experienced or were experiencing IPV represented a unique group with specific service and resource needs [34].

Study findings suggest that support workers perceived older and diverse women who had experienced IPV to be more dependent on their partners. Study participants felt that older and diverse women were not always aware that they had been abuse victims and were unacquainted with what resources and services were available and how to access them. Also, they shared that these women often did not have a lot of educational social support, and financial resources. They shared that these women were more at risk of being victimized by the legal system and socially isolated, especially if they were required to relocate from their homes in rural areas due to IPV. Study participants felt that more healthcare providers must conduct in-person educational sessions at centrally located places in the rural community or within their homes to overcome financial and transportation obstacles and ensure anonymity, dignity, and safe spaces. However, part of these educational sessions should involve asking questions about what is contextually and culturally relevant for women, including issues about safety and protection and how to access supportive healthcare and legal resources in and outside rural contexts.

4.3 Research implications

In this study sample, there was less representation of older and diverse women who had suffered IPV than support providers. However, there is a need to develop trusting relationships with community and organization leaders who identify or have access and trust with older and diverse women who have experienced IPV to avoid exploiting these women in the research process. Therefore, chosen research designs and methods to study IPV should centrally locate older and diverse women's voices and perspectives. Future research studies are needed using socio-ecological approaches and participatory research methods, such as photovoice and art ensure participants' visibility, engagement, and empowerment throughout the research process. Such research may help develop, implement, and evaluate future rural programs and services that reflect diverse women's voiced needs.

Acknowledgements

We want to acknowledge all members of The RESPOND ANORT research team for their contributions to this research and their valuable comments and feedback.

This research was supported by funding from the Justice Partnership and Innovation Program-Family Violence Initiative, Justice Canada.

Conflict of interest

The authors declare no conflict of interest.

Appendices and nomenclature

Please refer to **Table 1** for participant pseudonyms and descriptions.

Author details

Heather Helpard[1*] and Lori E. Weeks[2]

1 Saint Francis Xavier University, Antigonish, Nova Scotia, Canada

2 Dalhousie University, Halifax, Nova Scotia, Canada

*Address all correspondence to: hhelpard@stfx.ca

References

[1] Burczycka M. Police-reported intimate partner violence in Canada, 2018. In Family violence in Canada: A statistical profile, 2018 [Internet]. 2019. Statistics Canada Catalogue no. 85-002-X. Available from: https://www150.statcan.gc.ca/n1/pub/85-002-x/2019001/article/00018/02-eng.htm

[2] Weeks L, LeBlanc K. An ecological synthesis of research on older women's experiences of intimate partner violence. Journal of Women and Aging. 2011;**23**(4):283-304. DOI: 10.1080/08952841.2011.611043

[3] Pathak N, Dhairyawan R, Tariq S. The experience of intimate partner violence among older women: A narrative review. Maturitas. 2019;**121**:63-75. DOI: 10.1016/j.maturitas.2018.12.011

[4] Irwin P. Physical activity among older women living in rural areas of Canada: A scoping review. Journal of Population Ageing. 2022;**15**:755-801. DOI: https://doi-org.libproxy.stfx.ca/10.1007/s12062-022-09380-8

[5] Bierman A, Jaakimainen R, Abramson B, Kapral M, Azad N, Hall R, et al. Cardiovascular diseases. In: Bierman A, editor. Project for Ontario women's Health Evidence-Based Report. Toronto, Ontario, Canada: Keenan Research Center; 2009. pp. 1-15

[6] DesMeules M, Pong R. How Healthy are rural Canadians? An assessment of their health status and health determinants. Ottawa (ON): Public Health Agency of Canada; 2006

[7] Pong R, DesMeules M, Legace C. Rural-urban disparities in health: How does Canada fare and how does Canada compare to Australia? Australian Journal of Rural Health. 2009;**17**:58-64. DOI: 10.1111/j.1440-1584.2008. 01039.x

[8] Government of Canada. The Labour Market in Atlantic Canada. Ottawa (ON): Author; Ottawa, Ontario Canada; 2020. Available from: https://www.canada.ca/en/atlantic-canada-opportunities/services/researchstudies10.html

[9] Burczycka M. Section 2: Police-reported intimate partner violence in Canada [Internet]. Ottawa, Ontario Canada: Statistics Canada; 2017. Available from: https://www150.statcan.gc.ca/n1/pub/85-002-x/2018001/article/54978/02-eng.htm

[10] Statistics Canada. A Portrait of Canada's Growing Population Aged 85 and Older from the 2021 Census. Author; Ottawa, Ontario, Canada; 2021. Available from: https://www12.statcan.gc.ca/census-recensement/2021/as-sa/98-200-X/2021004/98-200-X2021004-eng.cfm

[11] Helpard H. Seeking self-worth: Physical activity behavior engagement in rural Nova Scotia women post-myocardial infarction: A constructivist grounded theory study [thesis]. Halifax, Nova Scotia: Dalhousie University; 2014. Available from: https://central.bac-lac.gc.ca/.item?id=TC-NSHD-50393&op=pdf&app=Library

[12] Leipert B. Rural women's health issues in Canada: An overview and implications for policy and research. Canadian Women's Studies. 2005;**24**(4):109-116. Available from: https://cws.journals.yorku.ca/index.php/cws/article/view/6074

[13] Sibley L, Weiner J. An evaluation of access to health care services along the rural-urban continuum

in Canada. BMC Health Services Research. 2011;**11**(20):online. DOI: 10.1186/1472-6963-11-20

[14] Boron J, Levett K, Pope M. Racial Inequities in Rural, Remote, and Northern Canadian Planning. Ottawa (ON): Canadian Institute of Planners; 2021. Available from: https://www.cip-icu.ca/getattachment/CIP-News/Latest-News/May-2022/Celebrating-National-Indigenous-History-Month-2022/PlanCanada_Spring2021_BoronLevettPope.pdf.aspx

[15] Pong R. Rural Health/Telehealth. Ottawa (ON): Minister of Public Works and Government Services; 2002. Available from: https://publications.gc.ca/collections/Collection/H13-6-2002-6E.pdf

[16] Troughton M. Redefining "rural" for the twenty-first century. In: Ramp W, Kulig J, Townsend I, McGowan V, editors. Health in Rural Settings: Contexts for Action. Lethbridge [AB]: University of Lethbridge; 1999. pp. 21-38

[17] Wilson C, Rourke J, Oandasan I, Bosco C. Progress made on access to rural healthcare in Canada. Canadian Journal of Rural Medicine. 2020;**25**(1):14-19. DOI: 10.4103/CJRM.CJRM_84_19

[18] Sarkki S, Torre C, Fransala J, Zivojinovic I, Ludvig A, et al. Reconstructive social Innovation cycles in women-led initiatives in rural areas. Sustainability. 2021;**13**:1-22. DOI: 10.3390/su13031231

[19] du Plessis V, Beshiri R, Bollman R, Clemenson H. Definitions of Rural. Ottawa [ON]: Statistics Canada, Agriculture and Rural Working Paper No. 61, Catalogue. No. 21-601-MIE; 2001

[20] Halfacree K. Locality and social representation: Space, discourse, and alternative definitions of the rural. Journal of Rural Studies. 1993;**9**(1):23-37. DOI: 10.1016/0743-0167(93)9000-3

[21] Hartley D. Rural health disparities, population health and rural culture. American Journal of Public Health. 2004;**94**(10):1675-1678. Available from: http://www.ncbi.nlm.nih.gov/pmc/articles/PMC1448513/

[22] Band-Winterstein T, Eisikovits Z. Aging out of violence: Multiple faces of intimate violence over the life span. Qualitative Health Research. 2009;**19**(2):164-180. DOI: https://doi-org.libproxy.stfx.ca/10.1177/1049732308329305

[23] Lundy M, Grossman S. Domestic violence service users: A comparison of older and younger women victims. Journal of Family Violence. 2009;**24**:297-309. DOI: 10.1007/s10896-009-9230-y

[24] McGarry J, Simpson C, Mansour M. How domestic violence affects the wellbeing of older women. Nursing Older People. 2010;**22**(5):33-37. DOI: 10.7748/nop2010.06.22.5.33.c7795

[25] McGarry J, Simpson C, Hinchliff-Smith K. The impact of domestic abuse for older women: A review of the literature. Health & Social Care in the Community. 2011;**19**(1):3-14. DOI: 10.1111/j.1365-2524.2010.00964.x

[26] Weeks L, Macquarrie C, Begley L, Gill C, LeBlanc K. Strengthening resources for midlife and older women who experience intimate partner violence. Journal of Women & Aging. 2016;**28**(1):46-57. DOI: 10.1080/08952841.2014.950500

[27] Weeks L, Stilwell C, Gagnon D, Dupuis-Blanchard S, Macquarrie C, Jackson L. Initiatives to support older women who experience intimate

partner violence. Violence Against Women. 2021;**27**(15-16):3011-3029. DOI: 10.1177.107780.220988355

[28] Waldron I, MacDougall E, Weeks L. Hear my cry: Breaking the code of silence around intimate partner violence among black women in and beyond midlife. Atlantis. 2021;**42**(1):17-30. DOI: 10.7202/1082013ar

[29] Charmaz K. Constructing Grounded Theory: A Practical Guide Through Qualitative Analysis. 1st ed. Thousand Oaks, CA: Sage; 2006

[30] Blumer H. Symbolic Interaction Perspectives and Methods. 1st ed. New Jersey: Prentice Hall; 1969

[31] Doucet S, Letourneau N, Stoppard J. Contemporary paradigms for research related to women's health. Health Care for Women International. 2010;**31**(4):296-312. DOI: 10.1080/07399330903518509

[32] Braun V, Clarke V. Using thematic analysis in psychology. Qualitative Research in Psychology. 2006;**3**(2):77-101. DOI: 10.1191/1478088706qp063oa

[33] Lincoln YS, Guba EG. Naturalistic Inquiry. 1st ed. Beverly Hills, CA: Sage; 1985

[34] Riddell T, Ford-Gilboe M, Leipert B. Strategies used by rural women to stop, avoid, or escape from intimate partner violence. Health Care for Women International. 2009;**30**(1-2):134-159. DOI: 10.1080/07399330802523774

[35] Williams I, Mattos M. We're still here: Addressing the diverse healthcare needs of older adults in rural areas. Public Policy and Aging Report. 2021;**31**(4): 126-128. DOI: 10.1093/ppar/prab017

Section 5

Health Financing: The Missing Piece to Universal Health Coverage

Chapter 14

Examining the Relationship between Access to Health Care and Socio-Economic Characteristics

Oluwafunmiso Adeola Olajide

Abstract

The link between good health and the ability to work effectively to meet livelihood needs is established but the economic implications of the reverse have often not been estimated; also how this plays out for different gender and socio-economic groups is often not estimated. The chapter examines the health care access that rural households have and examine how it relates to their education and employment in various sectors. The study used Nigeria as a case study as such the General Household Survey Data for wave 4 was used. The data were analyzed using descriptive, and Tobit regression model. The results showed that labour hours worked (in agricultural, non-agricultural and non-household activities) has a negative relationship with health care access. Age and literacy (ability to read) is important in health care access and have positive relationships with it. The policy implication of the study is that educational infrastructure must be developed along-side health policy initiatives.

Keywords: health care accessibility, infrastructure, income, employment, livelihoods

1. Introduction

A major target of the sustainable development goal three on good health and well-being includes achieving universal health coverage, which includes access to health services. This is relevant for developing countries and rural areas in particular where suffering and preventable diseases often lead to untimely death. Low insurance coverage, poverty and shortage of health care staff have been cited as deterrents to healthy lives in developing countries [1]; these can lead to increased out of pocket expenses which the vulnerable groups of the society may be unable to meet conveniently [2]. Hence, achieving the sustainable development goal three requires that the issue of access to health care and its socio-economic determinants like income, education, and gender be prioritized in policy and intervention strategy designs [1].

According to [3] access to health care means having "the timely use of personal health services to achieve the best health outcomes". Implicit in this definition is the thought that health facilities should be within the reach of all as at when needed; that it is utilized and positioned to render appropriate services from which users can achieve expected outcome. In reality many people lack access to adequate health care as a result of public policy failure which creates barriers such as poverty and other forms of inequality. On the other hand, there is the issue of self-selection as people show preferences for other 'medical' alternatives. However, health care system is a public policy issue and as such resources should be allocated to it to make it effective and efficient. Based on this, there is a need for empirical evidence that will support government planning and resource allocation with respect to the provider and the client.

To achieve this, appropriate definition of variables that define health care is important. In the literature [4, 5], some indicate that the ability to pay for services is a major determinant, in some case preferences indicated by clients' behavior in terms of perception of the illness, the options available are cited as playing important roles in health care access. There is also the gender dimension: poverty, religion, cultural values and norms are considered barriers to women's access [6]. Finally, there is the school of thought that lays emphasis on demographic and socio-economic factors as the determinants of health care access. The varied positions suggest the need to approach the question from a different perspective. This study defined an index for access to health care and used alternative set of variables which are particularly relevant to the clients' circumstance. The study focused on the rural areas of Nigeria and used hours worked, level of literacy as major covariates of health care access.

A focus on the rural area is apt because the poor are generally known to have less access to health care services. The continued disparity between the poor and the rich within the country, is the basis for research based evidence which will set the direction for approaches and interventions that will narrow the gap. Identifying the dimensions of healthcare deprivation in rural areas, the vulnerable and the hot spots for the disadvantaged can be a spring board for closing the gap. Based on this, the study examined the relationship between access to health care and socio-economic variables with the aim of suggesting evidence based policy options that will lead to improved personal health care system in rural Nigeria.

2. Methodology

2.1 Conceptual framework

Several organizations [3, 7] have given different definitions of health care access to include timeliness, coverage, a regular source of care and capable personnel. The word 'access' is also seen to have both quantitative and qualitative aspects which means that it may not be fully quantified while being evaluated. Some components used to assess and evaluate it in literature include 'being available', 'financial access', 'utilization', and 'barriers'. Part of the discourse on its measurement includes the capacity, demand [7] and geography or spatial dimension. But a common thread that runs through the literature is the need to have equity in health care access especially for planning and resource allocation at the macro level.

Figure 1 shows the conceptual framework which underlies this study. The definition of access to health care is taken from Penchansky and Thomas [8]. Access is grouped into five As: Affordability, Availability, Accessibility, Accommodation and Acceptability. These characteristics of health care access are defined to reflect provider and client's expectations and characteristics; and the fact that these need to fit. The framework shows that there are aspects of healthcare access which are easily influenced by the socio-economic status of the respondent. For example, the income generated by the

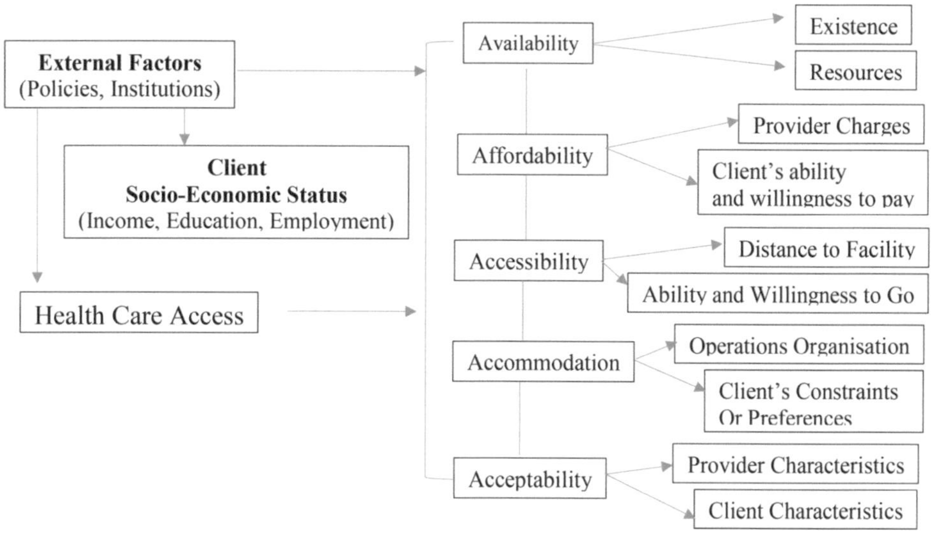

Figure 1.
Framework for health care access. Source: Author's Concept based on Penchansky and Thomas, [8] cited in McLaughlin and Wyszewianski [9].

client could influence not only the choice of the healthcare facility but also the ability to pay; also the resources of the facility especially in terms of personnel and technology may interact with the income level or socio economic status to determine health care access [10]. On the other hand, the level of access could impinge on the individual's continued ability to earn an income, improve the food security and livelihood status [11, 12]. Hence the relationships could be recursive in some cases. Also, the influence of external factors such as policies and institutions on elements of the framework can hamper or support clients' access to health care. The framework suggests the need for a holistic approach to improving rural people's access to healthcare so that it cuts across all socio-economic levels while not making any particular group worse off.

2.2 Analytical framework

2.2.1 The relationship between health care access and socio-economic status

The relationship of access to health care to socio-economic indices (Education, Income and Employment) was determined by first establishing an indicator of health care access. Rural people often have several health care options which may be formal or informal; also some combine different options in a bid to maintain a healthy life or restore themselves to health. This behavior reflects the different aspects of health care access, and may also be a reflection of what they feel comfortable with.

2.2.1.1 Measuring health care access

Health care access has been measured in different ways. The IOM [3] identified two quantifiable areas: utilization and outcomes. Indicators for both were then identified which could indicate problem areas as well as show when problems occur; these permitted a level of measurement but access was treated as an intervening variable to health care utilization and outcomes. A conditional logit model was proposed by Jang

S/N	Item	Indicator variables	Unit
1	Availability	The existence of a formal health care facility/Actually Visited The facility has some qualified personnel The facility is equipped	Yes/No Yes/No Yes/No
2	Affordability	No charges Client paid the charges and or bought medication	None Amount Spent in Naira Amount spent in Naira
3	Accessibility	Transportation cost to the nearest facility	Transportation cost in Naira
4	Accommodation	Wait time for consultation Walk-in possible	Minutes Yes/No
5	Acceptability	Actual Consultation made	Yes/No

Table 1.
Indicators for the measurement of access to health care.

[5]; the model combined a choice model with a Floating Catchment Area in such a way that the peculiarity of a client to use a hospital was captured. In this study, indicators were identified for each of the fives 'A's defined above. These were then used to generate an index using the Principal Component Analysis. The definition of the each A is relatively encompassing as such client and organizational peculiarities are included. The index generated was then used as the dependent variable in the regression model. The terms and the indicators are listed in **Table 1**. To examine the relationship between health care access and indicators of socio-economic variables [10], the people were classified as: (I) Able to read vs. Unable to read, (II) Male vs. Female (III) Hours worked in different jobs per week.

The PCA is a technique for reducing the dimensionality of large datasets, increasing interpretability but at the same time minimizing information loss [13]. It does so by creating new uncorrelated variables that successively maximize variance. Although for inferential purposes a multivariate normal (Gaussian) distribution of the dataset is usually assumed, PCA as a descriptive tool needs no distributional assumptions and, as such, is very much an adaptive exploratory method which can be used on numerical data of various types. Olajide, stated 'In mathematical terms, from an initial set of n correlated variables, PCA creates uncorrelated indices or components, where each component is a linear weighted combination of the initial variables. Mathematically, the transformation is defined by a set of p-dimensional vectors of weights or loadings (1) that map each row vector $\mathbf{X}_{(i)}$ of $\mathbf{X}$ to a new vector of principal component *scores* (2) given by (3).

$$W_k = (\omega_1, \dots, \omega_p)(k) \tag{1}$$

$$t_{(i)} = (t_i, \dots t_p)(i) \tag{2}$$

$$t_{k(i)} = X_{(i)} \bullet W_{(k)} \tag{3}$$

in such a way that the individual variables of $\mathbf{t}$ considered over the data set successively inherit the maximum possible variance from $\mathbf{x}$, with each loading vector $\mathbf{w}$ constrained to be a unit vector [14].

For example, from a set of variables X_1 through to X_n.

$$PC_1 = a_{11}X_1 + a_{12}X_2 + \dots + a_{1n}X_n \tag{4}$$
$$PC_m = a_{m1}X_1 + a_{m2}X_2 + \dots + a_{mn}X_n$$

Where:
a_{mn} represents the weight for the mth principal component and the nth variable [14].

2.2.1.2 Estimating the relationship between access to health care and selected indicators of socio-economic status

Since an index was generated to summarize the individual's access to health care, it means that it can be subject to a censoring effect. As such in order to examine the relationships between the variables, the Tobit model is used to avoid having a biased coefficient estimates [15]. The model is designed to estimate linear relationships between variables when there is either left- or right-censoring in the dependent variable. The Tobit Model presents a simple relation:

$$y_i^* = \beta_0 + \beta_1 x_{1i} + \varepsilon_i \tag{5}$$
$$y_i = 0, \quad \text{if } y_i^* = x_i^{`}\beta + \varepsilon_i \le 0 \tag{6}$$
$$= y_i^* = x_i^{`}\beta + \varepsilon_i \text{ if } y_i^* = x_i^{`}\beta + \varepsilon_i > 0 \tag{7}$$

The effect of the Xs on the probability that an observation is censored and the effect on the conditional mean of the non-censored observations are the same: β.

y_i * = HCA index (may be censored right or left).

β = Vector of parameters to be estimated.

x = Explanatory and control variables categorized into household head and household variables (sex, age, education, farm and non-farm income, employment type), household food security status. The model aimed at determining the partial effects of the x variables on the latent variable. The parameters of Eq. (5) are estimated by the maximum likelihood method. To examine the relationship between health care access and indicators of socio-economic variables, the people were classified as: (I) Able to read vs. Unable to read, (II) Male vs. female (III) Hours worked in different jobs per week.

2.3 Data

The paper used the wave 4 of Nigeria General Household Survey (GHS) data collected by the National Bureau of Statistics and the World Bank. The survey panel is implemented in collaboration with the World Bank Living Standards Measurement Study (LSMS) team as part of the Integrated Surveys on Agriculture (ISA) program. The data is nationally representative involving about 5000 households, and contains comprehensive data on socio-economic characteristics and welfare indicators. The households were selected through a random sampling procedure which ensured the distribution of EAs across the 6 geo-political zones (and urban and rural areas within) in the nation. The GHS consists of three panel questionnaires: Household, Agricultural and Community, which were administered using Computer Assisted Personal Interview (CAPI) in post planting and post-harvest periods. This study focused on the rural sector as a case study not only because it is the agricultural base of the country but also because additional empirical evidence is necessary for resource planning and policy implementation of improved health care delivery. It will also serve as a means of evaluating the current status of previously implemented rural programs in the nation. Individual level analysis was carried out using data for household heads in rural communities. All household heads were selected irrespective of sex leading to a total sample of 3433 individuals based in the rural areas but complete data for the variables of interest were found for 3217 people, so these were used in the analyses.

The Federal Republic of Nigeria is located in the south east of West Africa, with a coast at the Bight of Benin and the Gulf of Guinea. It lies between latitudes 4° and 14° N, and longitudes 2° and 15°E. It has a land area of 923,768 km^2 and a population of 192 million people. It has a tropical climate with variable raining and dry season periods. Agriculture, which is the main means of livelihood in the rural sector, contributes about 23.4 percent of the GDP. Health care delivery is the joint responsibility of the three tiers of the federal, state and local governments in the country. Since the Bamako Initiative of 1987, the country has made significant improvement in health care delivery and access using the community based approach. However, the sector is witnessing increasing emigration of skilled workers to the west. The rural population is about 47% the World Bank World Development Report, over 35 percent work in agriculture, in an environment that generally has low social infrastructure [16].

3. Results and discussion

3.1 Index generation

The Principal Component Analysis (PCA) indicated that the most important components in the index generated were those associated with the first 4 As: Availability, Affordability, Accessibility and Accommodation. Component 1 was responsible for about 32 percent of the variance as such it was used in the regression analysis. **Tables 2** and **3** indicate the bases for the acceptance of the model and confirms that a PCA could be carried out on it.

3.2 Relationship between HCA index and socio-economic variables

The HCA is the response variable predicted by the model. The tobit model was used because this response variable is censored. The tobit regression coefficients are interpreted in the same way as the OLS regression coefficients except that the linear effect is not on the observed outcome but on the latent variable. The expected HCA score or index will change for each unit increase in the corresponding predictors. As such an increase in hours worked is likely to reduce the probability of accessing health care while an increase in age could lead to an increase in health care access. The literacy status as a measure of educational level suggests that it could be a barrier to accessing health care. At $p < = 0.005$, labor hour in a week is the most significant variable, although negative, while Age and literacy status are significant at higher levels of the test statistic. Policy instruments that will encourage high literacy levels and create health care opportunities for the aged could increase personal access to health care in rural communities. Also, advocacy on the importance of balancing work with health could be necessary to encourage more visits even with a tight schedule (**Table 4**).

PCA Pattern Matrix[a]			
	Component		
	1	**2**	**3**
Actually consulted or visited	0.767		
Days Lost to illness			−0.938
Consultation fees (N)			
Transportation cost (N)			−0.908
Travel Time (minutes)	0.744		
Wait time (minutes)	0.600		
Cost of medicine purchased (N)	0.478		
Number of Nights Hospitalized		0.942	
Cost of Hospitalization (N)		0.936	

Extraction Method: Principal Component Analysis.
Rotation Method: Oblimin with Kaiser Normalization.
[a]Rotation converged in 7 iterations.

Table 2.
The component of the access to health care index.

KMO and Bartlett's test		
Kaiser-Meyer-Olkin measure of sampling adequacy.		0.647
Bartlett's Test of Sphericity	Approx. Chi-Square	8707.521
	df	36
	Sig.	0.000

Table 3.
Data sampling adequacy.

Tobit regression
Log likelihood = −2684.85

Number of obs = 3217
LR chi2(4) = 73.62
Prob > chi^2 = 0
Pseudo R^2 = 0.0135

HCA	**Coef.**	**Std. Err.**	**t**	**P > |t|**	**[95% Conf.]**	
Client is literate	0.234	0.12	1.93	0.054	−0.00374	0.470747
Hours worked/week	−0.14	0.02	−7.54	0	−0.17712	−0.104
Sex	0.22	0.15	1.43	0.15	−0.07955	0.510316
Age	0.01	0.004	1.85	0.065	−0.00043	0.014691
_cons	−1.78	0.28	−6.32	0	−2.3364	−1.23056
/sigma	2.53	0.0781			2.37461	2.680823

Obs. summary: 2490 left-censored observations at HCA < =0
727 uncensored observations
0 right-censored observations

Table 4.
Tobit regression results.

4. Conclusion

This study examined the relationship between health care access and some socio-economic variables. To achieve this, an index was generated based on several variables. The index showed that availability, affordability, accessibility and accommodation are really important as such policies that would enhance these should be pursued in order to improve rural health care system in terms of utilization and outcome. The policies should combine rural healthcare infrastructure development with rural health insurance schemes. The results also showed that labour hours worked (in agricultural, non-agricultural and non-household activities) has a negative relationship with health care access. Age and literacy (ability to read) is important in health care access and have positive relationships with it. The policy implication of the study is that educational infrastructure must be developed along-side health policy initiatives.

A. Appendix

A.1 Communalities

	Initial	Extraction
Consulted	1.000	0.555
Days Lost	1.000	0.805
Pay consult	1.000	0.340
Trans cost	1.000	0.845
Time Mins	1.000	0.599
Wait time minutes	1.000	0.334
Cost drug purchased	1.000	0.545
Number of nights admitted	1.000	0.865
Amount paid	1.000	0.843

Extraction method: Principal component analysis.

A.2 Total variance explained

Component	Initial eigenvalues			Extraction sums of squared loadings			Rotation sums of squared loadings[a]
	Total	% of variance	Cumulative %	Total	% of variance	Cumulative %	Total
1	2.877	31.966	31.966	2.877	31.966	31.966	2.193
2	1.687	18.741	50.707	1.687	18.741	50.707	2.057
3	1.168	12.974	63.681	1.168	12.974	63.681	2.206
4	0.927	10.303	73.984				
5	0.810	8.996	82.980				

Component	Initial eigenvalues			Extraction sums of squared loadings			Rotation sums of squared loadings[a]
	Total	% of variance	Cumulative %	Total	% of variance	Cumulative %	Total
6	0.553	6.149	89.129				
7	0.496	5.507	94.635				
8	0.277	3.082	97.717				
9	0.205	2.283	100.000				

Extraction method: Principal component analysis.

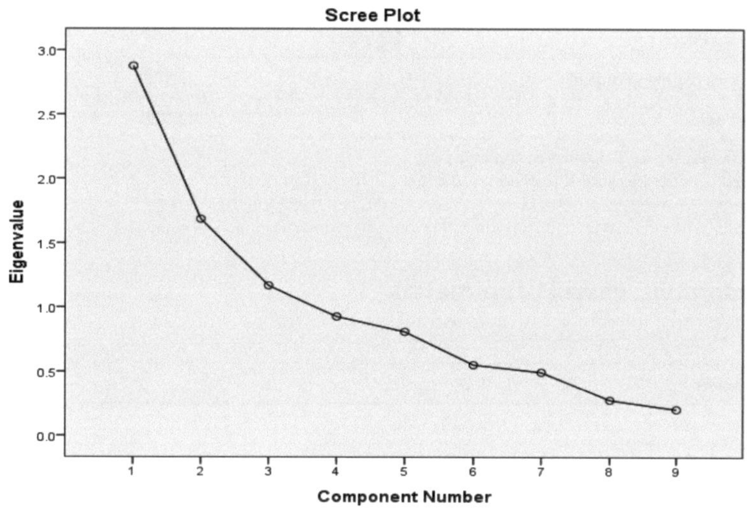

A.3 Component Matrix[a]

	Component		
	1	2	3
Consulted	0.523		0.499
Days Lost	0.595		−0.608
Pay consult	0.583		
Trans cost	0.706		−0.488
Time Mins	0.606		
Wait time minutes			
Cost Drug Purch	0.722		
Number of Nights admitted	0.466	0.804	
Amount paid	0.417	0.817	

Extraction method: Principal component analysis.
[a]3 components extracted.

A.4 Structure Matrix

	Component		
	1	2	3
Consulted	0.740		
Days Lost			−0.888
Pay consult	0.447		−0.442
Trans cost			−0.916
Time Mins	0.767		
Wait time minutes	0.567		
Cost Drug Purch	0.606	0.457	−0.451
Number of Nights admitted		0.928	
Amount paid		0.912	

Extraction method: Principal component analysis.
Rotation method: Oblimin with Kaiser normalization.

A.5 Component correlation matrix

Component	1	2	3
1	1.000	0.158	−0.329
2	0.158	1.000	−0.199
3	−0.329	−0.199	1.000

Extraction method: Principal component analysis.
Rotation method: Oblimin with Kaiser normalization.

Author details

Oluwafunmiso Adeola Olajide
Department of Agricultural Economics, University of Ibadan, Oyo, Oyo State, Nigeria

*Address all correspondence to: preciousfunso@yahoo.com; funso.olajide@ui.edu.ng

References

[1] Strasser R, Kam SM, Regalado SM. Rural health care access and policy in developing countries. Annual Review of Public Health. 2016;**37**:395-412. DOI: 10.1146/annurev-publhealth-032315-021507

[2] Adogu PO, Egenti BN, Ubajaka C, Onwasigwe C, Nnebue CC. Utilization of maternal health services in urban and rural communities of Anambra state, Nigeria. Nigerian Journal of Medicine: Journal of the National Association of Resident Doctors of Nigeria. 2014;**23**(1): 61-69

[3] Institute of Medicine, Committee on Monitoring Access to Personal Health Care Services. Access to Health Care in America. Washington, DC: National Academy Press; 1993 https://www.ncbi.nlm.nih.gov/books/NBK235882/

[4] Darin-Mattsson A, Fors S, Kåreholt I. Different indicators of socioeconomic status and their relative importance as determinants of health in old age. International Journal for Equity in Health. 2017;**16**:173. DOI: 10.1186/s12939-017-0670-3

[5] Jang HA. Model for measuring healthcare accessibility using the behavior of demand: A conditional logit model-based floating catchment area method. BMC Health Service Research. 2021;**21**:660. DOI: 10.1186/s12913-021-06654-3

[6] Puentes-Markides C. Women and access to health care. Social Science & Medicine (1982). 1992;**35**(4):619-626. DOI: 10.1016/0277-9536(92)90356-u

[7] Gulliford M, Figueroa-Munoz J, Morgan M, Hughes D, Gibson B, Beech R, et al. What does 'access to health care' mean? Journal of Health Services Research & Policy. 2002;**7**(3):186-188. DOI: 10.1258/135581902760082517

[8] Penchansky R, Thomas JW. The concept of access: Definition and relationship to consumer satisfaction. Medical Care. 1981:127-140

[9] McLaughlin CG, Wyszewianski L. Access to care: Remembering old lessons. Health Services Research. 2002;**37**(6): 1441-1443. DOI: 10.1111/1475-6773.12171

[10] Saif-Ur-Rahman KM, Anwar I, Hasan M, Hossain S, Shafique S, Haseen F, et al. Use of indices to measure socio-economic status (SES) in South-Asian urban health studies: A scoping review. Systematic Reviews. 2018;**7**(1):196. DOI: 10.1186/s13643-018-0867-6

[11] Melo A, Matias MA, Dias SS, Gregório MJ, Rodrigues AM, de Sousa RD, et al. Is food insecurity related to health-care use, access and absenteeism? Public Health Nutrition. 2019;**22**(17): 3211-3219. DOI: 10.1017/S136898001 9001885

[12] Ajayi OE, Adeola OO. Effect of healthcare accessibility on cocoa farmers' food security in Ondo State. Nigeria in Journal of Development and Agricultural Economics. 2021;**13**(3):248-255. DOI: 10.5897/JDAE2021.1288

[13] Jolliffe IT, Cadima J. Principal component analysis: A review andrecent developments. Philosophical Transactions of the Royal Society. 2016; **A374**:20150202. DOI: 10.1098/rsta.2015.0202

[14] Vyas S, Kumaranayake L. Constructing socio-economic status indices: How to use principal components analysis. Health Policy and

Planning. 2006;**21**(6):459-468. DOI: 10.1093/heapol/czl029

[15] Austin PC, Escobar M, Kopec JA. The use of the Tobit model for analyzing measures of health status. Quality Life Research. 2000;**9**:901-910. DOI: 10.1023/A:1008938326604

[16] World bank. World Development Report 2021: Data for Better Lives. Washington, DC: World Bank; 2021. DOI: 10.1596/978-1-4648-1600-0

Chapter 15

Out-of-Pocket Health Care Expenditures in Uzbekistan: Progress and Reform Priorities

Min Jung Cho and Eva Haverkort

Abstract

Over the past twenty years, Uzbekistan's health system changed drastically from the inherited Soviet health system. This research aims to examine the main aspects of the Uzbek health financing system and policy process that led to out-of-pocket (OOP) health care expenditures by using a mixed-method case study approach. Qualitative findings reveal that the covered basic benefit package is limited. Health care evaluation methods and accessible information on health quality are lacking. This leads to inefficient use of resources and a risk of using unnecessary or low-quality health services. Quantitative findings reveal that especially the chronically ill have high OOP. Furthermore, alcohol use, health status of the household head, money saved in the past and place of residence proved to be significant factors. This research showed that the limited benefit package, lacking evaluation methods, and inaccessible information on health care led to high OOP. Policies remain inefficient at addressing OOP due to limited civilian participation, lack of data, and limited evidence-based decision making. This research suggests that the benefit package should be expanded to cover the chronically ill.

Keywords: out-of-pocket expenses, chronic diseases, household budget, catastrophic health expenditure, health insurance, primary health care, health equity, Uzbekistan, Central Asia

1. Introduction

For a long time, the Uzbek health system was part of the Soviet health system, in which the state covered all health care services. After the Soviet Union's dissolution in 1991, Uzbekistan's government wanted to keep health care public [1, 2]. However, due to economic constraints, the state could no longer cover the use of all health care services. This meant that part of the health services had to be purchased directly by citizens: out of their own pocket. Hence the name, out-of-pocket expenditures (OOP) [3, 4].

Uzbekistan's large population of 33.6 million is struggling, both economically and health wise [5]. In 2013, 14% of the population lived under the poverty line. The fact that more recent data is not available proves one of Uzbekistan's challenges: there is a lack of monitoring and a lack of information management in their national statistical systems [6–9].

Furthermore, Uzbekistan is faced with double burden of infectious and non-communicable diseases, such as cancer and diabetes [5]. The average life expectancy in 2019 was 73 years for Uzbekistan compared to European countries' average life expectancy of 81 (in 2018) [10]. Infant mortality rate of 17 (in every 1000 children under five) in Uzbekistan compared to 5.11 in Europe also suggests a potential weakness in the health system. [11, 12].

OOP are a global phenomenon: all countries rely to some extent on OOP to fund their health care system. There are two general concerns about OOP. Firstly, the people with the greatest need and the people with the lowest income feel the financial burden the most. Secondly, patients may choose not to access necessary care to avoid this financial burden. Despite concerns, many countries have been shifting health care costs directly to patients [13].

This is also the case for Uzbekistan, which has been relying progressively on OOP [1, 3]. Between 2014 and 2018, the proportion of health expenditure that is paid out of pocket has been increasing from 45.41% in 2014 to 60.34% in 2018. Other Central-Asian countries have slightly different trends. Turkmenistan (76.34% in 2018) and Tajikistan (68.42% in 2018) have been gradually increasing their OOP proportion [14–16]. However, they have not experienced such a sharp increase as Uzbekistan. The Kyrgyz Republic's OOP proportion has been gradually decreasing, with a share of 52.44% in 2018. Kazakhstan seems to have been stabilising around 33%, much lower than the other countries [15, 16]. Thus, while other Central-Asian countries have alarming OOP rates, the sharp increase of Uzbekistan's OOP is concerning [17].

Trends may vary across Central-Asian countries because health financing reforms have also varied. Scholars have found that differentiation in success rates is, amongst other things, caused by variation in the type of pooling systems and the level of cooperation with international aid organisations [1]. Furthermore, the level of civilian involvement in policymaking and the level of evidence-based decision making may lead to varying success rates of health reforms. Uzbekistan, for example, has no national pooling system for health financing and limited international aid involvement [1, 3]. Furthermore, Uzbekistan stands out as a lower-middle income county. The average OOP of low-middle income countries is much lower than that of Uzbekistan. For years it has been around 36%, without many fluctuations [16].

Uzbekistan's government has implemented reforms targeting primary care, non-communicable diseases and project management and evaluation improvement. While these efforts have been made, partly in an attempt to reduce OOP, challenges remain and financial protection is not achieved [4]. The current policies are not effective in reducing OOP. Existing studies have already established that economic health shocks contribute to poverty in low-middle income country settings [3, 5, 18–20]. Addressing OOP is vital for improving the health of the population because high OOP is one of the first issues citizens encounter when accessing health care.

Studies have analysed health financing both in high income and low-middle income country contexts [21]. However, there are only a few studies that focus on Central Asian context [13, 22–24]. This research is motivated by providing evidence into an important policy debate on health financing by analysing what causes high OOP through examining Uzbekistan's health financing system and policy process.

2. Background

Uzbekistan is a democratic republic and has been independent of the Soviet Union since 1991. Since then, the public health care system is divided into three hierarchical levels: (1) the national (republican) level, (2) the regional (viloyati) level, and (3) the district (local tumanlar) levels. There are fourteen viloyati [1, 4]. Each viloyat exists out of smaller districts: cities or rural areas that are called tumanlar. The different hierarchical levels have different responsibilities in terms of regulation and financing of health services [25].

The formal actors in the public health sector are the President, the Cabinet of Ministers, the Supreme Assembly (Senate and Legislative Chamber), the Ministry of Health (MoH), the Ministry of Finance (MoF), viloyat health authorities and tuman (local) health authorities. In **Table 1**, presents an overview of all the actors and their tasks can be found.

The elected President, Shavkat Mirziyogyev (in power since 2016) determines the strategic course of health reforms in Uzbekistan [26, 27]. The direction for health care reform is co-determined by the Cabinet of Ministers and Parliament. They set priorities, formulate national health policies and determine means and sources of financing. The MoH and MoF are consulted before final policy documents are adopted, and they are involved in the policy development process [28, 29].

The MoH is also responsible for planning, organising and managing the health care system in general. It develops, implements and evaluates the policies, together with the Cabinet of Ministers. MoH also monitors the quality of care. Furthermore, it is directly responsible for managing and monitoring the national level hospitals, specialised medical centres, research institutions, medical schools and emergency care. The tasks of the Cabinet of Ministers and the MoH sometimes overlap, and they collaborate on many issues [30].

Subnational authorities have the responsibility to finance, manage and monitor sub-national hospitals, primary care units, sanitary-epidemiological services and ambulance services [4]. In general, the national government is more focused on specialised care, while the regional and local governments are more focused on primary care. Viloyat authorities are accountable to tuman or city health authorities and both are overseen by the MoH. Local governments can only implement policies that do not contradict national policies. Those are used as a regulatory tool [1, 4, 31].

Centralised decision-making remains mostly at the national level, but some administrative functions have been assigned to the viloyat, mostly budgetary responsibilities. There is to an extent cooperation between the different governmental levels, often those intersectoral approaches are donor-driven [30].

Although most health care is public, the private sector is gradually growing. The MoH has had to limit the private sector in the past due to unnecessary and unsafe care practices [4, 25]. However, the government has started to encourage private practices and clinics to mobilise resources and improve quality and efficiency. The private sector is now monitored better with unannounced inspections to private facilities [28]. Nevertheless, the private sector remains small.

It includes the supply of pharmaceuticals and other medical equipment. Moreover, some physicians have a private practice. Dental care is also privately provided. Many services cannot be provided in the private sector, either because the government does not allow it or because there are no private suppliers. Furthermore, government reimbursement is only possible in the public sector [32].

The role of international organisations and NGOs in the health system and policy process is small. Functions such as educational campaigns, free testing and treatment of AIDS/HIV are in many countries taken up by NGOs, but in Uzbekistan, the government has taken responsibility for this [2, 28]. Research has shown that many Central-Asian governments perceive NGOs to be politicising health care. Uzbekistan's government

Formal actors in the health system		
National level	President	• Develop a broad strategy for national health reform policies
	Cabinet of ministers	• Collaborate with the Ministry on developing detailed policies, implementation monitoring, evaluation and health information management • Supervise the activities of all government bodies concerned with health care
	Supreme Assembly/ Parliament	• Adopt legislation on health care • Approve national budget for health care and control its execution • Debate health care laws
	Ministry of Finance	• Formulates the budget and allocate funds to the MoH • Collaborate with the Ministry of health on developing detailed policies, implementation monitoring, evaluation and health information management
	Ministry of Health	• Develop, implement, monitor and evaluate detailed policies • Health information management • Determine standards for quality and prices of care • Manage research institutes and medical schools • Manage national health care institutions • Manage emergency centres • Issue licences for health care institutions and professionals • Coordinate international aid for the health sector
Regional level (viloyat)	Viloyat health authorities	• Collect government revenue (of which they keep a proportion) • Establish a work plan to implement national health policies • Manage and finance regional hospitals and health care • Directly provide sanitary-epidemiological services • Provide ambulance services, • Provide rehabilitation services for people with disabilities
District/ local level (city and tuman)	Tuman and local health authorities	• Manage local hospitals • Implement and ensure compliance with national guidelines • Ensure access to primary care • Control the quality of medical care through compliance with medical protocols • Provide pharmaceuticals • Create an environment that facilitates the development of the private sector

Table 1.
Tasks of formal actors in the health systems decision making.

has been pushing out most international donors and their projects since the mid-2000s. This is likely because they see non-state actors as a threat to state legitimacy [33, 34].

Local NGOs have been slowly growing and they have been trying to organise themselves better. Between 1999 and 2004, international donors have been helping to create a more autonomous NGO community with financial and technical support.

Nevertheless, the government keeps hindering their full development. To avoid governmental resistance, the term "social organisations", instead of non-governmental organisations, is sometimes used. This term sounds less as if the organisation is against the government [33, 34].

Uzbekistan receives disproportionally low amounts of aid money considering the disease burden. This is caused by bureaucratic governance and the lack of government-led aid coordination mechanisms. On top of that, aid actors are concerned with the "neglect of human rights issues, as well as cases of corruption" [29, 35]. Despite this resistance, President Mirziyogyev is slightly more willing to participate in international cooperation to improve his country's policies, as became appearant after his policy dialogue with the WHO [36]. Health reforms have targeted various areas of the health care system. Most recently, reforms have focused on improving primary care, reducing non-communicable diseases and improving project management and evaluation.

Furthermore, in 2019, the WHO has had policy dialogues with Uzbekistan to discuss the best practices for health financing reforms and effective policy instruments. Evidence-informed choices are in this way stimulated. Other topics discussed in this dialogue were establishing a single national pooling system for health financing, improving quality of health care, increasing equity and efficiency in resource allocation and designing a state-guaranteed benefit package with more clearly stated entitlements for recipients and obligations for care providers. These changes are aimed at achieving higher financial protection [36].

Finally, reforms have recently been made in the transparency of the policy process. The Parliament's visibility has been increasing, more fragments of their session are accessible, and the media covers the Parliament's work more often. Policy reforms suggested by the WHO are considered.

3. Methods

This study has a mixed-methods case study approach. This means that a single case (Uzbekistan) is studied, and both qualitative and quantitative methods are used to collect comprehensive data on the case. The mixed-methods case study approach can be used to find answers to a specific question about the case. It is commonly used to answer questions about the effectiveness and feasibility of a particular treatment, intervention or program [37–39]. The research aims to examine the governance system and policy process and examine these systems' effectiveness and functioning. Thus, a mixed-methods case study approach is a good fit. This approach is beneficial when it is impossible to obtain a sizeable homogenous sample of cases in similar conditions. This type of research is mostly exclusively relevant for the studied case and thus has intrinsic value for that case. Generalizability does not have priority [38, 39]. This applies in Uzbekistan's case study: it is not relevant whether this case is generalizable because every country has unique circumstances. Thus, this research mostly has intrinsic value for Uzbekistan and its policymakers.

The qualitative component is a comprehensive literature review. We searched MEDLINE, Econlit, CINAHL, Scopus, and Embase (from inception to June 2021), and grey literature sources using keywords relating to health policy, health finance, and Uzbekistan. In addition, the snowball sampling method was used [40]. This is a repeated process to identify relevant articles in the reference list of other relevant articles. A total of 27 references were used in the literature review. The inclusion and exclusion criteria that were used in selecting the references are shown in **Table 2**.

Inclusion criteria	Exclusion criteria
Articles about (health) governance	Articles about mental health
Articles about health financing schemes	Articles about specific treatments on the vertical level***
Articles about health insurance	Articles about hygiene status and water
Articles on epidemiological status	Articles on specific disease correlations
Articles on health status	Articles about the relationship between climate and health status
Articles on the relationship between national government and international agencies	Articles about sexual health status and health of sex workers
Articles about drug use and prescription practices*	Articles about nutritional status
Articles about differences between rural and urban**	Articles about environment health
Articles about unhealthy behaviours	
Articles about gender differences	
Articles about vaccination	

Table 2.
Inclusion and exclusion criteria literature review.

The quantitative part involves a linear regression analysis of cross-sectional secondary household survey data. The study was carried out using open data kit (ODK) in two districts- Olmalik and Kibray of the Tashkent province in Uzbekista. The lack of public statistics on the demographic, socio-economic, and health status of the population in the country made it challenging to stratify and randomise the sampling for the household survey. A simple random spatial sampling has been adopted to carry out a survey between July and October 2015. Further details of the study sampling strategy and survey data can be found in the Subramanian et al. (2018) study [41]. The study covered of 207 households in Olmalik and 200 in Kibray. Based on the survey responses, a linear regression analysis of each variable is performed. The software used to perform the statistical analysis is RStudio. Variables are considered significant when the p-value is lower than 0.05. Variables are considered significant if the p-value is lower than 0.05. After that, a model is proposed that includes all relevant variables and minimises the sum of squared errors. The objective is to predict the household OOPs based on a household's characteristics.

The variables in this expected model are based on what other studies into OOP have found to be significant. The response variable, health care expenditure in the last six months, is measured in Uzbekistan Sum, the local currency. Based on the exchange rate in 2015 and the average salary of an employed Uzbek citizen, the average proportion of household income spent on OOP is calculated.

Variables are considered significant if the p-value is lower than 0.05. To detect multicollinearity, a VIF test will be performed. Variables with a VIF between 5 and 10 are removed, as this is considered harmful.

The two methods provide comprehensive data on the constraints in the Uzbek health financing system and policy process. While the qualitative part provides a broader system overview, the quantitative part includes knowledge of what factors cause OOP on the household level and provides empirical evidence.

4. Results

4.1 Basic benefit package

Uzbekistan spends a relatively low proportion of gross domestic product (GDP) on health. In 2018, health expenditure, as a percentage of GDP, was 5.3% [42, 43]. This proportion has been increasing over the past decade, though it remains small. For comparison, countries in the European Union spent on average 9.9% of their GDP on health care. Almost half of Uzbekistan's total health care expenditure comes from private sources, such as OOP [15–17].

Funds for health financing are mostly raised at the sub-national level, mainly through taxes. In 2005, Uzbekistan received 87.7% of the government health expenditures from local taxes. Since there is variation in how much revenue sub-national units can raise, there is much geographical inequality. Moreover, the proportion of GDP spent on health care is higher in the richer than in the poorer areas. There is no national pooling system of health financing resources yet, although the WHO has organised policy dialogues with Uzbekistan to change that [2, 28, 32].

From the collected revenues, the government provides a basic benefits package. All citizens are covered. However, the range of benefits differs per group. For everyone, the package includes primary care, emergency care and care for socially significant and hazardous conditions. Uzbek's primary care includes initiatives in family, maternal and child health and preventive and sanitary-epidemiological activities [9, 28, 44]. The socially significant and hazardous conditions include specific respiratory, skin, intestinal, blood-borne infections (poliomyelitis, TB, leprosy, HIV/AIDS, syphilis), cancer and mental health. Pharmaceuticals for inpatient care are also included, but pharmaceuticals for outpatient care are not. In principle, primary health care is free and universal. Nevertheless, some tests have costs and some pharmaceuticals need to be paid out of pocket [1, 44, 45].

For certain people, the basic benefit package also includes outpatient pharmaceuticals and specialised care (secondary and tertiary). People with specific diseases, such as HIV/AIDS, or people belonging to particular groups, for example, war veterans, are included in the extra benefit. **Table 3** shows everyone with the right to extra benefit. Some uncertainty exists about the extent of the extra benefit. Moreover, reimbursed care cannot be higher than 20% of the institution's total budget [1, 45].

Vulnerable group eligible for extra benefit	
Disease groups	**Population groups**
Cancer	Single pensioners registered at the social services
Endocrinological and mental conditions	Participants of the 'labour front' in 1941–1945
Tuberculosis	People with incurred disabilities in WO II
Leprosy	People with disabilities as the results of the Chernobyl accident
HIV/AIDS	War veterans
Post-operated states related to cardiac interventions and transplantations	Retired military personnel who served in posts related to nuclear technology

Table 3.
Disease and population groups that receive extra benefit.

For example, for cardiac care, the treatment's expensiveness can form an access barrier as cardiac patients constrain their daily consumption because of high medical expenses [46].

To finance primary care, there is an increasing use of capitation-based payments for. They are paid for the covered population, adjusted for age and gender as a lump sum per year [45, 47]. Capitation rates are calculated at the viloyat level. This helps to spread the risk evenly and reduce income inequality [48]. The rates are set annually and are dependent on the size of the viloyat health budget. No protocol dictates a particular share of primary care of the total budget [49–51]. Another way in which the state covers health care services is through user fees, amounts of money that are paid by the government to the providers after they have performed a specific health service. Those are mostly used in secondary and tertiary care institutions [51, 52].

4.2 Financing outside the basic benefit package

For the largest part of the population, secondary and tertiary care, as well as outpatient pharmaceuticals, are not covered. Services that fall outside of the basic benefit package are expected to be paid for through other means, such as private health insurance, employer contributions, union funds and OOP [1, 3, 53]. In 2018, 60.3% of all health care expenses in the country were OOP, and this proportion has been increasing in the past years. Voluntary health insurance does not play a significant role. Nevertheless, it became more visible in recent years. Still, in 2012, it only accounted for 2.6% of total health ependiure [14, 16].

The government has been encouraging formal self-financing rather than the state budget. The price-setting process is regulated with price caps. The proportion of revenue coming from formally paid services has been gradually increasing in the past years [1, 54, 55]. Nevertheless, informal payments still occur, mostly in secondary and tertiary care [13, 56]. Despite self-financing options, physicians commonly accept informal payments to supplement their low income and keep care affordable to their patients. It is unclear if self-financing reforms have successfully [13, 56]. In 2007, a study showed that 42% of the respondents reported using informal expenditures [3]. Particularly the poor make informal payments: "patients from less affluent households are more likely to have to pay informal under-the-counter payments in health care settings" [57–59].

Informal payments are harmful because it is very hard to monitor the quality of care and manage data and information on informal services. Moreover, informal fees can become based on willingness to pay rather than on the service's quality. Furthermore, if informal payments make up a large part of the health care, it will formally seem like not many people need health care. This will result in lower investments in medical equipment or health care infrastructure [13, 24].

4.3 Consequences of OOP

The basic benefit package only covers part of health care results in OOP, which leads to high inequalities and catastrophic expenditures for households. The extra benefits for specific groups are a good initiative, but including those groups is not based on income necessarily [2, 28]. The burden remains particularly high for poor people because an OOP service takes up a larger proportion of the household income for poor households than for more affluent families [2, 28]. Fear of high OOP leads to various suboptimal behaviours related to health.

To begin with, financial constraints may cause delayed diagnosis [60]. If people cannot access health care when they need it, their health complaints may develop into larger problems that are harder and more expensive to treat. The costs may be much higher than they would have been if health care was accessed immediately.

So, fear of OOP leads to late diagnosis and also to starting the treatment later [60]. A study on the drugs for tuberculosis found that of the 146 patients that were interviewed, 79% experienced financial problems to get the diagnosis and treatment for tuberculosis. Some patients mentioned having to sell livestock and crops to pay for the treatment, and one patient felt forced to sell his house to cope with the financial burden [55, 61–63].

The treatment is sometimes started with cheaper services and medication, reducing its efficiency. Mostly routine outpatient medicines can be a drain on the patient and their family's resources [44]. Financial concerns thus lead to selecting low-quality drugs, and the treatments are even cut short [60]. Short treatments could mean that health complaints will return and care needs to be purchased again and this is possibly harmful to the patient's health long-term. Some physicians, when aware of the financial status of the patient, prescribe expensive medication, but also provide a cheaper (less effective) medication or they limit the number of drugs prescribed [55, 61–63].

The transition to increasing use of self-financing schemes will likely enlarge the problems of accessing services for poorer households. It encourages inappropriate use of health services, leading to a waste of resources [1, 2]. This improper use is an attempt at avoiding costs by trying to receive health care through services that are covered by the state, even if those services are not the most efficient way of obtaining the required care. For example, the fact that emergency services are free of charge leads to overuse of those services, while specialised centres would be more efficient in addressing the health complaints. Apart from efficiency loss, this inappropriate use limits access for those who really need emergency care [64, 65]. Additionally, using health services that are not adequate for the patient's condition may lead to the worsening of the condition, leading to higher OOP long-term.

Furthermore, patients will try to stay in the hospital, even if outpatient care would be more suitable. The inpatient pharmaceuticals are for free, while outpatient medications are paid out of pocket. There is a lack of financial support to promote outpatient care, even for diseases that are supposed to receive extra benefit [66]. This suggests, again, that patients are not correctly informed about their rights to coverage or that the regulations around coverage for the people who have a right to the extra benefit (see **Table 4**) are flawed.

The problem of inappropriate health care use of inpatient or ambulatory services is worsened because there is no clear pathway for patients, and the referral processes at each level of care are poorly regulated. Patients can refer themselves to secondary or tertiary care easily. There is a weak link between primary and specialised care, and GPs do not have the financial incentive to take a gatekeeper role [17]. With self-financing, the connection between primary care and inpatient care has grown weaker because accessing specialised care became more expensive through the health care institution's fees. In the private industry there is even less regulation of referrals. Not being referred to the proper type of care can again lead to higher OOP, since unnecessary care might be accessed or care needs to be accessed again in a different level of care [5, 17, 47].

		Olmalik (n = 207)	Kibray (n = 200)
Variable definition	**Categories**	**Average mean or % distribution**	**Average mean or % distribution**
	Socio-economic		
Household head gender	0 = female	19.3	30.5
	1 = male	80.7	69.5
Household members (size)	Average Mean	3.35 ± 1.6	5.04 ± 2.0
Household head education	1 = Primary education	6.1	7.8
	2 = Secondary vocational education	61.0	52.0
	3 = University	12.2	17.2
	4 = others (including graduate)	11.7	9.6
	5 = unknown	9.0	13.4
Households perceiving themselves as 'middle and above' income category (%)	0 = 'below middle'	6.3	7.0
	1 = 'middle or above'	93.7	93.0
No of Households having children under 10 years	0 = no	63.8	42.5
	1 = yes	36.2	57.5
Health related			
Chronic illness	0 = no	35.7	43.5
	1 = yes	65.3	56.5
Alcohol use	0 = no	61.3	45.0
	1 = yes	38.7	55.0
Money saved in the past to afford healthcare	0 = no	72.6	70.5
	1 = yes	27.4	29.5
Health status of the household head	0 = bad	5.8	6.5
	1 = fair	22.7	25.5
	2 = good	71.0	68.0

Table 4.
Description of household characteristics using categorical variables.

4.4 Caveats in health policy agenda setting

On the policymaking level, a lack of civilian participation, unavailability of data, low analytical skills, poor communication at the implementation phase and inadequate evaluation procedures are underlying causes for the persistence of policies that are inefficient at lowering OOP.

Civilian participation is limited, as issues that are most important to citizens, such as high OOP, may remain unprioritized. Uzbek citizens do not play an active role in the health policy process as there is no specific frameworks are in place to ensure public participation in the planning, purchasing and organisation of health services [1, 67, 68]. The role of civil society organisations is limited due to Uzbekistan's selective policies towards NGOs [33, 34, 69]. Finally, access to health information is generally only available to government agencies and not to the public. This limited transparency makes it even harder for citizens to know which issues are most important to them. One of the main shortcomings is that citizens are uninformed about their rights: policies about coverage have been made, but patients do not always know what services they can access free of charge. Moreover, there is too little information on what services are high-quality. This may inhibit the implementation of modern health policies further. Weak communication in the implementation stage means that even if a policy is in theory adequate in addressing OOP, it will be inefficient in practice.

The data information system is fragmented: public health facilities must collect data, but all data collection systems work independently from other collection systems (e.g., the national programs' data is not connected to the sanitary and epidemiological data system) [9]. The WHO reports that in various provinces, patients' needs were not monitored frequently enough [2, 32]. The data collection system is primarily focused on structural data, and there is little effort to collect process-related and qualitative data. It is not clear if any data is pooled at the different levels of data collection. Furthermore, the MoH provides data reports and shares these with the viloyat authorities for decision and policymaking. Meanwhile, there is very little attention to the local and tuman levels. Information on income, education and ethnicity are not part of the policy process. Data collection is only done in the public system [9, 28, 32]. Finally, the available data is not as useful due to weakness in policy makers' capacity to utilise such data. The inadequate evaluation tools lead to the wrong conclusion on whether a policy should be maintained, succeeded or terminated.

4.5 Challenges of health financing at the household level: Olmalik and Kibray

Olmalik is an old industrial township, and many households were small families or comprised of young migrant workers. On average, about three members (3.35) live in a household in this district compared to five members in Kibray (5.04). The socio-demographic characteristics are presented in **Table 4**. First, the majority of the households are male-headed in Olmalik (80.7) and Kibray (69.5). More than half (61.0% in Olmalik and 52.0% in Kibray) of the heads of household head have been educated up to secondary level and 13% do not have formal education. This shows the high level of literacy in the district as well as the educational requirement of the government. In Olmalik, most of the households (63.8) reported having no children in their homes, implying a worker population. Most of the households viewed themselves as being in the middle or above in terms of their income category (93.7% in Olmalik, 93% in Kibray).

The significant variables are 'number of household members with chronic illness', 'use of alcohol', 'saved money in the past', 'town of residence' and 'perceived health status household head'. The survey showed that none of the participants have health insurance. VIF statistics of the variables of the number of chronic disease, alcohol use, town of residence, money saved and perceived health status household head all turned out to have a value between 1 and 5 (average 1.054), which indicates a moderate correlation between the predictor variables, but not severe enough to require attention. Thus, the variables in the model do not create collinearity with the regression model. Finally, it was found that heteroskedasticity does not exist in the regression model above.

The adjusted R-squared of this model is 0.1099, with a p-value of 5.79e-10. This means that the model shows a significant correlation and the variables in the model explain about 11% of the variation in health care expenditures.

The variable 'perceived health household head' was significant. If the perceived health was 'good' the average OOP was 386,135 UZS, while if the health was considered fair, the average OOP was 655,000 UZS.

The mean amount of money spent by each household as out of pocket expenditures in the last six months is 418.373 UZS. Given the exchange rate, this would be 148,89 USD. Although there were far higher amounts reported too: 45 participants spent over a million (355,87 USD) in the last six months and the highest amount was 10 million (355,74 USD). For comparison, the GDP per capita in 2015 is 2.615,03. An Uzbek with a job earns 1307.52 USD in six months. In the sample population, 1.86 household members have a paid job. This means in 6 months there is an income of on average 2431,99 USD, with the average OOP, (355,87/2431,99*100=) 14% of the household income is spent on health care expenditures.

The finding that chronic illness is a strong predictor for high out of pocket expenditures is in accordance with other studies that have looked at OOP predictors. For example, a study in Bangladesh also found that chronic diseases are a strong predictor of high household health expenditures [70, 71].

Alcohol use could be the cause of specific disease and thus create out of pocket expenditures. However, drinking alcohol could also be a coping mechanism of dealing with the financial instability of out-of-pocket payments. The association between alcohol use and health care expenditure is not conclusive since it is impossible to determine the direction of the association. Only a longitudinal study could determine the relationship, while this was a cross-sectional study [72, 73].

Infectious diseases or diarrhoea individually did not show a significant correlation with OOP. This is likely because various infectious diseases fall within the extra benefit package (e.g. HIV or leprosy). Moreover, most care for infectious disease and diarrhoea often falls under primary care, while many chronic conditions require specialised care, which is not covered by the state [44].

Saved money in the past likely showed significance for the simple reason that people with more money saved have more money available to spend on health care, while people with less money saved have less money available to spend on health care. The reason that perceived health status household had was significant is also straightforward: household heads with a health status that is considered 'good' need less health care than household heads with a health status that is only perceived to be 'fair'.

It is unclear how the significance of the town of residence is caused. One hypothesis is that Olmalik has very different living conditions. Olmalik is much more industrial, which causes various health complaints, especially related to low air quality. However, it would be expected that the industrial environment has more health hazard, but the OOP is lower in Olmalik. As shown in **Table 5**, there are higher infectious and chronic disease rates in Kibray, but it is unclear how this is caused. Future research would be needed to be conclusive about the correlation. Survey participants expressed concerns with access to health care as well as quality of care as low quality can lead to high OOP.

	OOP (in SOEMS)	Chronic diseases sum household members	Infectious diseases sum household members	Household members with diarrhoea
Olmalik	303,449.3	1.81	0.78	0.45
Kibray	537,320	2.20	0.97	0.24

Table 5.
Difference in disease occurrence between Olmalik and Kibray.

4.6 Current progress on OOP reduction policy and universal health coverage

As of 2018, the Uzbekistan government declared to implement a mandatory health insurance (MHI) to move towards universal health coverage. The Presidential Decree No. 5590 was approved in December 2018 under the name of "About complex measures for radical enhancement of health care system of the Republic of Uzbekistan", to introduce mandatory health insurance (MHI) for population coverage of essential health services and pharmaceuticals [74]. The decree states that the state will lay out mechanisms and stages of implementation for compulsory medical insurance. It also plans to determine the subjects of compulsory medical insurance as well as authorised entity on regulation for its legal scope, rights, and obligations. It also states the state will sought out sources of financing for programs of compulsory medical insurance. The Ministry of Foreign Affairs of the Republic of Uzbekistan planned to take measures for the organisation of interaction with the World Health Organisation and the international financial institutions for ensuring technical assistance in case of implementation of this Decree, including carrying out the feasibility statement on actions for implementation of compulsory medical insurance [74].

Departing from the existing health financing structure, as implementation of this new strategy was the introduction of a new single-payer state health insurance organisation: the State Health Insurance Fund. Amid the COVID-19 pandemic, in November 2020, Presidential Decree No. 4890 was approved to formally established the State Health Insurance Fund as a national purchasing agency to be financed through the central government budget to purchase health services defined in a new state-guaranteed benefits package, which will be available to the whole population [75]. Starting from June 1, 2021, in the Syrdarya region of Uzbekistan, a pilot project was launched to introduce a new model of healthcare delivery. Furthermore, the feasibility study by WHO (2021) recommended general taxation as the most effective way to pool funds and risks, to redistribute resources in an equitable manner and to support progress towards universal health coverage [76, 77].

Based on this recommendation, the State Medical Insurance Fund mainly receive funds from the state budget for basic compulsory medical insurance along with targeted deductions from excise taxes on tobacco products, alcohol, high sugar foods, trans fats and other products that are harmful to health (introducing the so called "sin taxes" as the first nation in Central Asia) as well as voluntary contributions and grants from international organisations. From 2023, state health insurance is planned to be introduced in Karakalpakstan, Tashkent, Samarkand, Navoi, Surkhandarya and Fergana regions, and from 2025 – throughout the entire Uzbekistan [78].

5. Conclusion

The basic benefit package only covers primary care, emergency care and inpatient pharmaceuticals. Extra care is provided for some, but this selection is not necessarily based on income. The specialised care and outpatient pharmaceuticals need to be financed in other ways. Since there is almost no public or private health insurance, most care that is not in the basic benefit package needs to be paid out of pocket. The regression model suggests that having a chronic illness is an important factor in high OOP.

Additional aspects of the health financing system that lead to high OOP are a lack of qualitative, patient-centred evaluation methods. What is more, there is no publicly available information on quality, prices or types of health services. This large information asymmetry makes it easy for physicians to provide low-quality or unnecessary services. Moreover, the patient's referral pathways are poorly regulated. Attempts to avoid OOP lead to delay in diagnosis and delay in treatment. Furthermore, some patients seek informal care, where quality is even less regulated. These behaviours lead to higher OOP long-term.

The policy process is constrained by the limited civilian participation, which is partly due to socio-political factors such as resistance towards NGOs and the limited transparency of the policy process. In the implementation of policies, clear communication is lacking. Finally, the lack of qualitative data and analytical skills negatively impact almost all phases of the policy process. Uzbekistan is dealing with a capacity problem in data collection and analysis. Evaluation and information management is also important for improving the policy cycle. If more data is available and policymakers are additionally trained in analytical skills, evidence-based policymaking will become easier. Policymaking can be further improved by increasing civilian participation, for example, through civil society organisations. For meaningful civilian participation, more transparency about the policymaking is also needed.

Based on the findings, recommendations on improving the health (financing) system and policy process can be made. These are broad recommendations that need more research before they can be used in policies. In short, improving monitoring and evaluation procedures can help reduce the information asymmetry between the providers and citizens and between the providers and policymakers. Information on price, type and quality of services should be provided to patients. Additionally, patients should be made aware of their rights in terms of coverage. Finally, the benefit package should be expanded. This research suggests that expansion should include chronically ill. Uzbekistan has rolled out its pilot state funded compulsory health insurance for the first time in the nation [79, 80]. Based on the pilot project, it aims to design a benefits package of free medical services and medicines guaranteed by the state as well as to strengthen disease prevention, organising regular screening examinations of various categories of citizens [78]. Hence, prioritising health insurance coverage for the vulnerable as well as earmarking a coverage for chronic illness may be necessary.

Additionally, it would be relevant to understand what specific services were purchased with OOP by households. This could give insight into whether or not the guaranteed basic benefit package is serving the population's needs and what services outside of the package form the biggest drain on households. Finally, the examined variables in this research only explained 11% of the variation in OOP. Thus, future research should examine additional variables.

6. Limitations

Most of the secondary data was not very recent and thus up-to-date information on the health system's financing status and policy process is lacking. The WHO and news articles provide more current information on certain issues such as ongoing reforms, but there is a lack of recent academic literature. Furthermore, while a combination of primary and secondary qualitative data would have been ideal, the time and COVID-19 pandemic-related constraints only made secondary data accessible.

The method of snowballing literature has a risk of neglecting relevant articles due to the exclusion of articles that are not relevant but form a useful connection to other papers [40]. Additionally, the inclusion and exclusion criteria, as well as terminologies used in health financing systems and health policy, overlap with other terminologies which may lead to different literature search results. Only English articles were included, meaning that Russian or Uzbek articles were not used, even if they would have contained a relevant approach or relevant information.

There is a limitation in the quantitative data collection because all participants came from the same region in Uzbekistan. While there were no other options due to resource constraints, it forms a limitation in nation-wide generalizability. Thus, if specific factors are found to be relevant, additional research is needed before recommendations to change nation-wide policy can be made. Nevertheless, the research can provide a broad view based on which detailed research can be recommended.

In this research, the range of aspects explored in the qualitative part may be broader than the range of aspects examined in the quantitative part. However, it should be noted that each part provides different types of information that complement each other. While the qualitative component may be able to point out broader aspects on a large-scale, the quantitative data can point out factors leading to high OOP that are experienced on the household-level.

Acknowledgements

The authors are grateful to Dr. Saravanan Veluswami Subramanian for his support in concluding this research work.

Conflict of interest

The authors declare no conflict of interest.

Author details

Min Jung Cho* and Eva Haverkort
Faculty of Global Governance and Affairs, Global Public Health, Leiden University College, Hague, Netherlands

*Address all correspondence to: m.j.cho@luc.leidenuniv.nl

References

[1] Ahmedov M, Azimov R, Mutalova Z, Huseynov S, Tsoyi E, Rechel B. Uzbekistan: Health system review. Uzbekistan Health system review [Internet]. 2014;**16**(5):43. [cited 2022 Dec 12]. Available from: https://apps.who.int/iris/handle/10665/151960

[2] Rechel B, Ahmedov M, Akkazieva B, Katsaga A, Khodjamurodov G, McKee M. Lessons from two decades of health reform in Central Asia. Health Policy Plan [Internet]. 2012;**27**(4):281-287. [cited 2022 Dec 12]. Available from: https://academic.oup.com/heapol/article/27/4/281/604711

[3] Kulzhanov M, Rechel B. Uzbekistan: Health System Review. 2007;**9**(7). [cited 2022 Dec 12]. Available from: https://apps.who.int/iris/handle/10665/107847

[4] World Health Organization. Health Care Systems in Transition: Uzbekistan. 2001 [cited 2022 Dec 12]. Available from: https://apps.who.int/iris/handle/10665/108417

[5] Ahmedov M, Ravshan A, Zulkhumor M, Shahin H, Elena T, Asmus H, et al. Challenges to universal coverage in Uzbekistan. Eurohealth (Lond). 2015;**21**(2):17-19 [Internet] [cited 2022 Dec 12]. Available from: https://apps.who.int/iris/bitstream/handle/10665/332790/Eurohealth-21-2-17-19-eng.pdf

[6] The World Bank in Uzbekistan: Development news, research, data | World Bank [Internet]. [cited 2022 Dec 12]. Available from: https://www.worldbank.org/en/country/uzbekistan

[7] Statistical Capacity Indicators | DataBank [Internet]. [cited 2022 Dec 14]. Available from: https://databank.worldbank.org/source/statistical-capacity-indicators

[8] Uzbekistan's National Statistical System to Modernize with World Bank Support [Internet]. [cited 2022 Dec 14]. Available from: https://www.worldbank.org/en/news/press-release/2022/02/16/uzbekistan-s-national-statistical-system-to-modernize-with-world-bank-support

[9] Ahmedov M, de Haan S, Sarymsakova B. Strengthening Health Research Systems in Central Asia: A System Mapping and Consultative Process. Working paper 2. Geneva: Council on Health Research for Development; 2007. [Internet] [cited 2020 Jan 12]. Available from: http://www.cohred.org/downloads/cohred_publications/wp2_CentralAsia.pdf

[10] Life Expectancy at Birth, Total (years) - Europe & Central Asia | Data [Internet]. [cited 2022 Dec 12]. Available from: https://data.worldbank.org/indicator/SP.DYN.LE00.IN?locations=Z7

[11] Mortality Rate, under-5 (per 1,000 live births) - Europe & Central Asia | Data [Internet]. [cited 2022 Dec 12]. Available from: https://data.worldbank.org/indicator/SH.DYN.MORT?locations=Z7

[12] Mortality Rate, under-5 (per 1,000 live births) - Uzbekistan | Data [Internet]. [cited 2022 Dec 12]. Available from: https://data.worldbank.org/indicator/SH.DYN.MORT?locations=UZ

[13] Belli P, Gotsadze G, Shahriari H. Out-of-pocket and informal payments in health sector: Evidence from Georgia. Health Policy (New York). 2004;**70**(1):109-123 [Internet] [cited 2022 Dec 12]. Available from: https://pubmed.ncbi.nlm.nih.gov/15312713/

[14] Out-of-Pocket Expenditure (% of Current Health Expenditure) - Uzbekistan, Kazakhstan, Kyrgyz Republic, Tajikistan, Turkmenistan | Data [Internet]. [cited 2022 Dec 12]. Available from: https://data.worldbank.org/indicator/SH.XPD.OOPC.CH.ZS?end=2018&locations=UZ-KZ-KG-TJ-TM&start=2000&view=chart

[15] Out-of-Pocket Expenditure (% of Current Health Expenditure) - Uzbekistan, Low & Middle Income | Data [Internet]. [cited 2022 Dec 12]. Available from: https://data.worldbank.org/indicator/SH.XPD.OOPC.CH.ZS?end=2018&locations=UZ-XO&start=2000&view=chart

[16] Out-of-Pocket Expenditure (% of current health expenditure) - Uzbekistan | Data [Internet]. [cited 2022 Dec 12]. Available from: https://data.worldbank.org/indicator/SH.XPD.OOPC.CH.ZS?locations=UZ

[17] Health Systems in Action: Uzbekistan [Internet]. 2021 [cited 2022 Dec 14]. Available from: https://eurohealthobservatory.who.int/publications/i/health-systems-in-action-uzbekistan

[18] Jeon WC, Kim HJ, Park J, Kim KH, Shin DW, Park JM, et al. The importance of preliminary evaluation in developing ambulance staff training curriculum for developing countries: A survey in Uzbekistan. Ulusal Travma ve Acil Cerrahi Dergisi. 2020;**26**(1):9-14 [Internet] [cited 2022 Dec 12]. Available from: https://europepmc.org/article/MED/31942745

[19] World Health Organization. Uzbekistan [Internet]. [cited 2022 Dec 12]. Available from: https://www.who.int/countries/uzb/

[20] Asadov DA, Aripov TY. The quality of care in post-soviet Uzbekistan: Are health reforms and international efforts succeeding? Public Health. 2009;**123**(11):725-728 [Internet] [cited 2022 Dec 12]. Available from: https://pubmed.ncbi.nlm.nih.gov/19889431/

[21] Chang AY, Cowling K, Micah AE, Chapin A, Chen CS, Ikilezi G, et al. Past, present, and future of global health financing: A review of development assistance, government, out-of-pocket, and other private spending on health for 195 countries, 1995-2050. The Lancet. 2019;**393**(10187):2233-2260

[22] Nessipbayeva O, Dalayeva T. Developmental perspectives of higher education in the post-soviet countries (for the cases of Kazakhstan, Uzbekistan, Kyrgyzstan, Tajikistan and Turkmenistan). Procedia - Social and Behavioral Sciences. 2013;**89**:391-396 [Internet] [cited 2015 Apr 6]. Available from: http://www.sciencedirect.com/science/article/pii/S1877042813029960

[23] van Assche K, Shtaltovna A, Hornidge AK. Visible and invisible informalities and institutional transformation in the transition countries of Georgia, Romania, and Uzbekistan. Informality in Eastern Europe: Structures, Political Cultures and Social Practices, Peter Lang, Bern. 2013;**11**:89-118

[24] Baumann E. Post-soviet Georgia: It's a long, long way to 'modern'social protection.... Economies et Sociétés Série Développement. Croissance et Progrès. 2012;**46**:259-285 [Internet] [cited 2015 Aug 27]. Available from: http://georgica.tsu.edu.ge/files/02-Economy/Development/Baumann-2002.pdf

[25] Balabanova D, Roberts B, Richardson E, Haerpfer C, McKee M. Health care reform in the former Soviet Union: Beyond the transition. Health Services Research. 2012;**47**(2):840-864. [Internet]

[cited 2016 Jan 2]. Available from. DOI: 10.1111/j.1475-6773.2011.01323.x

[26] Gel'Man V. Post-soviet transitions and democratization: Towards theory-building. Democratization. 2003;**10**(2):87-104

[27] Ider BE, Adams J, Morton A, Whitby M, Clements A. Infection control systems in transition: The challenges for post-soviet bloc countries. Journal of Hospital Infection. 2012;**80**(4):277-287 [Internet] [cited 2015 Aug 27]. Available from: http://linkinghub.elsevier.com/retrieve/pii/S0195670112000485

[28] Mohir Ahmedov. Health Systems in Transition Uzbekistan: Health System Review. 2014 [cited 2015 Feb 23]. Available from: http://www.euro.who.int/__data/assets/pdf_file/0019/270370/Uzbekistan-HiT-web.pdf?ua=1

[29] Ulikpan A, Mirzoev T, Jimenez E, Malik A, Hill PS. Central Asian post-soviet health systems in transition: Has different aid engagement produced different outcomes? Global Health Action. 2014;**7**(1):24978 [Internet] [cited 2015 Jan 6]. Available from: http://www.ncbi.nlm.nih.gov/pubmed/25231098

[30] Aminova M, Jegers M. Informal structures and governance processes in transition economies: The case of Uzbekistan. International Journal of Public Administration. 2011;**34**(9):579-590. [Internet] [cited 2015 Feb 21]. Available from:. DOI: 10.1080/01900692.2011.588436

[31] Ilkhamov FA, Jakubowski E. Healthcare System in Transition. 2001 [cited 2015 Jan 6]. Available from: http://www.euro.who.int/__data/assets/pdf_file/0006/96423/E73067.pdf

[32] Ahmedov M, Kennedy A, IJsselmuiden C. Governance and policy frameworks for health research in 38 countries. In: Forum on Higher Education, Research and Knowledge: Global research seminar: sharing research agendas on knowledge systems. Paris: United Nations Educational, Scientific and Cultural Organization; 2008. [cited 2015 Feb 23]. Available from: http://portal.unesco.org/education/es/files/58048/12246671755Ahmedov.pdf/Ahmedov.pdf

[33] Johnson E. Non-state health care provision in Kazakhstan and Uzbekistan: Is politicisation a model? Europe-Asia Studies. 2014;**66**(5):735-758 [Internet]. [cited 2022 Dec 12]. Available from: https://www.tandfonline.com/doi/abs/10.1080/09668136.2014.906935

[34] Johnson E. State-NGO Relations in Health Care in Central Asia. 2008 [cited 2015 Apr 6]. Available from: http://kms2.isn.ethz.ch/serviceengine/Files/RESSpecNet/91697/ipublicationdocument_singledocument/697A7FF3-5E61-4A16-A716-50F8D52527D3/en/Report_Erica_eng.pdf

[35] Arazmuradov A. Can development aid help promote foreign direct investment? Evidence from Central Asia. Economic Affairs. 2015;**35**(1):123-136 [Internet]. [cited 2015 Dec 26]. Available from: http://doi.wiley.com/10.1111/ecaf.12102

[36] World Health Organization. Policy Dialogue to Support Development of Health Financing Strategy in Uzbekistan [Internet]. 2019 [cited 2022 Dec 12]. Available from: https://www.who.int/europe/news/item/30-04-2019-policy-dialogue-to-support-development-of-health-financing-strategy-in-uzbekistan

[37] Creswell J, Plano Clark V, Gutmann M, Hanson W. Advanced mixed methods research designs. Handbook of Mixed Methods in

Social and Behavioural Research. 2003:1(240):209-240

[38] Creswell JW, Clark VLP. Designing and conducting mixed methods research. Thousand Oaks Sage; 2007

[39] Onghena P, Maes B, Heyvaert M. Mixed methods single case research: State of the art and future directions. Journal of Mixed Methods Research. 2019;**13**(4):461-480

[40] Wohlin C. Guidelines for snowballing in systematic literature studies and a replication in software engineering. Proceedings of the 18th International Conference on Evaluation and Assessment in Software Engineering. [Internet]. Vol. 1. 2014. pp. 1-10. [cited 2022 Dec 14]. Available from: https://dl.acm.org/doi/10.1145/2601248.2601268

[41] Subramanian SV, Cho MJ, Mukhitdinova F. Health risk in urbanizing regions: Examining the nexus of infrastructure, hygiene and health in Tashkent Province, Uzbekistan. International Journal of Environmental Research and Public Health. 2018;**15**(11):4-7. [Internet]. [cited 2022 Dec 12]. Available from: https://pubmed.ncbi.nlm.nih.gov/30453679/

[42] Current Health Expenditure (% of GDP) - European Union | Data [Internet]. [cited 2022 Dec 12]. Available from: https://data.worldbank.org/indicator/SH.XPD.CHEX.GD.ZS?locations=EU

[43] Current Health Expenditure (% of GDP) - Uzbekistan | Data [Internet]. [cited 2022 Dec 12]. Available from: https://data.worldbank.org/indicator/SH.XPD.CHEX.GD.ZS?locations=UZ

[44] Ahmedov M, Green J, Azimov R, Avezova G. Addressing the Challenges of Improving the Quality of primary Care for Chronic Heart Failure in Uzbekistan: A Qualitative Study. curatiofoundation.org [Internet]. [cited 2016 Jan 2]. Available from: http://curatiofoundation.org/projects/uploads/pdffiles/doc%20 10%20chf%20paper%20uzbek%20 case%20study.pdf

[45] Ahmedov M, Rechel B, Alimova V, Azimov R. Primary health care reform in Uzbekistan. The International Journal of Health Planning and Management. 2007;**22**(4):301-318 [Internet]. [cited 2015 Jan 13]. Available from: http://www.ncbi.nlm.nih.gov/pubmed/17726712

[46] Han S, Choi S, Heo J, Park J, Kim WH. Evaluation of a ten-year team-based collaborative capacity-building program for pediatric cardiac surgery in Uzbekistan: Lessons and implications. Annals of Global Health. 2020;**86**(1):1-11 [Internet].[cited 2022 Dec 12]. Available from: http://www.annalsofglobalhealth.org/articles/10.5334/aogh.2883/

[47] Organization WH. Primary Care Quality Management in Uzbekistan. 2008 [cited 2022 Dec 12]. Available from: https://apps.who.int/iris/handle/10665/350278

[48] Cashin CE, Borowitz M, Zuess O. The gender gap in primary health care resource utilization in Central Asia. Health Policy and Planning. 2002;**17**(3):264-272 [Internet]. Available from: http://www.ncbi.nlm.nih.gov/pubmed/12135992

[49] Primary Care and Disease Prevention Become Priorities in Uzbekistan [Internet]. [cited 2015 Feb 14]. Available from: http://www.worldbank.org/en/news/feature/2014/02/12/primary-care-and-disease-prevention-become-priorities-in-uzbekistan

[50] Menlikulov PR. Organizational forms of primary health care in

Uzbekistan. Problemy Sotsial'noi Gigieny, Zdravookhraneniia i Istorii Meditsiny. 2001;**1**(4):31-32. [Internet] Available from: http://www.ncbi.nlm.nih.gov/pubmed/11593816

[51] Pavin M, Nurgozhin T, Hafner G, Yusufy F, Laing R. Prescribing practices of rural primary health care physicians in Uzbekistan. Tropical Medicine & International Health. 2003;**8**(2):182-190 [Internet] [cited 2022 Dec 12]. Available from: https://onlinelibrary.wiley.com/doi/full/10.1046/j.1365-3156.2003.00992.x

[52] Kalucy L, Jackson-Bowers E, McIntyre E, Reed R. The feasibility of determining the impact of primary health care research projects using the Payback Framework. Health Research Policy and Systems. 2009;7:1-10. [Internet] [cited 2020 Jan 12] DOI: 10.1186/1478-4505-7-11

[53] Tursunov KZ. Perinatal and neonatal mortality (according to the data of republican Pathoanatomic Center of the Ministry of health of Uzbekistan). Likars'ka Sprava / Ministerstvo Okhorony Zdorov'ia Ukraïny [Internet]. 2004;**2**:85-88. Available from: http://www.ncbi.nlm.nih.gov/pubmed/15208885

[54] Mishra V, Arnold F, Semenov G, Hong R, Mukuria A. Epidemiology of Obesity and Hypertension in Uzbekistan. 2005 [cited 2015 Feb 23]; Available from: http://www.popline.org/node/257212

[55] Hasker E, Khodjikhanov M, Sayfiddinova S, Rasulova G, Yuldashova U, Uzakova G, et al. Why do tuberculosis patients default in Tashkent City, Uzbekistan? A qualitative study. The International Journal of Tuberculosis and Lung Disease. Sep 2010;**14**(9):1132-1139 [Internet]. Available from: http://www.ncbi.nlm.nih.gov/pubmed/20819258

[56] Rasanayagam J. Informal economy, informal state: The case of Uzbekistan. Polese A, editor. International Journal of Sociology and Social Policy. 2011;**31**(11/12):681-696 [Internet] [cited 2015 Feb 23]. Available from: http://www.emeraldinsight.com/doi/abs/10.1108/01443331111177878

[57] Urinboyev R, Svensson M. Corruption, social norms and everyday life in Uzbekistan. In: Kubbe I, Engelbert A, editors. Corruption and Norms. Vol. 1. Palgrave Macmillan, Cham: Political Corruption and Governance. 2018. pp. 187-210 [Internet] [cited 2022 Dec 12]. Available from: https://link.springer.com/chapter/10.1007/978-3-319-66254-1_10

[58] Urinboyev R, Svensson M. Living law, legal pluralism, and corruption in post-soviet Uzbekistan. The Journal of Legal Pluralism and Unofficial Law. 2013;**45**(3):372-390. [Internet] [cited 2015 Apr 5] DOI: 10.1080/07329113.2014.867752

[59] Urinboyev R, Svensson M. Corruption in a Culture of Money: Understanding Social Norms in Post-Soviet Uzbekistan [Internet]. In: Baier M editor. Social and Legal Norms. Vol. 1. Rochester, NY: Aldershot, Ashgate; 2013. pp. 267-284. [cited 2015 Nov 24]. Available from: http://papers.ssrn.com/abstract=2197792

[60] Belkina TV, Khojiev DS, Tillyashaykhov MN, Tigay ZN, Kudenov MU, Tebbens JD, et al. Delay in the diagnosis and treatment of pulmonary tuberculosis in Uzbekistan: A cross-sectional study. BMC Infectious Diseases. 2014;**14**(1):3-6. [Internet] [cited 2022 Dec 12]. Available from: https://pubmed.ncbi.nlm.nih.gov/25421106/

[61] Hasker E, Khodjikhanov M, Usarova S, Asamidinov U, Yuldashova U, van der Werf MJ, et al. Drug prescribing

practices for tuberculosis in Uzbekistan. The International Journal of Tuberculosis and Lung Disease. 2009;**13**(11):1405-1410. [Internet] [cited 2022 Dec 12]. Available from: https://www.ingentaconnect.com/content/iuatld/ijtld/2009/00000013/00000011/art00016

[62] Hasker E, Khodjikhanov M, Usarova S, Asamidinov U, Yuldashova U, van der Werf MJ, et al. Default from tuberculosis treatment in Tashkent, Uzbekistan; who are these defaulters and why do they default? BMC Infectious Diseases. 2008;**8**:97 [Internet]. Available from: http://www.ncbi.nlm.nih.gov/pubmed/18647400

[63] Lalor MK, Greig J, Allamuratova S, Althomsons S, Tigay Z, Khaemraev A, et al. Risk factors associated with default from multi- and extensively drug-resistant tuberculosis treatment, Uzbekistan: A retrospective cohort analysis. PLoS One. 2013;**8**(11):e78364 [Internet]. Available from: http://www.ncbi.nlm.nih.gov/pubmed/24223148

[64] Gafurov BG, Zakhidov AI. [An experience of intra-arterial thrombolytic therapy of ischemic stroke in Uzbek republic center of emergency care]. Zhurnal Nevrologii I Psikhiatrii Imeni SS Korsakova/Ministerstvo Zdravookhraneniia I Meditsinskoĭ Promyshlennosti Rossiĭskoĭ Federatsii. Vserossiĭskoe Obshchestvo Nevrologov [i] Vserossiĭskoe Obshchestvo Psikhiatrov. 2005;(**Suppl 15**):28-31. [Internet]. Available from: http://www.ncbi.nlm.nih.gov/pubmed/16447550

[65] McGuire M, Silvia C. The effect of problem severity, managerial and organizational capacity, and agency structure on intergovernmental collaboration: Evidence from local emergency management. Public Administration Review. 2010;**70**(2):279-288 [Internet] [cited 2015 Mar 4]. Available from: http://onlinelibrary.wiley.com/doi/10.1111/j.1540-6210.2010.02134.x/abstract

[66] Kohler S, Asadov DA, Bründer A, Healy AS, Khamraev AK, Sergeeva N, et al. Ambulatory tuberculosis treatment in post-Semashko health care systems needs supportive financing mechanisms. International Journal of Tuberculosis and Lung Disease. 2014;**18**(12):1390-1395

[67] Kohler S, Asadov D, Bründer A, Healy S, Khamraev A, Sergeeva N, et al. Health system support and health system strengthening: Two key facilitators to the implementation of ambulatory tuberculosis treatment in Uzbekistan. Health Economics Review. 2016;**6**(1):1-11. [Internet] [cited 2022 Dec 12]. Available from: https://healtheconomicsreview.biomedcentral.com/articles/10.1186/s13561-016-0100-z

[68] Ibraimov A, Manzhieva E, Kyrgyzstan BR. Health Care Systems in Transition: Uzbekistan. 2001 [cited 2022 Dec 12]. Available from: https://apps.who.int/iris/handle/10665/108417

[69] Johnson E. Authoritarian Survival and Health Care Provision in Post-Soviet Central Asia. 2011 [cited 2015 Apr 6]. Available from: http://academiccommons.columbia.edu/item/ac:139576

[70] Walugembe DR, Kiwanuka SN, Matovu JKB, Rutebemberwa E, Reichenbach L. Utilization of research findings for health policy making and practice: Evidence from three case studies in Bangladesh. Health research policy and systems/BioMed Central. 2015;**13**(1):26 [Internet] [cited 2015 Dec 26]. Available from: http://www.health-policy-systems.com/content/13/1/26/abstract

[71] Molla AA, Chi C, ALN M. Predictors of high out-of-pocket healthcare

expenditure: An analysis using Bangladesh household income and expenditure survey, 2010. BMC Health Service. 2017;**17**(1):1-8 [Internet] [cited 2022 Dec 12]. Available from: https://pubmed.ncbi.nlm.nih.gov/28143517/

[72] Estabrooks CA, Derksen L, Winther C, Lavis JN, Scott SD, Wallin L, et al. The intellectual structure and substance of the knowledge utilization field: A longitudinal author co-citation analysis, 1945 to 2004. Implementation Science 2008;3:49. [Internet]. Available from: http://www.ncbi.nlm.nih.gov/pmc/articles/PMC2621243/pdf/1748-5908-3-49.pdf

[73] Innstrand S. Positive and negative work-family interaction and burnout: A longitudinal study of reciprocal relations. Work and Stress %M. 2008;**22**:1-15. DOI: 101080/02678370801975842

[74] Presidential decree of the Republic of Uzbekistan. About Complex Measures for Radical Enhancement of Health Care System... UP-5590: Presidential Decree Of The Republic Of Uzbekistan; 2018 [Internet]. Available from: https://cis-legislation.com/document.fwx?rgn=112101

[75] Resolution of the President of the Republic of Uzbekistan. About Measures for Implementation of New Model of the Organization of Health Care System and Mechanisms... About measures for implementation of new model of the organization of health care system and mechanisms of national health insurance in the Syr Darya region; Uzbekistan. 2020. p. 4890 [Internet] [cited 2020 Jan 12]. Available from: https://cis-legislation.com/document.fwx?rgn=128595

[76] Aiypkhanova A. Feasibility Study is Published about the Introduction of Mandatory Health Insurance in Uzbekistan | P4H Network [Internet]. 2021 [cited 2023 Jan 14]. Available from: https://p4h.world/en/news/feasibility-study-published-about-introduction-mandatory-health-insurance-uzbekistan

[77] World Health Organization. Feasibility Study for the Introduction of Mandatory Health Insurance in Uzbekistan [Internet]. Copenhagen: WHO Regional Office for Europe; 2021 [cited 2023 Jan 14]. Available from: https://www.who.int/europe/publications/i/item/WHO-EURO-2021-2317-42072-57915

[78] Aiypkhanova A. State Health Insurance Fund of Uzbekistan has Announced Piloting State Health Insurance for the First Time in the Nation | P4H Network [Internet]. 2021 [cited 2023 Jan 14]. Available from: https://p4h.world/en/news/state-health-insurance-fund-uzbekistan-has-announced-piloting-state-health-insurance-first

[79] State Health Insurance Fund of Uzbekistan has Announced Piloting State Health Insurance for the First Time in the Nation | P4H Network [Internet]. [cited 2022 Dec 14]. Available from: https://p4h.world/en/news/state-health-insurance-fund-uzbekistan-has-announced-piloting-state-health-insurance-first

[80] Uzbekistan to Introduce Mandatory Health Insurance System in 2021 [Internet]. [cited 2022 Dec 14]. Available from: https://gratanet.com/news/uzbekistan-to-introduce-mandatory-health-insurance-system-in-2021

Chapter 16

Investing in Health Education to Reduce Rural Health Disparities

Jean Ross, Samuel Mann and Kate Emond

Abstract

The global rural population accounts for almost half of the total global population. Access to health care for these rural populations is reduced, leading to increased health disparities. Nurses play a critical role in reducing health disparities but with limited models to guide their practice. The Community Health Assessment Sustainable Education model is a practical teaching and learning solution, which has been developed to engage student nurse learners in a health promotion philosophy for rural areas. Nurse learners assess and gather data to progress community development and navigate the holistic landscape of health. In this chapter, we describe how this approach integrates the sociopolitical, cultural, sustainable, economic, and environmental aspects of rural communities' health. Our focus is on preparing nurse learners to improve the health of rural populations globally and reduce health disparities. The CHASE model enables nurse learners to influence and change policy and legal responsibilities at local, national, and global levels, while community development aims to address nurses' role in advocacy that requires them to act on behalf of communities from a social justice perspective as they prepare for registered nurse practice.

Keywords: rural, health, education, CHASE model, nurses

1. Introduction

Improving the quality of life in rural areas requires investment in rural health. While such investment often involves spending on physical infrastructure, we focus on the education of nurse learners in preparation for registered nurse practice in rural contexts. Nursing in rural areas is not the same as urban centers. Rural nurses must combine their clinical skills with that of community developers. In this chapter, we describe how the Community Health Assessment Sustainable Education (CHASE) model is used for introducing nurse learners to this complex nature of rural health [1, 2].

Rural nurses must be prepared for situations that are outside their usual lived experience and outside the textbook of clinical practice. Even for rural nurses who work in their home districts, we need them to be able to step back and look at the rural communities as if through the eyes of geographers or perhaps as strategic designers. These capabilities as community change agents will not come about through the usual clinically focused placements alone. We need to invest in the difference, that is, rurality. The CHASE model, therefore, enables nurse learners to influence and change policy and legal responsibilities at local, national, and global levels, while community development aims to address nurses' role in advocacy that requires them to act on behalf of communities from a social justice perspective as they prepare for registered nurse practice.

After canvassing the challenges of rural health education, we outline the development and nature of the CHASE model. We then describe an international collaboration of investment in rural health education using the CHASE model. We commissioned the production of a film of the rural village of Bishop's Castle (Shropshire, UK) to enhance the learners' engagement and critical thinking and questioning of this community to enhance their community profiling and assessment.

The purpose of this chapter is to add to the growing debate of improving the provision of rural health care and equally rural workforce planning. Our focus is on preparing nurse learners to enhance the health of rural populations globally. To achieve this, we demonstrate the value of engaging with a research framework guiding our collaborations as we collaborate with rural communities. This project is explored using ethnographic reflections of the participating academics (authors), as we engage with an authentic teaching practice to consider the success of the CHASE model in preparing nurse learners for rural practice.

2. Background

Nurses make up the largest segment of the global health care profession [3] and play a critical role in assessing the health care of rural populations while working collaboratively with rural community residents to reduce rural health disparities [4]. In consideration of nurses' positionality as community development practitioners, it is therefore imperative that an understanding of this joint role—of assessing and collaboration—is passed onto nurse learners. The demand of educating nurse learners for rural areas goes beyond the clinical, to provide them also with the opportunity to practice as community development practitioners a term derived by the International Association of Community Development (IACD) who note the inclusivity of all people whether in unpaid or paid work who offer their services to improve community welfare are considered community development practitioners [5].

The challenges of practicing within the contexts of rural geographical locations are numerous, which add to the complexity of practicing nursing in rural locations. Rural locations are widely dispersed and often isolated. Nurses practice health care in these contexts at times as solo practitioners, as a member of an intradisciplinary, interdisciplinary, or multidisciplinary teams in small hospitals, community venues, residents' homes, schools, recreation facilities [4] the outback, a village, the bush, or an open space [6]. Equally, these practitioners care for rural residents and visitors from birth to death and experience all manner of health care eventualities. In addition to the clinical practice of all nurses, the scope of practice of rural nurses includes the complexities of living rural, the economic factors, isolation; limited transportation and communication and the variety of occupations including engaging with nature; and agriculture and farm life, including animals; farmed space; domesticated; and wild [7].

The rural resident population accounts for 44 percent of the total global population [8]. People in rural areas experience similar rural health issues yet often suffer more than urban communities because of a lack of access to health care including affordability [9]. The provision of health care services in rural locations are under threat with centralization (hence urbanization) of services [10]. The provision of rural health care services is of global concern and has been recognized as such for the past two decades [11–13]. Despite the huge differences between developing and developed countries, access to health care is the major issue in rural health around the world [14]. The provision of health care within rural communities remains a global challenge [15].

The state of rural health is one of the disparities and inequities [16]. This recognition acknowledges that the health of rural people experiences numerous health disparities and suffers more than their suburban and urban counterparts. A lack of access to health care is in turn related to the lack of health providers including the availability of specialists [9]. Further, the reduced numbers of rural health care practitioners have led to the lack of availability and recruitment of experienced health practitioners and a corresponding lack of rural planning and dedicated funding. Rural health care practitioners include doctors, nurses, midwives, and pharmacists, who make up most of current practicing rural professionals to improve access for the provision of health care and to highlight these issues to health planners, regulators, and governments, globally [17]. Rural nurses are one of the main contributors of this action [18].

Rural nurses need to have the capability of working with rural communities to gather and analyze population-level data, promote wellness and disease prevention, assist in adopting and disseminating best practices for population health, and identify patients who are at greater risk of disparities, necessitating greater outreach efforts [18]. Therefore, nurses need broad-based knowledge to succeed with this endeavor and more importantly to ensure that they are prepared and competent to practice successfully in rural contexts. There is no better time to engage with nurse learners about community development and the practice of "nursing a community" to improve health care. Student nurse learners can be immersed in community development, to enable them to develop the professional competence to contribute to solution-focused and sustainable health care. It is therefore imperative that nurse educators expose, facilitate, and provide their experience of practicing community development, for the future endeavors of rural health care as nurse learners prepare for registered nurse practice.

3. CHASE model

The purpose of this chapter is to add to the growing debate of improving the provision of rural health care and equally rural workforce planning. Our focus is on preparing nurse learners to enhance the health of rural populations globally, in keeping with the vision of the Global Rural Nursing Exchange Network (GRNEN) [19] which is discussed in relation to the student nurse learners project grant, later in this chapter. To achieve this, we demonstrate the value of engaging with a research framework guiding our collaborations as we collaborate with rural communities.

The Community Health Assessment Sustainable Education (CHASE) model is used for introducing nurse learners to rural health [1, 2]. CHASE provides a consolidated structure that immerses nurse learners in community development practice and involves them to be active in their own learning in partnership with their team peer members, community organizations, community key stakeholders, and educational supervisors. CHASE guides learners through ethical, cultural, professional, and critical thinking, verbal and written communication, and visual presentations. CHASE enables nurse learners to influence and change policy and legal responsibilities at local, national, and global levels.

It is therefore imperative that student nurse learners experience community development work, as part of their primary health care clinical placements. Students are guided by the CHASE model to create opportunities for improved community health among rural population groups. Learners use both primary and secondary data collection to describe the community, map resources, uncover inequities, and listen to stories of community resilience. Health needs are identified between learners and community members, and sustainable responses evolved in the form of solution-focused strategies and resources and disseminated within the community to improve well-being.

3.1 CHASE engagement

CHASE stands for Community Health Assessment Sustainable Education model. CHASE was developed in 2017 to assist nurse learners (as a component of their Bachelor of Nursing (BN) degree program from the School of Nursing, Otago Polytechnic, Dunedin, in New Zealand) to undertake community development projects. These projects related to clinical practice experience and received ethical approval in 2021–2024 to proceed by the School of Nursing, Ethics Committee, Otago Polytechnic, Dunedin, New Zealand, for learners to profile and assess the rural community, take action, and design and develop health promotion messages and resources to improve the health of the identified population associated with that rural community. CHASE consists of two preparatory stages: a pre-engagement stage and pre-orientation, an orientation stage and six phases [1].

The **pre-engagement** stage is extremely important, where the facilitator or the lecturer engages with the community.

The **orientation** stage offers learners the opportunity to become acquainted with team members (nurse learners) whom they participate with throughout this 4-week project, the supervising lecturers, and the rural geographical location to which they have been assigned to conduct the community development project.

Phase one commences with the planning stage to undertake the community assessment associated with the identified rural geographical location. The community assessment is guided by an adapted version of Anderson and McFarlane's community-as-partner wheel [20], which enhances the collection of both secondary and primary data including the demographics and social, political, and economic services aligned with the community. One of the outcomes is to "get to know the community better"; therefore, developing a film of the community was recognized as beneficial and could assist the students to experience visually, the community.

Phase two requires learners to prepare a draft written report for verbal and visual presentation in consultation with the supervising lecturers and community stakeholders and identify health disparities and health needs.

Phase three learners work in smaller teams and progress their individual component of the wider project. Additional consultation may occur with community members specific to the learners focus on the agreed (with the community) identified health need and population group. A detailed evidence-based literature review is completed related to this health need.

Phase four learners continue to work collaboratively and progress with their written report and engage with the Ottawa Charter [21] and design and develop evidence-based resources that match the health need for the identified population group.

Phase five learners present back to the identified community partners the final completed published written report, the health promotion resources, and presentation.

Phase six learners initially assessed the health promotion resources designed to improve the health of the identified population 3–6 months following completion of phase five.

4. Investment in action

In the collaborative nature of rural practice, CHASE is not just a teaching device. The model is one of co-design, research, evaluations, education and ongoing and future collaborations, and community development. We illustrate this working research framework [22] with an example of a community development project connected to the rural community of Bishop's Castle, Shropshire, England, United Kingdom. This community development project commenced in February 2020, revisited in 2021 and 2022. We are showcasing the 2022 project in this chapter, while the community development projects 2020 and 2021 provide an informative background to the 2022 project. Our overall focus in this chapter is to share the collaboration between the Bishop's Castle community stakeholders, the educators from La Trobe Rural Health School, Victoria, Australia, (LRHS) the School of Nursing, Otago Polytechnic, Dunedin, New Zealand, and the funders of the GRNEN project grant. This GRNEN international learning grant partnered this collaborative venture between these education institutions, the rural community Bishop's Castle, Shropshire, United Kingdom.

This international project offered a platform for meaningful conversations and encouraged global diversity for rural student nurse learners to improve decision-making and progress on issues that matter most to rural nurses and rural communities around the globe. The goal for this endeavor was to advance nurse learners' community development practice and to provide an opportunity for learners to engage with each other to:

- participate and engage with rural communities;
- undertake community assessment to identify issues;
- plan community development;
- assist with change as necessary;
- build leadership and teamwork;
- challenge policy if relevant.

Beyond the community development goals and learning experiences for learners, the project had research goals to:

- **foster** interactive virtual global relationships and collaboration between nine New Zealand and nine Australian Year 3 BN nursing students, as they engaged with this interactive project and shared their knowledge from their own countries associated with rural community development and public health focused on the mental health of rural youth and COVID-19 lockdowns;

- **improve** the understanding, of the local-global connections, unique cultural relationships, similarities, and differences associated with rural locations, rural locale, and rural sense of belonging among the Year 3 BN nursing students;

- **engage** with the CHASE model to enhance the New Zealand and Australia BN Year 3 nursing students' engagement and understanding of the rural village of Bishop's Castle, Shropshire, United Kingdom community profile and health needs assessment through film;

- **incorporate** the CHASE model (supported with the film of Bishop's Castle the identified rural community) as the Australian and New Zealand BN Year 3 nursing students progressed their involvement and contributions to improve the health care of this community from an illness-focused perspective to one that incorporates sustainability and holism and have increased their awareness of health inequities for vulnerable population groups.

Thus, the project had the following objectives that integrated the educational, community development, and research goals:

- to **share** the students' learning journey and communication/collaboration along the way with GRNEN, the following mediums were engaged with Higher Logic including film, videos, photography, art, or poems. These mediums were aimed to support virtual connections *via* Zoom including videoconferencing, collaboration tools for co-creating and updating documents that would support collaboration and communication among the students, and the residents of the rural village, and the nurse educators that support social networking and create online communities;

- to **promote** awareness of mental health, mental ill health, and mental well-being, build positive behavior constructs, and destigmatize mental health among the community residents of Bishop's Castle while progressing the nurse learner's engagement and understanding, especially when confronted with different cultural groups;

- to **stimulate** self-esteem, empowerment, and self-actualization for the community residents and identified population groups residing in Bishop's Castle;

- to **combat** loneliness and social isolation for the community residents of Bishop's Castle;

- to **kindle** team building and networking among the nursing students associated with La Trobe Rural Health School and School of Nursing, Otago Polytechnic, Dunedin, New Zealand, and together work on the project virtually together;

- to **enhance** individual learning development and showcase community knowledge and share ideas;

- to **create** cohesion between the partnering universities and foster ongoing virtual relationships among students and educators.

This project, therefore, provides an example of investing in nurse learners' education as a mechanism for addressing rural health disparities. The collaboration that occurs across stakeholders and education providers offers learnings and resources that would not otherwise be available to nursing students. Investing in nursing education with a focus on rural health and rural communities provides students with the opportunity to genuinely understand the health disparities that occur between metropolitan, regional, and rural areas. Engaging with rural communities is a key characteristic of building a sustainable health workforce [17]; therefore, incorporating this into undergraduate nursing curricula at a university rural health school is vital.

4.1 Investment in community story

We engaged with a local professional filmmaker from Bishop's Castle to film the community. To achieve this, we set a task for the filmmaker to engage with a foot-survey template in looking at the different aspects of how the students were going to profile and assess this community. The foot-survey encourages students to review, for example, housing, roading, safety, transportation, education, recreation, economics, and health care services based on the original Anderson and McFarlane's community-as-partner wheel [20]. This assisted the filmmaker in creating the story line and then producing the film (**Figure 1**).

4.2 Investment in virtual platform

A virtual platform is developed using a platform within a Learning Management System (LMS—"Moodle"). This Moodle shell allowed us to retain resources and information, offer direction and discussion, and support for teams of nurse learners locally, regionally, nationally, and internationally. The Moodle shell is a working space and resource for students and staff and in the future will accommodate community users. All relevant content organized into a cohesive Moodle course, including

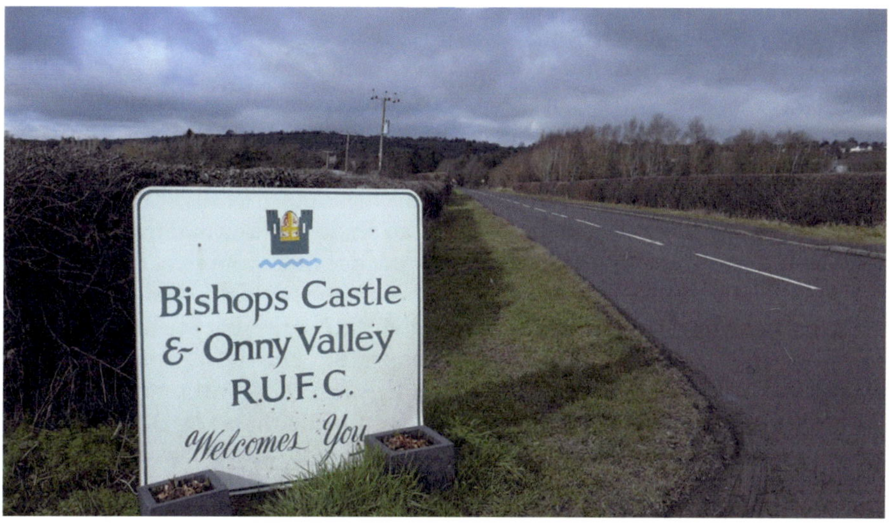

Figure 1.
Rural community Bishop's Castle. Source: John Keeley (published with permission).

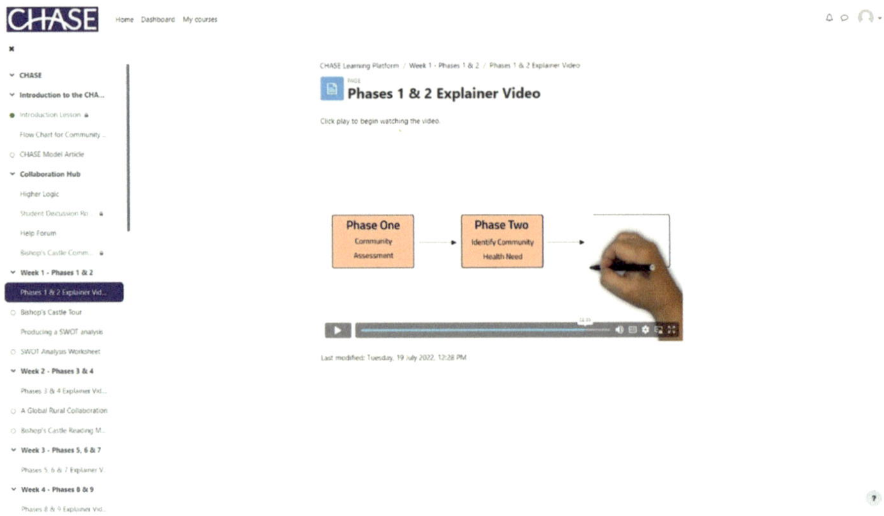

Figure 2.
Moodle shell CHASE whiteboard animations. Source: Authors.

downloading documents/materials including videos to include virtual conference rooms and whiteboard animations with narration (**Figure 2**). Interactive lessons outlining the platform and how to use Moodle and forums as required for student groups and community were provided. Technical support and ongoing revisions were also provided. The content and direction provided in the Moodle shell has showcased through numerous community case studies engaged by the learners, in which all CHASE model phases are exemplified. The CHASE model enhances collaborative relationships in the global landscape and further contributes to inform nursing curricula and teaching and learning pedagogy internationally. CHASE supports the community development project, and the LMS is the means to achieve this.

4.3 Engaging with rural health

There was a total of 4 weeks of collaboration between the universities in New Zealand and Australia during 2021. The New Zealand students shared their community profile assessment and analysis presentation comprising phases one and two of CHASE of Bishops Castle in the United Kingdom to the Australian students. Following this, the New Zealand and Australian students discussed together using GRNEN virtual platform for student correspondence (a requirement of the GRNEN grant) and the mental health of youth and other members of the community from their own countries' perspective while critiquing and reviewing the literature related to the information that would be relevant to assist the United Kingdom of Bishop's Castle, youth community. The academic team invested time and communicated regularly with students to assess their progress, ensuring there was a strong alignment in their thinking and their progress of their piece of work with community needs, making sure that it was continually coming back to the information that they received about Bishop's Castle and the challenges and then lifting that up to think about the global context as well and what was going on in this community. There was an emphasis on mental health and appreciating where we were at in terms of the globe and coming out of the COVID-19 pandemic, and it is not surprising that mental health was high on everyone's agenda and an area that was worth paying some attention to.

Nursing students from both Australia and New Zealand interacted with the virtual networking and collaboration tools that were created, and by using these platforms and engagement opportunities they were able to right from the commencement of the community development project, connect with each other, and share in different ways and at different points of time, through the project and also draw the project to completion.

4.3.1 Reflection on learning

(First author reflection): *Community Assessment – Getting to know the community.*

The film we created to assist the students to assess and get to know the community certainly had that desired effect. What we found was that the students who watched the film both from Australia and in New Zealand, could start to really understand the complexity of this medieval village. What we as lecturers and registered nurses are facilitating through this learning are the complexities of the landscapes of the village. The changing British seasons that the film identified included a snow scene; a spring scene and a summer scene, those changes in weather patterns, the trained eye of a registered nurse would consider, how these seasonal changes impact on the village residents which further stimulates the registered nurse to consider the services local to the village, for example is there an ambulance service? is there a hospital service?, how do people get from one place to the other, especially during seasonal changes which could impact the residents on accessing services. Being introduced to these complexities through the medium of image (film) we found that the students could ask more significantly in-depth questions to the community stakeholders (via Zoom meetings and emails) to gather and be able to develop a much better comprehensive assessment of the community, which enhanced their understanding as they progressed with the CHASE phases.

(Third author reflection): *Community Engagement – Increasing Awareness.*

Our nursing students did impressive work, and the feedback from them revealed they felt the CHASE model and engaging in this program was beneficial to their practice, in that it could be used to inform a health promotion message, or an event endorsed by health promotion to a real rural community, rather than exploring these concepts theoretically. They were pleased with identifying the strengths of the rural community and offer to build a health promotion message based on that strength [23]. Nursing students reported an enhanced understanding of the local-global connections, unique cultural relationships, similarities, and differences associated with rural locations and rural sense of belonging of rural communities, their people, and their health. At the completion of the project, they developed a mental health promotion recommendation for the community. This project increased their awareness and knowledge of mental health needs in rural communities and how important it is to engage communities in health promotion for sustainable outcomes.

(Third author reflection): *Collaboration – CHASE in Action.*

The information about the rural community via film was really important. The communication channel that was established between students and facilitators with time differences, had some challenges there but it was not something that we couldn't negate or overcome and that was part of the students' learning as well in terms of when you're collaborating with colleagues overseas. The skills developed in terms of teamwork stemmed from creating that sense of team in an online interface, and that's where the structure that's provided in the CHASE model gave the students a great sense of shared understanding of the point of collaboration and their role in what they were going to contribute.

5. Implications of the investment in rural health education

We invested in the community development project by embedding it into curriculum. When learning opportunities are part of an undergraduate curriculum, the engagement of students is high [24].

Engaging with this global research project supported with the film of the rural village of Bishop's Castle enhanced the nursing students across international universities' engagement and understanding of the rural community. Nurse learners profiled and assessed this community's health and identified the health needs with a strong focus on mental health of the rural community (**Figure 3**).

(First and third authors reflections): *community Assessment – Film as Asset.*

We are keen to explore the possibilities of linking similar films of rural communities together in the future and even aspire to growing a regional, national and global network of rural communities and making sure that extends to student nurses and their learnings and how they've engaged with the CHASE model. This will enhance this way of working and could promote international collaboration, and unique learning opportunities, and also enable students to have global connections and foster relationships with other students but also then connect with the community case study. This is a focus on the work of GRNEN and we hope to collaborate further with them in this endeavor. This would also lend itself to being able to research the way that students are connecting and groups of nursing students and nurse educators relative to the healthcare discussions from their respective countries because it's been quite interesting in terms of what's been revealed.

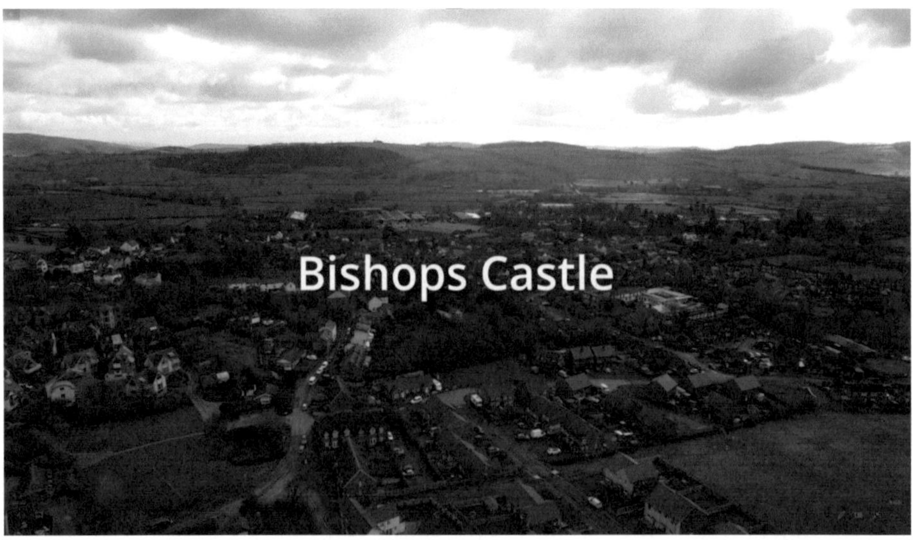

Figure 3.
Screen shot introduction to film. Source: Authors.

(Third author reflection): *creative Learning – Being Courageous.*

When learning opportunities are part of an undergraduate curriculum the engagement of students is high, so it was really important for us to be able to create an alternate assessment for nursing students and gain approval from La Trobe's Academic Board. This approval was a significant milestone because we weren't adding to students' work, this was part of their learning embedded in a third-year mental health subject. In terms of the implementation that the information about the rural community via video was really important and the communication channel that was established between students and facilitators with time differences, there were challenges there but it was certainly not something that we couldn't negate or overcome and that was part of the students' learning as well in terms of when you're collaborating with colleagues overseas, how do you actually create that sense of team and that's where the structure that's provided in this piece of work really gave the students a great sense of shared understanding of the point of collaboration and their role in what they were going to contribute.

In terms of monitoring, we were in touch and communicating regularly with students' progress and also making sure that there was a strong alignment in their thinking and their progress of their piece of work with community needs, so making sure that it was continually coming back to the information that they received about Bishop's Castle and the challenges, and then lifting that up to think about the global context as well and what was going on in this community.

(Third author reflection): *collaboration – Responding Virtually.*

An interesting finding engaging in the project for students at that point in time coming out of the COVID-19 pandemic, was to think about collaboration using these online platforms, because the expectations of the students with working online via different online mediums was actually quite low because they have become so used to it over COVID, they're used to using technologies, they're used to working with other colleagues even within their cohort via Zoom and via different platforms, so in terms of where they were sitting with expectations they were really quite open to this way of learning. Feedback from the students was that they really enjoyed the experience, time zones, that was a bit challenging and we needed to think about our timeframe, appreciating that they're all enrolled in other subjects as well, so really making sure that we were providing resources in a timely manner and the expectations of participation were realistic; and the other thing too is it was really interesting for students at this point in time to think about collaboration using these platforms, because the expectations of the students with working online via different online mediums was actually quite low because they've got so used to it over COVID-19 lockdowns, they're used to using technologies, they're used to working with other colleagues even within their cohort via Zoom and via different platforms, so in terms of where they were sitting with expectations they were really quite open to this way of learning.

5.1 Implications of the project to improve health disparities

Our approach to this project was cyclic, aligning with a quality assurance approach. The implications of undertaking community development as a component of the wider collaborative research project were evaluated between the two educational institutions and the community stakeholders of Bishop's Castle, Shropshire,

United Kingdom, who assessed that the project was meeting its goals and objectives (introduced above) on three monthly intervals and at the completion of the project.

(First author reflection): *community Development – Improving Health Disparities.*

A positive impact of the project and engaging with CHASE was demonstrated by the students' commitment to improve health disparities. The students stayed in regular connect with the community stakeholders supported with regular facilitation and guidance by the lecturers. This was achieved through live virtual meetings such as Zoom and email correspondence they were able to update the community and liaise with them around the identified health issues and latterly as the project developed the health promotion messages and then in partnership with this community, they were able to focus on designing and producing the health promotion resource benefitting the health of the population of Bishop's Castle youth.

(Third author reflection): *community Development – Working Together.*

La Trobe nurse learners offered a significant and a wonderful focus of mental health and youth within their own community to actually share with the students of New Zealand, and they focused on the Rainbow community.

The students from New Zealand presented their findings on Bishop's Castle by using nursing frameworks, they incorporated the framework of Te Whare Tapa Whā [25] which is the New Zealand indigenous population framework, into their presentation by using a holistic approach to discuss all four aspects of the health needs – physical, mental, social and spiritual [25]. They also used the framework of the community -as-partner wheel by Anderson and McFarlane [20] this allowed them to develop a comprehensive display of all relevant health issues disparities within the community, together with these frameworks enabled them to give the Australian students an extensive insight into the health needs of Bishop's Castle which they picked up on and it became evident that they successfully communicated this information after La Trobe students produced a presentation to the students of New Zealand in return which contained and expanded all that they had developed.

(First author reflection): *community Development – Sustainable Practice.*

Developing and maintaining ongoing relationships, and model development partnership collaboration and communication are very important to maintain sustainability between the three groups and with GRNEN. Sustainability included meeting with the stakeholders where we could discuss with the local health professionals including general practitioners, and district nurses, and from our conversations we were able to reflect upon the position Bishop's Castle was in with the closure through COVID-19 pandemic of their community hospital and how it had affected health outcomes for those with more serious conditions and medical events that required very prompt medical response. Through this we discovered that there were five district nurses that covered 10 rural communities in the Shropshire region, and therefore there was an empathy towards those district nurses and how they were expected to work with the closure of that hospital and with the increase in social isolation of older people and the mental ill-health of youth.

6. Conclusion

In this chapter, we have described how the CHASE model works to engage learners and provide benefits for rural community despite geographic separation. These students were positioned to act as community development practitioners with the aim to reduce health disparities in partnership with community stakeholders.

A challenge of educating nurses for rural health is directly related to the nature of rural health. The isolation, complexity, and diversity of health needs mean it is challenging to provide authentic learning experiences that cover the breadth of rural health. Added to this is the need for learners to experience and learn the integrated nature of clinical practice and what might be called community development needed for rural practice.

Herrington et al. [24] laid out a set of situated learning principles for authentic learning. Key elements include a real-world problem that is ill defined at the beginning; the learners need to incorporate multiple perspectives to first understand the problem, and then propose and select from a diversity of solutions that are seamless integrated into the real world. The development requires complex activities over time to deliver polished products that are whole and valued; and all takes the leaners outside their comfort zones, with work across subject boundaries and into diverse roles; and much of the learning is through reflection. The application of the CHASE model as a framework for rural-nurse learning meets all of these objectives. The learners engaged with a community without preconceived or predetermined ideas of what the problem is. They used the tools of CHASE to engage with the community to understand the health of the community as a system and to identify a pressing health need that could be addressed in the relatively short time available. The learners engaged with each other through virtual platforms and pitched their potential solutions to the community and delivered actual useful resources.

Thus, CHASE can be seen to be operating in a sweet spot. The model enables learners to navigate the complexity of learning rural practice. The project mirrors rural nursing practice; in that, it is unavoidably purposeful, collaborative, and relationship-based.

This has resulted substantial positive impact on improving the understanding, local-global connections, unique cultural relationships, similarities and differences associated with rural locations and rural communities, their people, and their health, among nine BN Year 3 students from New Zealand and nine from Australia. The use of the film to provide the context of the community and their health is new, as is the learners being part of an international collaboration with learners from two countries in partnership with a community in a third.

We intend to do further research on these aspects of collaboration between international nurse learners. Anecdotally, these discussions helped with the reflective process and helped learners with the challenges of identity formation as to what it means to be a rural nurse.

All three locations involved in the CHASE project described here are from the Global North (despite the southern positioning!). Previous applications of CHASE have involved rural communities in the Global South – primarily Small Island States in the Pacific (or "Large Ocean States") [26, 27], but with New Zealand as the source of nurse learners. It would be interesting to flip this and have LOS nurse learners.

Remote collaboration is enabled by virtual networking and collaboration tools. Further research will be to explore the value of a film as part of the CHASE model and to enhance the collaboration tools within the networking environment. These international collaborations will foster global connections and deeper research as the groups of nursing students and nurse educator(s) will launch rural/remote health care discussions from their respective countries. We share a community of academics situated in Australia, New Zealand, and the United Kingdom who are involved in this project and are positioned to examine the process, outcomes, and evaluation of this initiative so that the results can be shared locally and globally through GRNEN.

Given the cost of producing films for every community, it would be interesting to explore whether we could link or group similar interactive films of rural communities together in the future, perhaps to grow a regional, national, and global network. Or would this defeat the purpose of an introduction to each specific rural community?

Acknowledgements

The authors wish to acknowledge the Global Rural Nursing Exchange Network (GRNEN) learning grant which stimulated and supported this international learning protect. The authors also thank the community stakeholders and residents from Bishop's Castle, Shropshire, United Kingdom, for their time and engagement with the nursing learners. The authors also thank the Latrobe University, Victoria, Australia COIL Programme Funding, La Trobe Rural Health School, Victoria, Australia final-year Bachelor of Nursing students 2022 for their engagement, commitment, and feedback with this project work. The authors also thank the Otago Polytechnic, Dunedin, New Zealand Contestable Research Funding, and the School of Nursing, Otago Polytechnic, Dunedin, New Zealand Year 3 Bachelor of Nursing students' 2022 engagement with community development and virtual platform communication and learning. The authors also thank Associate Professor Mel Bish for her commitment to this learning project from its inception to completion.

Author details

Jean Ross[1]*, Samuel Mann[1] and Kate Emond[2]

1 TePukenga, Dunedin, New Zealand

2 La Trobe, Rural Health School, Victoria, Australia

*Address all correspondence to: jean.ross@op.ac.nz

References

[1] Ross J, Crawley J, Mahoney L. Sustainable community development: Student nurses making a difference. Scope Learning and Teaching. 2017;**4**:8-16

[2] Ross J, Whiddon K, Mann S, Page D. Case study 4 – New Zealand/UK: Engaging with the CHASE model to enhance community wellbeing. In: McConnell C, Muia D, Clarke A, editors. International Community Development Practice. New York: Routledge; 2022. pp. 105-108

[3] Haddad LM, Annamaraju P, Toney-Butler TJ. Nursing shortage Treasure Island. FL: StatPearls Publishing; 2022

[4] Ross J. 'Place' matters to rural nurses [thesis]. Dunedin, New Zealand: University of Otago; 2016

[5] McConnell C, Muia D, Clarke A, editors. International Community Development Practice. New York: Routledge; 2022

[6] Halfacree K. Rural space: Constructing a three-fold architecture. In: Cloke P, Marsden T, Mooney P, editors. Handbook of Rural Studies. London: Sage Publications; 2006. pp. 44-62

[7] Woods M. Rural. London, England: Routledge; 2011

[8] World Bank. Rural population%. 2022. Available from: data.worldbank.org/indicator/SP.RUR.TOTL.ZS.

[9] Jones CA, Parker TS, Ahearn M, Mishra AK, Veriyam JN. Health Status and Healthcare Access for Farm and Rural Populations. Washington, DC: US Department of Agriculture; 2009

[10] University of Central Lancashire. A Tale of Two Countrysides: Remote and Rural Health and Medicine. Lancashire, UK: University of Central Lancashire; 2020

[11] Australian Institute of Health and Welfare. Nursing and midwifery workforce. Canberra: Australian Institute of Health and Welfare; 2015

[12] Scheil-Adlung X. Global Evidence on Inequities in Rural Health Protection New Data on Rural Deficits in Health Coverage for 174 Countries. Geneva, Switzerland: International Labour Office; 2015

[13] Hughes C. Rural health. In: Germov J, editor. Second Opinion: An Introduction to Health Sociology. Victoria, Australia: Oxford University Press; 2009. pp. 197-218

[14] Couper I, Strasser R, Rourke J, Wynn-Jones J. Rural health activism over two decades: The WONCA working party on rural practice 1992-2012. Rural and Remote Health. 2015;**15**(3):3245

[15] Wilson NW, Couper ID, De Vries E, Reid S, Fish T, Marais BJ. A critical review of interventions to redress the inequitable distribution of healthcare professionals to rural and remote areas. Rural and Remote Health. 2009;**9**:1060. DOI: 10.3316/informit.496326474031125

[16] Thomas TL, DiClemente R, Snell S. Overcoming the triad of rural health disparities: How local culture, lack of economic opportunity, and geographic location instigate health disparities. Health Education Journal. 2014;**73**(3):285-294

[17] Dolan-Nolan F, Ross J, Johnson R, Birks M, Francis K, Mills J. Rural nursing in Aotearoa New Zealand and Australia:

Embracing strategic foresight to sustain tomorrow's workforce. Scope Health & Wellbeing. 2019;**4**:58-62. DOI: 10.34074/scop.3004018

[18] Ross J, Crawley J. Stories of Nursing in Rural Aotearoa: A Landscape of Care. Dunedin, New Zealand: Rural Health Opportunities; 2018

[19] Ross J, Vander Woude D, Snyder A, Merwin E, Hamilton Kilgore C, Feller LM. Global rural nursing student exchange: Engaging with the CHASE model and fostering worldview intelligence towards solution-focused community wellbeing. Scope Health & Wellbeing. 2019;**4**:82-87. DOI: 10.34074/scop.3004014

[20] Anderson E, McFarlane J. Community as Partner: Theory and Practice in Nursing. 6th ed. Philadelphia: Lippincott Williams & and Wilkins; 2008

[21] World Health Organization. Ottawa Charter for Health Promotion. Geneva: World Health Organization; 1986

[22] Ross J, Mann S, Whiddon K. Collaboration enhances community wellbeing: A collaborative development research framework. Scope Health & Wellbeing. 2020;**5**:60-64. DOI: 10.34074/scop.300509

[23] Onnis LL. What is a sustainable remote health workforce? People, practice and place. Rural and Remote Health. 2016;**16**(3):1-13

[24] Herrington J, Reeves TC, Oliver R. Authentic tasks online: A synergy among learner, task, and technology. Journal of Distance Education. 2006;**27**(2):233-247

[25] Durie M. Whaiaora - Maori Health Development. Auckland, NZ: Oxford University Press; 1994

[26] Chan N. "Large ocean states": Sovereignty, small islands, and marine protected areas in global oceans governance. Global Governance: A Review of Multilateralism and International Organizations. 2018:537-555

[27] Hume A, Leape J, Oleson KLL, Polk E, Chand K, Dunbar R. Towards an ocean-based large ocean states country classification. Marine Policy. 2021;**134**:104766. DOI: 10.1016/j.marpol.2021.104766